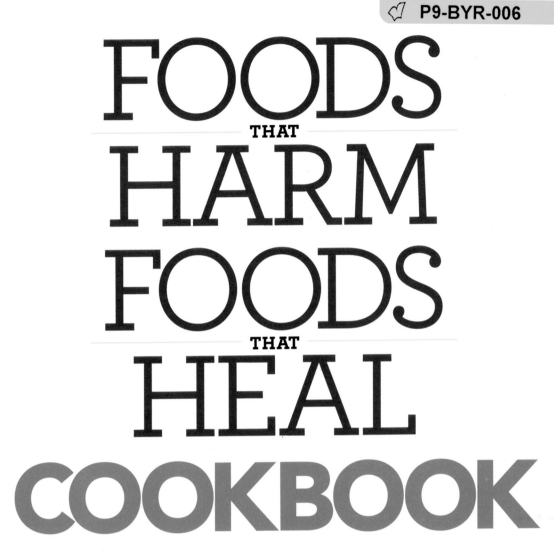

# FOODS THAT HARM FOODS THAT HEAL

# COOKBOOK

*More Than 250 Delicious Recipes
to Beat Disease and Live Longer*

**CONSULTANTS:** FRAN BERKOFF, RD, AND KATHLEEN HANUSCHAK, RD

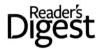

Reader's
Digest

The Reader's Digest Association, Inc.
New York, NY · Montreal

A READER'S DIGEST BOOK

Library of Congress Cataloging-in-Publication Data
Foods that harm, foods that heal cookbook : 250 delicious recipes to beat disease and live longer /
from the editors at Reader's Digest.
    pages cm
  Includes index.
    Summary: "Each recipe also does double or even triple duty, being suitable for healing multiple
ailments. Sample meal plans for almost 100 ailments: For each of common ailments, from acne to
cataracts to kidney disease, a complete daily meal plan using recipes from the book shows readers
how to combine all the healing foods into an easy-to-follow sample meal plan. There is also tips on
making the most of healing foods: An A-Z summary of healing foods gives buying and storing tips for
the almost 100 healing foods, plus information on how to cook them to best preserve their nutrients.
For instance, eating apricots raw gives you the most vitamin C but cooked apricots deliver more beta
carotene"-- Provided by publisher.
    ISBN 978-1-62145-058-0 (pbk.) -- ISBN 978-1-62145-060-3 (epub)
  1. Diet therapy--Popular works. 2. Cooking--Popular works. 3. Health--Popular works. 4. Nutrition-
-Popular works. 5. Functional foods--Popular works. 6. Menus--Planning--Popular works. I. Reader's
digest.
    RM219.F66 2013
    615.8'54--dc23
                                    2013001773

ISBN 978-1-62145-058-0

We are committed to both the quality of our products and the service we provide to our customers.
We value your comments, so please feel free to contact us.
        The Reader's Digest Association, Inc.
        Adult Trade Publishing
        44 South Broadway
        White Plains, NY 10601

For more Reader's Digest products and information, visit our website:
        www.rd.com (in the United States)
        www.readersdigest.ca (in Canada)

Printed in the United States of America

1 3 5 7 9 10 8 6 4 2

## NOTE TO OUR READERS
The information in this book should not be substituted for, or used to alter, medical therapy without
your doctor's advice. For a specific health problem, consult your physician for guidance.

Eating eggs or egg whites that are not completely cooked poses the possibility of salmonella food
poisoning. The risk is greater for pregnant women, the elderly, the very young, and persons with
impaired immune systems. If you are concerned about salmonella, you can use reconstituted powdered egg whites or pasteurized eggs.

# contents

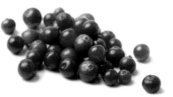

# PART 2
# Recipes

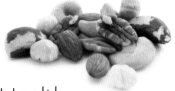

## 250 Delicious Recipes for Good Health

# Salads

# Entrées

## Sides

## Snacks

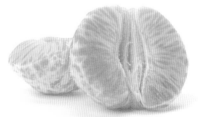

# PART 3
# Ailments
## Daily Meal Plans to Heal What Ails You

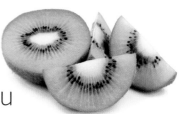

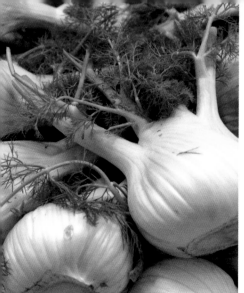
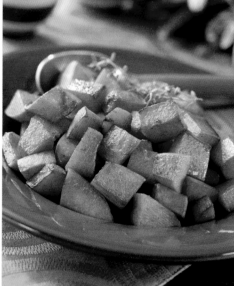
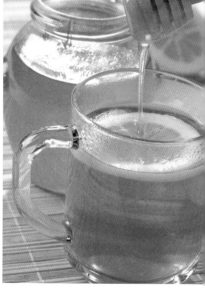
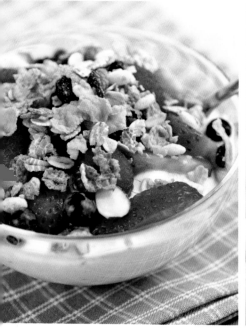
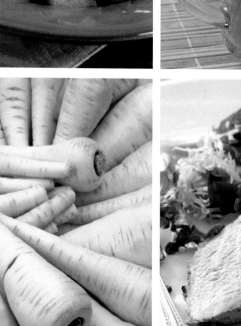
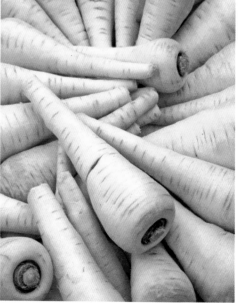
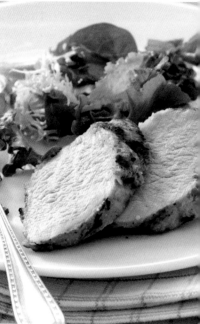
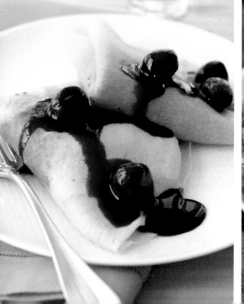
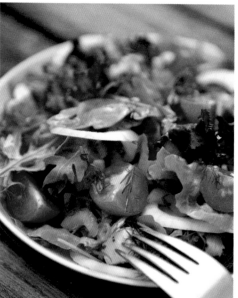
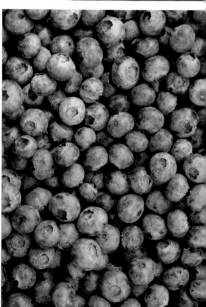

# ABOUT THIS BOOK

## An all-new cookbook companion to the mega-selling food guide

Welcome to *Foods That Harm, Foods That Heal Cookbook!* This companion to the best-selling *Foods That Harm, Foods That Heal* will help you take all of its knowledge about nutrition, healing foods, and harmful foods and put it to use every day, so you and your family can lead healthier, happier lives.

The first edition of the pioneering *Foods That Harm, Foods That Heal,* published in 1997, introduced readers to the explosion of research on the links between nutrition and health and the benefits of whole foods. Subsequent editions—including the latest, published in 2013—expanded on that information to highlight new healing compounds as well as introduce you to new foods and explore the connections that certain foods have to specific ailments.

Knowledge is power, but it only goes so far. You need to know how to put that knowledge to work for you, and that's where *Foods That Harm, Foods That Heal Cookbook* comes in. It is your practical, daily guide. Loaded with 250 recipes plus meal plans for more than 100 ailments, this cookbook gives you the tools you need to get more "foods that heal" into your diet and "foods that harm" out of it.

*Foods That Harm, Foods That Heal Cookbook* is divided into three sections: Foods, Recipes, and Ailments. The first part of the book is an A-to-Z directory of almost 150 foods along with selected lists of "What They Heal," "How They Harm," and the nutrients they provide. You'll find serving sizes and calorie amounts (for your information only—no need to measure, count, or calculate!), along with advice on how to buy the best products, keep them fresh, and prepare them simply. You'll also find special sidebars about foods that you should enjoy "In Moderation Only," along with tips on how to make them healthier when you do indulge.

Recipes make up the next section. Organized by categories, including Breakfasts, Soups and Stews, Sandwiches and Light Meals, Salads, Entrées, Sides, Snacks, Desserts, and Drinks, they are quick, easy-to-make, and delicious. Each recipe features at least three healing foods and a list of some of the ailments it can heal.

In the third section, you'll find an alphabetical listing of more than 100 ailments—from a common sore throat to debilitating conditions such as multiple sclerosis. For each ailment, we show you which foods can cause or exacerbate that condition, and which can help prevent or treat it. For example, those with arthritis should seek out foods rich in omega-3s, such as fish and flaxseed, but avoid red meat, butter, and other foods with saturated fat. The centerpiece of each entry is a sample daily meal plan with recipes. You'll see exactly what to eat, how to eat it, and when to eat it to maximize the healing benefits. In addition, we provide a list of more healing food recipes and eating tips (in the order they appear in the book) to make it easy for you to plan future menus.

So what are you waiting for? Get out your measuring cups, preheat the oven, and start to cook up a healthier diet.

# INTRODUCTION: COOKING TO HEAL WHAT AILS YOU

Cooking up healthier meals starts with an understanding of basic nutrition. In this section, you'll get an overview of what you need to know. From there, you'll learn tips to perfect your cooking techniques and get advice on choosing the healthiest method for the foods you're preparing.

# Nutrition Know-How

Are fats all bad for you? Is vitamin D a cure-all? And what are phytochemicals, anyway? New research is published every day about the effects of nutrients on our health, and it's easy to become confused by all the details. But the basics are simple. We need two main types of nutrients: macronutrients (carbohydrates, fat, and protein), which we need in large amounts; and micronutrients (vitamins, minerals, and other substances), which we need in smaller amounts. Here's a breakdown of the nutrients you'll hear more about throughout the book.

## Carbohydrates

Despite the bad rap they've gotten over the years—thanks to low-carb diets such as Atkins and South Beach—carbs are your body's primary source of energy. They should make up 45% to 65% of children's, teens', and adults' total calories; pregnant and lactating women need even more. Breads, pastas, and cereals are what most people think of as carbohydrates; however, fruits and vegetables (including beans) are carbs, too.

All carbohydrates are made up of different types of sugars that the body breaks down into glucose or blood sugar. Glucose is essential for the proper functioning of your brain, nervous system, muscles, and various organs. Carbohydrates are divided into two groups: simple and complex.

**Simple carbohydrates,** or sugars, are made of just one or two sugars. They form a short chain that breaks down quickly for a burst of energy that doesn't last long. Some simple sugars are naturally occurring, such as those found in a variety of fruits, some vegetables, and honey. Processed sugars include table sugar, brown sugar, molasses, and high-fructose corn syrup. Sodas, baked snacks, jams, ice cream, and sweets all contain simple carbs that add calories but don't offer much, if anything, in the way of nutrition.

**Complex carbohydrates,** or starches, are made of longer chains of sugars. These types of carbohydrates are harder to break down and provide longer-lasting energy. Starches are naturally found in most grains, vegetables, and legumes. Unprocessed whole grains are the healthiest; they retain fiber and other major nutrients that can help reduce your risk of heart disease. Refined grains—such as white bread, sugary cereal, white rice, and white pasta—lack fiber and many essential nutrients, and boost heart attack risk by up to 30%. You should aim to make at least half of the grains you eat whole grain. Look for products with at least 3 g of fiber per serving and for the first ingredient to be a whole grain such as:

- Bran
- Brown rice
- Bulgur
- Kasha
- Oats
- Quinoa
- Rye
- Whole wheat

In addition to unprocessed grains, get plenty of legumes, beans, and raw or slightly cooked vegetables and fruits.

## Fats

They're not all bad; in fact, fats are essential to health. They are necessary for growth and development in children, the production of sex hormones and prostaglandins (chemical messengers), the formation and function of cell membranes, and the transport and absorption of fat-soluble vitamins such as A, D, E, and K. Some fats, like those found in fish and olive oil, actually lower your risk of heart disease. But the key is to choose the right fats and limit your consumption. Adults should restrict their fat intake to 20% to 35% of each day's calories.

As with carbohydrates, the type of fats you eat is more important than the total amount. Fats fall into two main categories: saturated and unsaturated. Most foods naturally contain both but are higher in one. Many commercially produced foods are made with trans fats, which are rarely found in nature.

**Saturated fats** generally come from animal sources and include meat, poultry, butter, cheese, and coconut and palm oils. A diet high in saturated fats can raise your risk for heart disease and some types of cancer. Experts recommend that no more than 10% of your daily calories come from saturated fat, especially animal fats.

**Unsaturated fats** tend to be healthier and may lower cholesterol and blood pressure. Unsaturated fats are divided into two groups: monounsaturated and polyunsaturated. Polys are further broken down into omega-3 and omega-6 fats. Each type affects your health in different ways.

- **Monounsaturated fats:** MUFAs, for short, should be the predominant source of fat in your diet. They improve cholesterol levels, thus lowering your risk of heart disease. Major food sources include olives, nuts, avocados, and olive, canola, and peanut oil.
- **Omega-3 fats:** These are another healthy fat that should be a part of your regular diet. Research shows that people who consume just 1 or 2 servings of omega-3-rich fish per week lower their risk of a fatal heart attack by an average of 36%.

These fats are also important for proper brain function. Omega-3s are found in fatty fish—including salmon, mackerel, herring, and sardines—as well as flaxseed, walnuts, canola oil, and some newer products such as omega-3-rich eggs.

- **Omega-6 fats:** These types of fats can have an opposite effect, increasing your risk of heart disease and some types of cancer if you consume too much. Omega-6 food sources include safflower, sunflower, and corn oils, and some nuts and seeds. While opinions vary on the optimal ratio of omega-3 to omega-6, experts agree that we tend to eat far more omega-6 fats than we need and too few omega-3s.

**Trans fats** are man-made fats created when a vegetable oil undergoes hydrogenation, a process that lengthens the shelf life of food. The result is that polyunsaturated vegetable oils act like saturated fats, raising LDL (bad) cholesterol levels. Experts recommend that you consume as few trans fats as possible. Trans fats are found in products that list partially hydrogenated vegetable oils in their ingredient lists, such as margarines, crackers, cookies, and commercially fried foods.

## Proteins

They are the building blocks that every cell in the human body requires for growth or repair. The antibodies that protect us from disease, the enzymes needed for digestion and metabolism, and hormones like insulin are all proteins. While protein is linked to so many essential functions, you need only 10% to 12% of your daily calories to come from proteins to meet your body's requirements.

Proteins are made up of amino acids. The human body requires 20 different amino acids to build all the proteins it needs. Of those, 11 can be made in the body, but the other nine, referred to as essential amino acids, must come from the diet. With the exception of oils and pure sugar, all foods contain at least some protein, but its quality varies according to the amino acids it provides. Animal protein provides all nine essential amino acids and is therefore referred to as complete, or high-quality, protein. Unfortunately, many animal proteins also come with relatively high amounts of saturated fat. Plant proteins lack one or more of the essential amino acids. To get complete proteins from plants, you need to combine foods such as a grain with a legume. Most North Americans, though, eat too much protein rather than not enough.

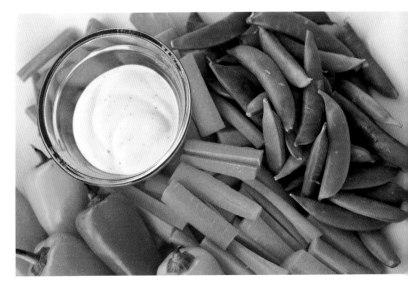

## Vitamins

To date, 13 vitamins essential to human health have been discovered. They are classified as fat- or water-soluble, according to how they are absorbed and stored in the body. Fat-soluble vitamins (A, D, E, and K) need fat in order to be absorbed. Because the body can store fat-soluble vitamins in the liver and fatty tissue, toxic amounts may build up if a person takes high doses of these supplements. Overdosing is unlikely to happen if you get your vitamins from food. The B vitamins and C are water-soluble so they are more easily absorbed. However, the body stores only a small amount and excretes the rest in urine, so they need to be consumed more often.

## Minerals

All minerals are vital to health. Because the body is unable to make them on its own, they must be provided by food. Some minerals, such as calcium, phosphorus, and magnesium, are needed in greater quantities and your body is able to store larger amounts. Others, such as iron, fluoride, selenium, iodine, zinc, and potassium, are stored in small amounts and you don't need as much of them.

## Phytochemicals

These plant chemicals include antioxidants, polyphenols, flavonoids, and a whole host of hard-to-pronounce substances. While they are not technically nutrients, research has shown that many phytochemicals play a critical role in your health. Polyphenols that include the subgroup flavonoids may help prevent heart disease and cancer and lower blood pressure. Carotenoids, such as beta-carotene, lycopene, and lutein, may reduce the risk of some cancers and have powerful antioxidant effects. Allyl sulfides, found in garlic and onions, help strengthen the immune system.

> **QUICK TIP: Get a vitamin boost**
> Add shredded or pureed veggies to pasta sauces or soups for an extra dose of nutrients.

While phytochemicals play a wide variety of roles in the body, most research has focused on their potential as antioxidants, which are molecules that stabilize free radicals. Free radicals, unstable molecules that can damage healthy cells, are created every time a cell in your body uses oxygen to derive energy from digested food. Thus, by neutralizing free radicals, antioxidants help prevent cardiovascular disease and cancer, among other ailments. Researchers have identified hundreds of substances that act as antioxidants in our foods, including vitamins C and E, selenium, and carotenoids such as beta-carotene and lycopene.

In order to get all of these nutrients without going overboard on calories, the key is to choose nutrient-dense foods—those with a high proportion of nutrients to calories—and keep your portions reasonable. (See "Portion Patrol" at left.) Remember, even when we list a particular food as being healing for a condition, that doesn't mean you should eat as much as you can of that food.

## Smart Shopping

Now that you know the basics of good nutrition, it's time to start shopping. In Part 1 of this book, Foods, you'll see specific buying tips for each food to ensure that you choose the freshest and most nutritious items. You'll also learn how to store each food to prevent it from spoiling and losing nutrients. Here are some general guidelines on how to find the healthiest foods.

### What to Avoid

For our ancestors, getting food was fraught with danger, whether they were hunting wild animals or gathering plants they hoped weren't poisonous. Luckily, our modern-day food supply is generally safe. But there are still a few things you may be concerned about.

**Pesticides and other chemicals,** including fertilizers used on crops, antibiotics

### PORTION PATROL

In our supersized world, the portions you serve yourself or see on your plate in restaurants can be as much as four or five times larger than the recommended serving sizes that are best for your health. Follow these guidelines on appropriate servings and how to eyeball them to maximize your nutrients while minimizing your calories.

- **Sliced cheese and meat:** About 2 to 3 oz is the equivalent of a stack of three CDs.

- **Beans and hot cereal:** About ½ cup equals two golf balls.

- **Meat, chicken, and salmon:** 3 to 4 oz equals a deck of cards.

- **Rice, pasta, and cereal:** About 1 cup equals a baseball.

- **Rolls, potatoes, and starches:** About ⅔ cup equals a tennis ball.

- **Cheese:** One oz equals four dice.

- **Medium baked potato:** Roughly equal to a personal-size bar of soap.

- **Peanut butter:** Two Tbsp is the size of a ping-pong ball.

- **Salad dressing:** Two Tbsp equals a shot glass.

- **Juice:** Six oz equals the size of a small yogurt container.

and hormones given to livestock, and environmental pollutants such as mercury and PCBs (polychlorinated biphenyls), may cause birth defects, neurological damage, and even cancer in high doses. In the United States and Canada, these chemicals are heavily regulated, and the trace amounts found in our food are unlikely to be enough to affect our health. But it's not a bad idea to limit your exposure to them as much as possible.

**Additives** include preservatives to prevent spoilage; emulsifiers to prevent water and fat from separating; thickeners; vitamins and minerals (either to replace nutrients lost in processing or to increase nutritional value); sweeteners (both natural and artificial); salt; flavorings to improve taste; and dyes to make everything from candies to soft drinks more visually appealing. Additives are carefully regulated and generally safe to eat, but they are rarely nutritious. The most common additives are sugar, corn syrup, sodium, and trans fats, which can contribute to obesity, high blood pressure, heart disease, and many other health problems. And some additives, such as artificial colorings and saccharin, have been identified by the Center for Science in the Public Interest and other nonprofit groups as ones that may be linked to cancer. So it's best to avoid additives, especially artificial ones, as much as possible.

**Foodborne pathogens** such as bacteria, viruses, parasites, and toxins can cause different diseases, and food can be contaminated at any point from harvesting to transporting to processing to displaying for sale. While farms, food manufacturers, and restaurants are all subject to inspection by government agencies, it's impossible to completely avoid contamination. But proper food storage and preparation can reduce your risk.

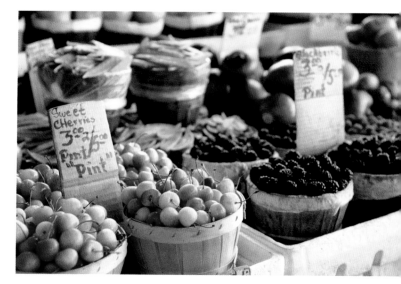

## What to Look for

While the lists of pesticides, additives, and other chemicals to avoid can sound very scary, just a few precautions can help to lower your exposure:

**Eat a wide variety of foods.** Doing so helps keep you from overeating any one type of food that may have high levels of a particular chemical.

**Eat plenty of fresh fruits and vegetables.** They're rich in fiber and antioxidants that may help protect the body from carcinogens.

**Eat whole foods with minimal processing.** The less that's been done to get a food from the farm to your table, the fewer additives and other chemicals it's likely to have. In addition to fresh fruits and vegetables, choose fresh fish and meats rather than canned or boxed foods. (Frozen foods, on the other hand, frequently are free of additives.)

**Read food labels.** Look for shorter ingredient lists and those with ingredients you recognize. And choose products with the lowest amounts of trans fats, saturated fats, sodium, and sugar (which can often be listed as "corn syrup" or any ingredient that ends in "-ose").

**Consider buying organically grown foods.** Organic foods are grown or processed without the use of any synthetic chemicals. (See "Organic Foods" below.)

## How to Store Foods

Of all the potential dangers lurking in your food, bacteria, viruses, and other foodborne pathogens are the most likely to cause acute illnesses like food poisoning. Luckily, there are many things you can do to protect yourself.

### ORGANIC FOODS

Organic foods are typically more expensive, so it makes sense to shop selectively. Although there is no evidence that fruits and vegetables with higher residues of pesticides or other chemicals (as identified by nonprofit research groups such as Consumers Union and the Environmental Working Group) pose a hazard, selecting the organic versions of these foods is a logical place to start:

- Apples
- Strawberries
- Spinach
- Imported grapes
- Potatoes
- Lettuce
- Celery
- Peaches
- Imported nectarines
- Sweet bell peppers
- Domestic blueberries
- Kale and collard greens

These foods tend to have a low residue so you don't need to buy organic:

- Onions
- Pineapples
- Asparagus
- Mangoes
- Cabbage
- Sweet potatoes
- Mushrooms
- Avocados
- Sweet peas
- Eggplants
- Cantaloupes
- Kiwis
- Watermelons
- Grapefruits

Finally, consider organic meat. While most people worry about produce, animals actually accumulate residues from the foods they eat, which is stored in their fat. So you may want to buy organic hamburger, steak, pork chops, and lamb to avoid a more concentrated exposure.

- Refrigerate or freeze all perishables within two hours of purchase. If the weather is hot, reduce that time to one hour and use a cooler if possible for high-risk foods, which include meat, fish, shellfish, poultry, eggs, dairy products, mayonnaise mixtures, and moist foods such as poultry stuffing.
- Store grains, flours, and nuts in plastic, metal, or glass containers with tight-fitting lids. Whole grain flours and nuts should be stored in the refrigerator or freezer; other flours and grains should be stored in a dry place between 50°F and 70°F (10°C to 21°C).
- Store tightly sealed oils in a dark cupboard or the refrigerator.
- Most produce is best stored at about 50°F (10°C). If refrigerated, put it in the crisper section.
- Cook frozen vegetables straight from the freezer; don't thaw them first.
- Store meats and fish in the coldest part of the refrigerator, or freeze them. Defrost frozen meat, poultry, and fish on the bottom shelf of the refrigerator. If using the microwave to defrost, cook immediately.
- Fresh milk and cream should be stored in paper cartons, rather than plastic or glass, and should be tightly sealed.
- Store spices and dried herbs in tightly sealed containers in a dark place away from sunlight.
- To store fresh herbs, wash them and stand them upright in a glass containing 1 to 2 in (2.5 to 5 cm) of cold water. Cover with a plastic bag and refrigerate.

# Healthy Cooking Basics

You could choose the healthiest foods possible, but depending on the method you use to cook them, you could negate many or all of their benefits. Eating a diet rich in foods that heal requires learning to cook in the healthiest ways possible to maximize the benefits. Forget frying, and give some of these methods a try for your next meal:

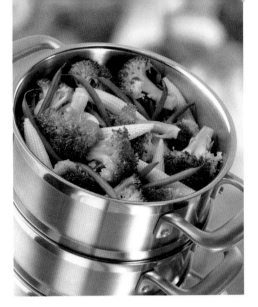

## Steaming

It takes just as long as other cooking methods and retains more nutritional goodness and flavor from foods. A Chinese study found that broccoli retained more vitamin C when it was steamed as compared to microwaving, boiling, or stir-frying.

**Use a flat steamer basket.** You'll have more space for food. Bring the water to a rolling boil and spread the vegetables out in a single layer. Cover with a tight-fitting lid to retain the heat. Be sure that the pan containing the water doesn't boil dry.

**Try it for fish and chicken.** Steaming isn't just for veggies. It's an ideal cooking method for delicate foods like fish, too. You can line the basket with cabbage leaves to prevent sticking.

**Don't use salt.** Although food can be seasoned before steaming, wait until it's done before sprinkling on the salt, as it will draw out the moisture and nutrients.

**Add flavor.** Toss thick slices of onions, chopped vegetables such as celery or fennel, lemon slices, or fresh herb sprigs into the boiling water. Their flavors will waft upward and seep into the food as it cooks.

**Put it in a packet.** You can steam foods in a packet made from parchment paper or aluminum foil. Load your ingredients (traditionally some fish, vegetables, and seasonings of your choosing) into the packets, crimp the edges, and grill or bake until done. The packets will puff up due to steam generated as the food cooks, so open carefully and examine contents for doneness before serving.

**Use your microwave.** Place freshly washed vegetables in a glass bowl and cover with plastic wrap that has a few holes poked into it. Cooking times will vary depending on the power level and quantity of food, so follow the manufacturer's instructions.

## Boiling

Like steaming, boiling is a good method to cook vegetables, meats, and fish quickly without adding any extra fat. Unfortunately, boiling can cause foods, especially vegetables, to lose nutrients. Here's how to preserve them:

**Leave skins on root vegetables.** Vitamins and minerals are often concentrated in and near the skin. Just make sure you scrub vegetables thoroughly before cooking.

**Think big.** Chop and slice vegetables into larger pieces to reduce the surface area exposed, thereby minimizing nutrient loss. Cook vegetables whole whenever possible, then slice or chop them after cooking if needed.

**Use little water.** Cook vegetables in the minimum amount of water. Water-soluble vitamins leach out into cooking water and vanish down the drain when the water is discarded.

**Be quick.** Cook vegetables only as long as necessary. Long cooking times destroy vitamins that are susceptible to heat.

**Give veggies the right dunk.** Root vegetables such as potatoes should be covered with cold unsalted water and simmered to cook them through. Leafy green vegetables should be plunged into a large quantity of boiling water and cooked just until their color is bright, to preserve taste and nutrients.

**Skip the salt.** If you're not in a rush, don't add salt before boiling water. Salted water boils at a slightly higher temperature than plain water so food cooks faster, but increases sodium in your dish.

> **QUICK TIP: Spray sparingly**
>
> A 1 to 3 second spray from an oil mister is all you need to lightly coat pans. Spraying more than that can add a lot more calories and fat to dishes. Here's an alternative to oil-misting devices: Dip the corner of a paper towel in oil and wipe your skillets, baking sheets, or muffin tins with a light layer of oil.

## Braising

Braising is a moist-heat cooking method that requires food to be browned first, and then cooked low and slow in a heavy pot with a tight-fitting lid either on a stovetop or in the oven. Slow cookers are another option for delivering similar results. Whatever equipment you choose, this method is a foolproof way to lock in flavor and render lean cuts of meat tender and delicious when you follow these key rules:

**Avoid peeking.** Braised dishes lose a lot of heat when you take the top off. Instead, rely on a timer to make sure you're stirring at regular intervals and not extending the cooking time longer than necessary.

**Use minimal liquids.** Follow recipes closely and don't add extra liquid. Most vegetables and meats give off their own liquids, and the braising process retains moisture. Too much liquid will dilute the flavor.

**Cook ahead if you can.** Refrigerating your dish overnight will make it easy to remove fat; simply scoop off congealed fat before reheating. Most braised dishes, especially those with complex spices, actually taste better the next day.

## Stir-frying

Lean cuts of meat and poultry are perfect for stir-frying, as are firm-textured fish, shellfish, vegetables, and cooked rice and noodles. Because cooking is quick, the flavors, colors, and nutrients are retained. As long as you use only a little oil, stir-frying is a healthy way to prepare foods.

**Choose the right oil.** You need to use oil that can withstand a high cooking temperature. Good choices are peanut, corn, canola, or sunflower oils. Don't use olive oil because it has a low smoke point and will burn. For the same reason, toasted sesame oil should be sprinkled over a stir-fry toward the end of cooking.

**Make your own seasoning.** Avoid pre-made stir-fry sauces because they are often high in sodium and added sugars, as well as preservatives. To make your own sauce, whisk together ½ cup homemade chicken stock, 3 Tbsp reduced-sodium soy sauce, 1 Tbsp rice wine vinegar, 1 tsp toasted sesame oil, 1 tsp minced garlic, 1 tsp minced ginger and ½ tsp red pepper flakes. If you want the sauce to thicken as it cooks, dissolve 1 tsp cornstarch in 1 Tbsp of cold water and add it to the mix before using.

**Be prepared.** Stir-fries cook quickly, so it's essential to have all your ingredients cut up, measured, and marinated before you start cooking.

**Heat first.** Get a wok or large, deep-based frying pan very hot before adding oil to ensure an even heat. Use about 1 to 2 Tbsp of oil and swirl it around. When it starts to sizzle, you're ready to start cooking. Because hot oil can spit, use a long-handled spatula for stirring.

**Go in order.** Cook protein foods first and transfer to a plate before cooking vegetables. Start with veggies that require the longest cooking time, such as carrots, and add tender ones, such as bean sprouts, last. In the final few minutes of cooking, toss cooked protein and seasoning sauces into the wok and mix gently until ingredients are thoroughly combined and heated.

## Grilling

This popular summertime activity gives intense flavor to meat, vegetables, and even fruit because of grilling's very high temperatures—four to six times higher than can be reached in an oven. The high heat, however, can cause the outside of food to become charred before the inside is cooked through. That's why grilling is best for quick-cooking foods, such as fish, as well as thin cuts of meat and poultry. It is also an excellent method of preparing many vegetables, including eggplant, onion, zucchini, peppers, and mushrooms, and even fruits like peaches, mangoes, pineapple, and bananas. In general, pregrill preparation requires little more than a light brushing of oil to prevent food from sticking to the grill or drying out. Marinating food before grilling also helps and adds flavor without much fat. One downside: Cancer-causing substances can form when fat from meat drips onto hot coals; the resulting smoke deposits those substances on the food. To minimize risks, take the following steps:

**Defrost first.** Trying to cook frozen meat tends to burn the surface and can lead to dry and tough results.

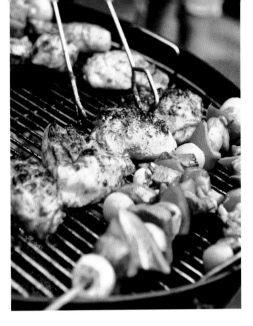

**Avoid chill.** If time allows, let meat sit at room temperature for a half hour or so before putting it on the grill, for more even cooking.

**Trim the fat.** Choose lean cuts and trim all visible fat from meat. Keep meat portions thin so they don't have to spend as long on the grill.

**Cover the grill with punctured aluminum foil.** The foil protects food from smoke and flames.

**Grill for a finishing touch.** You can avoid the struggle of making sure your meat is properly cooked through if you partly bake the food in the oven beforehand. Finish it off with a few minutes on the grill for a crusty exterior and succulent interior.

**Rely on indirect heat.** Don't place the heat source directly under the meat. For example, place coals slightly to the side so the fat doesn't drip on them. When using a gas grill, turn one set of burners off, place meat over the cool side, and cover to cook. Indirect heat is also a good way to ensure more even cooking.

**Avoid flare-ups.** Burning juice or fat can produce harmful smoke. If smoke from dripping fat is heavy, move the food to another section of the grill or reduce the heat.

**Slice off charred parts.** It's not always possible to cook meat until it is done without charring it. When that happens, just don't eat those pieces.

## Roasting

Roasting is a term for a dry-heat cooking method that can be done at either high or lower temperatures in the oven. It browns food and produces a distinct caramelized flavor, and it's a good option for meat, poultry, and vegetables.

**Use the convection.** With a fan designed to circulate the air inside, a convection oven allows you to roast foods at a lower temperature with faster results. To convert recipes developed for a conventional oven, lower the heat about 50°F (10°C) and expect your dish to be done about 25% sooner.

**Flip the bird.** When roasting poultry, consider starting your bird breast side down for juicier results.

**Coat lightly.** To help foods brown properly and to lock in rich, intense flavors, lightly coat them with oil beforehand. For vegetables and cut meat, place in a plastic bag with oil, seal, and toss to coat.

**Use a rack.** Elevate meat or poultry on a rack in the pan so it doesn't simmer in the fat drippings. Also, consider using wine or lemon juice to baste the meat instead of pan drippings.

**Skim the drippings.** If you want to make a quick pan gravy, use a bulb baster to extract the flavorful drippings from the pan. Simply insert the tip beneath the layer of fat that floats on the surface. To remove fat from pan drippings, drop an ice cube into the cooled liquid. The fat will harden around the ice cube and can be easily removed.

**Give it a rest.** To ensure your finished roast or poultry is moist and juicy, cover your dish loosely with foil and let sit for 15 minutes before slicing or carving. This allows time for the natural juices to seep back into the meat or bird. Carve any earlier and the resulting slices are far more likely to be tough and dry.

## Microwaving

There's a lot more that you can do with a microwave beyond heating leftovers and making popcorn. Some models now have built-in sensors that measure the amount of steam in the oven to gauge how long your food needs to cook. Others have incorporated convection oven technology to provide better roasting options. Regardless of these advances, even the most basic microwave ovens are great for boiling water, softening butter and cream cheese, and steaming vegetables. Here's how to make your microwave work for you:

**Cook in glass.** Or use other microwave-safe dishes.

**Opt for undercooking.** When in doubt, always slightly undercook the food, then stir (if appropriate) and allow it to rest for a few minutes. You can always return it to the microwave if it needs a little more cooking.

**Keep it covered.** Most food heats more evenly in microwave ovens when it is covered, and plastic wrap is ideal for that job. It also prevents food from drying out or splashing the inside of the oven.

**Don't let plastic wrap touch your food.**
Poke a few holes in the top before cooking to release the steam; otherwise, the plastic will deflate onto the food as the steam escapes.

## Baking

For healthier versions of cakes, cookies, and pies, you can usually cut the amount of fat in recipes by at least one-third and sugar by up to one-half without substantially jeopardizing texture and flavor. Here are more ways to bake up healthier treats:

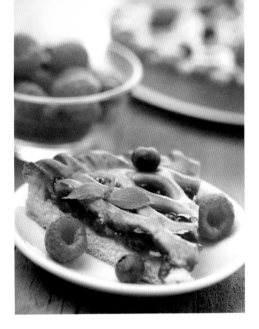

**Use fruit.** You can substitute applesauce, strained prunes, mashed bananas, and other pureed fruits for at least some of the fat in cookie and cake recipes without affecting the taste and texture. While adapting your particular recipes may require some trial and error, in general you should plan to replace the butter you remove from a dish with half as much fruit puree. For example, if you are taking ⅔ cup of butter out, use ⅓ cup of fruit puree instead. When oil is called for, use ¾ of the amount in fruit puree. Since the fruit is sweet, you may be able to use less sugar, too.

**Swap sugar for spices.** Fruit contains its own sugar, so you can use even less added sugar in fruit pies and other fruit-filled baked goods. Experiment to see how low you can go. For more flavor without the calories, add an extra dash of ground cinnamon or allspice.

**Use two flours.** Replace half of the all-purpose flour in recipes with the same amount of whole wheat pastry flour for a fiber boost. If you don't have whole wheat pastry flour, try replacing ⅓ of the all-purpose flour with rolled oats in recipes that don't already call for oats. Whirl the flour and oats together in a food processor for a finer texture.

**Consider crust options.** One easy way to cut the fat content in a crusty dessert is to use a low-fat graham cracker crust or make a deep-dish crustless pie or cobbler. If you can't bear to part with a flaky crusted pie, make a single-crust pie versus a double. For a real change of pace, put the crust on top instead of the bottom.

**Cut the yolks.** In general, you can safely replace half the egg yolks. This increases protein and decreases fat and cholesterol. One exception: any recipe that calls for you to beat the yolks and whites separately.

**Lighten up toppings and fillings.** Substitute condensed skim milk for cream in frostings and pie fillings. Similarly, try strained yogurt cheese instead of high-fat cream cheese for toppings and fillings. Fruit and fruit sauces are good low-calorie toppings.

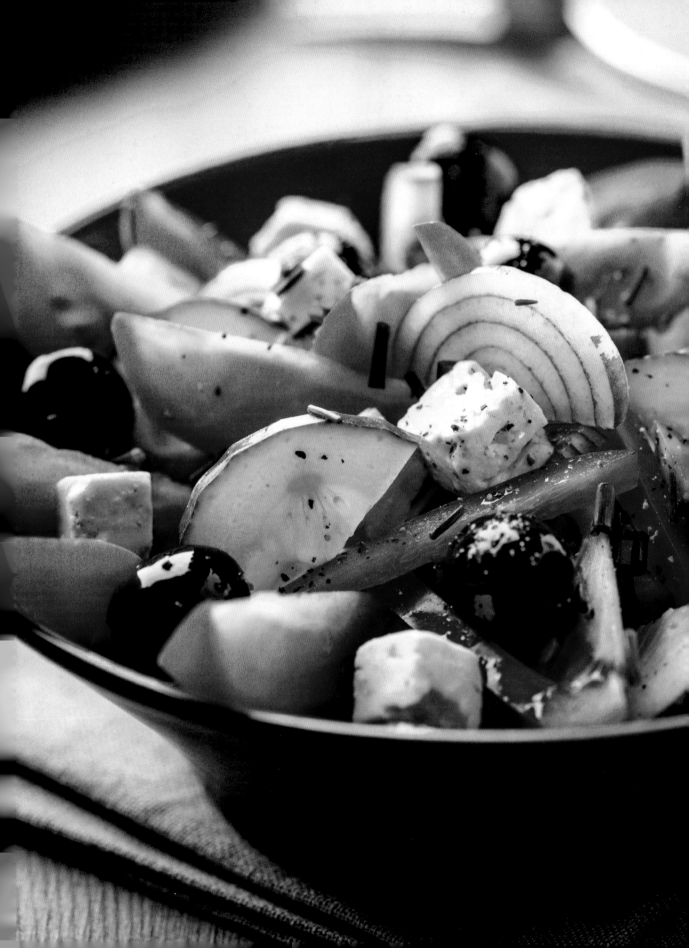

# 1

# FOODS

## An A-to-Z Guide to Healing Foods

Most of us tend to eat the same foods over and over again. Even if they're healthy choices, the wider the variety of foods you eat, the more healthy compounds you're likely to get and the more enjoyable eating will be. This section is going to introduce an array of new foods and, along with your old favorites, help you pinpoint the ones that can boost your health and heal any ailments you may have.

Each entry includes a list of the ailments or the parts of your body that the food may affect. These lists are not meant to be comprehensive—some foods, like beans and legumes, are jam-packed with anti-inflammatory compounds that protect against cancer, heart disease, and diabetes. But they also stop food cravings, help build bone, boost immunity, and offer many other benefits we couldn't fit on these pages. The ailments that a food may heal or harm are listed roughly in order of how much they may boost or hurt health. This treatment allows you to weigh the possible ben-

efits of a food versus its potential risks. One such example: One such example: Spinach is rich in anti-oxidants that may help prevent cancer, blindness, and birth defects. However, it can also contribute to kidney and bladder stones and interfere with blood-thinning drugs.

In addition to the healthful and potentially harmful effects of specific foods, you'll get calorie info based on typical serving sizes (just to give you an idea, no need to measure!) and find out how to buy and store foods to maintain freshness. (Most foods are available year-round but if there's an optimal time to buy fresh produce, we've noted it here.) Plus, you'll see important food-drug interaction warnings and get ideas on quick and easy ways to incorporate each food into your diet, including delicious recipes from Part 2 to try.

So, get ready to take your taste buds on an exciting adventure as you discover new foods and new ways to prepare your favorites for better health!

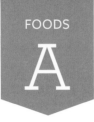

# ACORN SQUASH

*See* Squash, page 108

# ALMONDS

*See* Nuts and Seeds, page 76

# APPLES

**Typical serving size:** 1 medium (182 g), 95 calories

## HOW THEY HARM

Pesticide residues

Bacterial infection

Allergies

## WHAT THEY HEAL

Alzheimer's disease

Colon cancer

High blood pressure

Weight gain

Blood sugar swings

Cardiovascular disease

High cholesterol

Teeth and gums

## NUTRIENTS

Fiber

Flavonoids (antioxidants)

Procyanidins (cancer-fighting antioxidant)

Quercetin (antioxidant)

Vitamin C

### QUICK TIP:
**Bake your way healthy**

Golden Delicious, MacIntosh, and Granny Smith are some of the favored varieties for baking. Save Red Delicious and Gala for snacking.

## BUYING

Choose apples that are:
- smaller
- firm with no soft spots

Avoid apples that are:
- larger
- discolored
- have soft spots, bruises, or worm holes

## STORING

**Where:** Refrigerator.
**How:** In plastic bags. Remove any that begin to decay immediately.
**For how long:** 6 weeks.

## COOKING

- Layer apple slices with cashew butter on a toasted whole wheat English muffin.
- Serve apple wedges on a vegetable crudités platter.
- Roast apple chunks with chicken wings.

## RECIPES TO TRY

- Pasta with Cabbage, Apples, and Leeks
- Herbed Chicken and Apple Burgers
- Fruity Brussels Sprouts

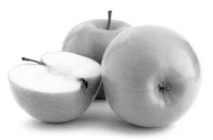

# ALCOHOL, BEER, AND WINE

While studies show there are some benefits to moderate drinking, alcohol is addictive, and overindulging can negate those benefits or worse. It may increase your risk of developing cancer or heart disease, cause liver damage, and affect blood sugar in people with diabetes. Pregnant women should avoid alcohol because of potential adverse effects on the unborn child. Drinking too much may also interfere with vitamin and mineral absorption, as well as provoke mood swings, aggression, and hangovers.

To enjoy some of the benefits alcohol has to offer—relaxation, higher HDL (good) cholesterol levels, less chance of having a heart attack, and maybe even stronger bones—stick to about 8 servings a week (no more than two a day for men, one for women).

### KEEP IT HEALTHY

**Avoid mixing alcohol and medication.** It can cause a host of symptoms, including drowsiness, fainting, nausea, vomiting, and headaches.

**Chase a drink with water.** If you're out for the evening and know you're going to have several drinks, sip a glass of water in between. You'll drink less and being well hydrated may curb any aftereffects.

**Don't drink on an empty stomach.** It can cause spikes in blood sugar.

**Choose low-cal mixers.** Diet sodas or juices, club soda, or sparkling water will cut your calorie and alcohol intake.

## WHAT'S IN THE GLASS?

You'll make smarter drinking decisions when you have a little information. The drinks below are organized from least healthy to healthiest.

| | SERVING SIZE | ALCOHOL VOLUME | CALORIES | BOTTOM LINE |
|---|---|---|---|---|
| Frozen drinks such as piña coladas, daiquiris | 10 oz (300 mL) | 10% | 375-770 | A low alcohol content, but a serious calorie wallop |
| Creamy mixed drinks like white Russians, mudslides | 5 oz (150 mL) | 17.7% | 275-465 | Basically these are desserts in a glass |
| Martini | 4 oz (120 mL) | 43% | 220-260 | Get a dose of healthy fats by adding olives |
| Margarita | 8 oz (225 mL) | 10% | 280-340 | Syrups or homemade blends can add sugar and calories |
| Clear drinks like vodka tonics | 6 oz (180 mL) | 14% | 150-175 | Calorie-free mixes like tonic cut calories and alcohol |
| Sparkling wine/champagne | 5 oz (150 mL) | 13% | 105-120 | Similar benefits as red and white wine |
| Stouts/dark beer | 12 oz (355 mL) | 7% | 130-190 | More flavonoids, but also more calories than lighter beer |
| Mimosa, Bloody Mary | 5 oz (150 mL) | 6% | 90-120 | Vitamin C and minerals from juice mixers |
| Regular beer | 12 oz (355 mL) | 5% | 150 | Some healthy compounds |
| Light beer | 12 oz (355 mL) | 5% | 95-140 | Some healthy compounds and fewer calories |
| White wine | 5 oz (150 mL) | 11.5% | 90-120 | Healthy flavonoids |
| Red wine | 5 oz (150 mL) | 11.5% | 95-125 | Resveratrol and 8 times more healthy flavonoids than white |
| Wine spritzer | 8 oz (225 mL) | 6% | 75-100 | Healthy flavonoids with fewer calories |

# APRICOTS

**Typical serving size:** 3 medium (115 g), 51 calories; ¼ cup dried (33 g), 78 calories

## HOW THEY HARM

Allergies

Cavities

## WHAT THEY HEAL

Cancer

High cholesterol

High blood pressure

Nerves and muscles

Eyes

## NUTRIENTS

Beta-carotene

Iron

Pectin (soluble fiber)

Potassium

Vitamin C

## BUYING

Choose apricots that are:
- plump
- golden orange
- slightly soft

Avoid apricots that are:
- pale yellow or greenish-yellow
- very firm
- shriveled
- bruised

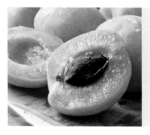

## QUICK TIP: Skip the pit

Doctors warn that apricot pits in any form should not be ingested because eating them could cause cyanide poisoning.

**Best time to buy:** summer

When buying dried apricots, avoid ones that are brown, which means they've been treated with sulfites.

## STORING

**Where:** Refrigerator when ripe. To help them ripen, place apricots in a paper bag with an apple.

**How:** Unwashed, in a paper or plastic bag.

**For how long:** 2 days.

## COOKING

- Broil halves sprinkled with brown sugar and cinnamon; top with Greek yogurt.
- Toss chopped dried apricots into a wild rice pilaf.
- Mix all-fruit apricot spread with grated ginger as a glaze for grilled shrimp.

## RECIPES TO TRY

- Turkey Bacon and Apricot Bites
- Wheat Berry Salad with Dried Apricots
- Fruit Salad with Spiced Coconut

# ARTICHOKES

**Typical serving size:** 1 medium, cooked (120 g), 64 calories

## HOW THEY HARM

Allergies

## WHAT THEY HEAL

Skin cancer

Indigestion

### NUTRIENTS
Fiber

Folate

Silymarin (anticancer compound)

## BUYING

Choose artichokes that:
- are firm without "give"
- are compact and heavy for their size
- have thick, green, fresh-looking scales
- squeak when squeezed

Avoid artichokes that have:
- thin stalks
- large areas of brown on the scales
- spreading scales
- grayish-black discoloration
- mold
- worm injury

**Best time to buy:** spring

## STORING

**Where:** Refrigerator.

**How:** Unwashed, in a plastic bag.

**For how long:** 1 week. For maximum taste and tenderness, cook as soon as possible.

## COOKING

- Toss thinly sliced raw baby artichokes into a mixed green salad.
- Top bruschetta with sliced marinated artichoke hearts and grated parmesan.
- Stir frozen artichoke hearts into a chicken stew about 10 minutes before the end of cooking time.

## RECIPES TO TRY

- Orange Chicken with Artichokes and Sun-Dried Tomatoes
- Artichokes with Lentils and Lima Beans
- Warm Artichoke and Bean Dip

# ASPARAGUS

**Typical serving size:** ½ cup cooked (90 g), 20 calories

## HOW IT HARMS
Gout

## WHAT IT HEALS
Cancer

Aging

Cognitive decline

Edema

Stress

## NUTRIENTS
Asparagine (natural diuretic)

Chromium

Folate

Vitamin C

Vitamin K

## BUYING

Choose asparagus that are:
- firm, yet tender
- smooth and round
- deep green on the stalks
- purplish on closed, compact tips
- narrow in diameter (thicker ones are less tender)

Avoid asparagus with:
- open and spread-out tips
- mold or decay
- ridges up and down the spear
- excessive sand

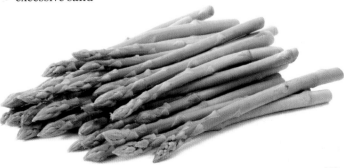

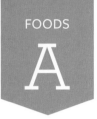

**A**

**QUICK TIP: Limit fridge time**

Asparagus is best eaten the day it is purchased, because the flavor lessens with each passing day.

**Best time to buy:** early spring

## STORING

**Where:** Crisper drawer of refrigerator.
**How:** Store stalks with bottoms wrapped in a damp paper towel. If you don't have a crisper, put them in plastic bags and place them in the coldest part of the refrigerator.
**For how long:** 3 to 4 days.

## COOKING

- Grill lightly oiled spears until browned.
- Stir-fry pieces until crisp-tender, drizzle with Thai peanut sauce.
- Bake spears coated with olive oil and grated parmesan cheese.

## RECIPES TO TRY

- Asparagus, Egg, and Ham Sandwiches
- Asparagus and Chicken Stir-Fry
- Salmon and Asparagus Farfalle with Walnut-Feta Sauce
- Open-Faced Grilled Vegetable Sandwich
- Beef, Scallion, and Asparagus Roll-Ups

# AVOCADOS

**Typical serving size:** ½ cup cubed (75 g), 120 calories

## HOW THEY HARM

Weight gain
Allergies

## WHAT THEY HEAL

High cholesterol
Cardiovascular disease
Cancer
Blood sugar swings
Insulin resistance
Hair

## NUTRIENTS

Fiber
Folate
Magnesium
Monounsaturated fat
Potassium
Sterols (cholesterol-lowering compounds)
Vitamin B6
Vitamin E

## BUYING

Choose avocados that are:
- slightly firm, but yield to gentle pressure if you're planning to use immediately
- firm if you're planning on using them later

Avoid avocados with:
- bruises
- hard or soft spots

## STORING

**Where:** At room temperature to ripen; in the refrigerator when ripe.

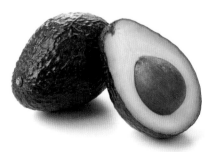

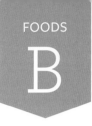

**How:** In a paper bag to ripen, uncut.
**For how long:** 2 to 5 days to ripen; 2 to 3 days in fridge.

To retain a fresh green color, avocados should either be eaten immediately or should be sprinkled with lemon or lime juice or white vinegar.

## COOKING

- Avocados are best eaten raw.
- Serve sliced avocado with huevos rancheros.
- Layer slices with sliced red onion, tomato, and lettuce on whole grain toast.
- Stuff avocado half with chicken salad dressed with salsa.

## RECIPES TO TRY

- Individual Breakfast Tortilla
- Shrimp Seviche with Avocado and Pumpkin Seeds
- Papaya and Avocado Salad

# BANANAS

**Typical serving size:** ½ cup sliced (75 g), 67 calories; 1 medium (7 to 8 in or 17 to 20 cm long) (118 g), 105 calories

## HOW THEY HARM

Allergies

## WHAT THEY HEAL

Stress, anxiety, and depression
High blood pressure
Blood sugar swings
Muscles
Teething pain
Sleeplessness

## NUTRIENTS

Fiber
Potassium
Tryptophan
Vitamin B6
Vitamin C

## BUYING

Choose bananas that are:

- firm
- free of bruises
- solid yellow and speckled with brown if you're planning to use immediately
- unripe (with green tips or practically no yellow color) if you're planning to use later

Avoid bananas that:

- have brown spots
- are very soft
- have a strong odor

## STORING

**Where:** Refrigerator when ripe. To ripen, leave at room temperature for a couple of days.
**How:** In the peel. The peel may turn brown in the refrigerator, but the fruit will not change.
**For how long:** 3 to 5 days.

## COOKING

- Top sliced bananas with low-fat yogurt and a sprinkle of low-fat granola.
- Add slices to chicken curry.
- Drizzle lengthwise halves with honey, cinnamon, and chopped walnuts.
- Serve chunks atop mango sorbet.

## RECIPES TO TRY:

- Grilled Fruit en Brochette
- Cauliflower Salad with Cashews
- Banana-Peanut Bread
- Chocolate Banana Soufflés

# BARLEY

*See also* Grains, page 57

**Typical serving size:** ½ cup cooked (79 g), 97 calories

### HOW IT HARMS

Allergies

### WHAT IT HEALS

Cardiovascular disease
Weight gain
Blood sugar swings
Anemia
Muscles and nerves

### NUTRIENTS

Fiber
Niacin
Selenium
Thiamine

### BUYING

Choose:

- pearl, scotch, or pot barley for use in soups and casseroles
- scotch or pot barley for more dietary fiber
- barley meal when making breads
- whole barley for the nutrition (you can often find whole, hull-less barley in the natural foods section)

### STORING

**Where:** Refrigerator or freezer.
**How:** In an airtight container.
**For how long:** 6 months.

### COOKING

- Toss cooled cooked barley with chopped canned beets, red onion, and a dollop of plain yogurt.
- Serve warm cooked barley with honey and milk for breakfast.
- Toss ¼ cup cooked barley into banana bread batter for extra nutrients and fiber.

### RECIPES TO TRY

- Barley and Beet Salad
- Broccoli and Pearl Barley Salad

# BEANS AND OTHER LEGUMES

*See also* Lentils, page 70; Peanuts and Peanut Butter, page 88; Peas and Pea Pods, page 89; Soy, page 105

**Typical serving size:** ½ cup (86 to 128 g), 108 to 143 calories

### HOW THEY HARM

Nutrient absorption
Gout
Favism (in susceptible people)
Allergies
Drug interaction
Flatulence

### WHAT THEY HEAL

Cardiovascular disease
High cholesterol
Cancer
Diabetes
Weight gain

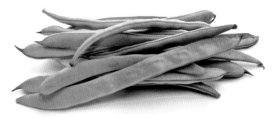

## NUTRIENTS

Calcium

Copper

Fiber

Folate

Iron

Isoflavones (phytochemical that protects against heart disease)

Magnesium

Manganese

Phosphorous

Phytosterols (anticancer and cholesterol-lowering compounds)

Potassium

Protein

Saponins (cholesterol-lowering compounds)

Thiamin

Zinc

## BUYING

Choose beans that:

- are firm, clean, and whole (dried)
- have a bright color and slight sheen (dried)

Avoid beans that are:

- cracked or chipped (dried)
- in cans with dents
- past the sell-by date

## STORING

**Where:** Cool, dry place away from direct sunlight.

**How:** In an airtight container.

**For how long:** Up to 1 year.

### BEAN COUNTING

When planning meals with beans, here's how to judge the amount of beans you'll need:

15 oz (425 mL) canned beans = 1½ cups cooked beans, drained

1 lb dry beans = 6 cups cooked beans, drained

1 lb dry beans = 2 cups dry beans

1 cup dry beans = 3 cups cooked beans, drained

You can store cooked beans in an airtight container in the refrigerator for up to 3 days or in the freezer for several months.

## COOKING

- Soak dried beans in water for at least 12 hours before cooking.
- Rinse canned beans before using.
- Simmer brown lentils in vegetable broth with carrots, celery, and onions for a quick soup.
- Toss drained and rinsed cannellini beans with canned tuna, scallions, olive oil, and lemon juice.

## RECIPES TO TRY

- Italian White Bean Spread
- Lentil Soup with Canadian Bacon
- Couscous-Stuffed Peppers

# BEAN SPROUTS

**Typical serving size:** 1 cup (104 g), 31 calories

## HOW THEY HARM

Bacterial infection

Lupus

## WHAT THEY HEAL

Cancer

## NUTRIENTS

Calcium

Fiber

Iron

Protein

Sulforaphane (anticancer compound)

Vitamin C

**WARNING!**
**FOOD-DRUG INTERACTION**

If you take a monoamine oxidase (MAO) inhibitor to treat depression, you should avoid fava beans; the combination can raise blood pressure.

## BUYING

Choose sprouts that:
- are crisp with the buds attached
- have firm, white roots that are slightly moist

Avoid sprouts that are:
- musty smelling
- slimy
- dark

## STORING

**Where:** Crisper drawer of refrigerator.

**How:** Wash the sprouts thoroughly with water to remove any dirt, then place them in a plastic bag.

**For how long:** 3 days. Rinsing daily under cold water may extend their life. Sprouts can be frozen for up to 1 year if you're going to cook them in the future.

## COOKING

- Add bean sprouts to coleslaw.
- Sprinkle sprouts on chili.
- Blend a handful of sprouts in a smoothie.

## RECIPES TO TRY

- Crab and Avocado Salad
- Sesame Greens and Bean Sprouts

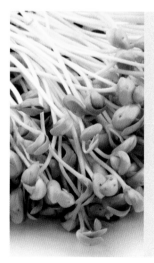

### QUICK TIP:
### Avoid sprouts if indicated

Children, the elderly, and people with weak immune systems should avoid eating sprouts because they have been associated with outbreaks of salmonella and *E.coli* infection. Alfalfa sprouts can also prompt a flare-up of symptoms in people with lupus. You can reduce risk of illness by cooking sprouts before eating them.

# BEEF AND VEAL

**Typical serving size:** 3 oz (90 g), calories vary depending on the cut (see charts on page 23 and 24)

## HOW THEY HARM

Cardiovascular disease
Cancer
Bacterial infection
Hormones

## WHAT THEY HEAL

Anemia
Weight gain
Bones, muscles, cartilage, skin, and blood

## NUTRIENTS

Iron
Phosphorous
Potassium
Protein
Selenium
Vitamin B6
Vitamin B12
Vitamin D
Zinc

## BUYING

- When buying raw meat, select it just before checking out at the register.
- If available, put the packages of raw meat in disposable plastic bags, to contain any leaks.

Choose:
- lean cuts (see charts on pages 23 and 24)
- bright red beef (maroon if vacuum packed)
- whitish veal with pink highlights
- beef and veal that is firm to the touch

# WHAT'S IN THE BEEF?

Choose the leanest cuts for the dish you want to make. The following all contain 10 grams or less of total fat per 3-oz (90-g) serving, and are organized first by cooking method, then from least to most fatty.

| CUT | CALORIES & FAT PER 3-OUNCE (90-G) PORTION | | AVERAGE SIZE | TOTAL TIME | BEST COOKING METHOD | DONENESS GUIDELINE |
|---|---|---|---|---|---|---|
| Top round steak | 169 | 4.2 g | ¾-1 in (1.5-2.5 cm) | 1¼- 1¾ hr | Braise by covering with liquid, covering dish, and either simmering on stove top or baking in 325°F (160°C) oven | Cook until beef is fork-tender |
| | | | 1-1½ in (2.5-3.5 cm) | 1¾ - 2½ hr | | |
| Shank cross cuts | 171 | 5.4 g | Varies | Varies | | |
| Arm pot roast | 179 | 6.5 g | 2½-4 lb (1.25-2 kg) | 2-3 hr | | |
| First half of a brisket | 181 | 6.8 g | 2½-3 lb (1.25-1.5 kg) | 2½-3 hr | | |
| Top sirloin steak | 156 | 4.9 g | ¾ in (1.5 cm) | 9-12 min | Broil; position broiler pan so that meat is approximately 3-4 in (7.5-10 cm) from the heat | Cook until internal temperature reaches 145°F (63°C) (medium-rare) or 160°F (71°C) (medium) |
| | | | 1½ in (3.5 cm) | 26-31 min | | |
| T-bone steak | 150 | 6.3 g | ¾ in (1.5 cm) | 10-13 min | | |
| | | | 1 in (2.5 cm) | 15-20 min | | |
| Top loin steak (such as strip or New York steak) | 164 | 6.5 g | ¾ in (1.5 cm) | 9-11 min | | |
| | | | 1 in (2.5 cm) | 13-17 min | | |
| Tenderloin steak | 160 | 7 g | 1 in (2.5 cm) | 13-16 min | | |
| | | | 1½ in (3.5 cm) | 18-22 min | | |
| Flank steak | 172 | 7.9 g | 1½-2 lb (750 g-1 kg) | 13-18 min | | |
| Shoulder steak (chuck tender) | 160 | 8 g | ¾ in (1.5 cm) | 10-13 min | | |
| | | | 1 in (2.5 cm) | 16-21 min | | |
| Rib-eye steak | 170 | 10 g | 1 in (2.5 cm) | 14-18 min | | |
| Eye-round roast | 142 | 4.1 g | 2-3 lb (1-1.5 kg) | 1½ - 1¾ hr | Roast at 325°F (160°C) | Remove from oven when internal temperature reaches 145°F (63°C) (medium-rare) or 160°F (71°C) (medium) |
| Round tip roast | 154 | 6.4 g | 4-6 lb (2-3 kg) | 2-2½ hr (medium-rare) | | |
| | | | | 2½ hr (medium) | | |
| Tri-tip roast | 184 | 9.2 g | 1½-2 lb (750 g-1 kg) | 30-40 min (medium-rare) | Roast at 425°F (220°C) | |
| | | | | 40-45 mins (medium) | | |
| 95% lean ground beef | 154 | 6.4 g | Varies | 10-15 min | Pan-brown | Until completely brown |

Avoid:

- ground beef that contains pink slime (listed on labels as Lean Finely Textured Beef)
- products with damaged packaging or excess moisture

## STORING

**Where:** Refrigerator or freezer.

**How:** In original packaging if possible. Otherwise, tightly wrap in plastic wrap or freezer paper. If freezing longer than 2 months, overwrap these packages with airtight heavy-duty foil, plastic wrap, or freezer paper or place the package inside a plastic bag.

**For how long:** 1 to 2 days for fresh hamburger, ground beef or veal, and stew meats (3 to 4 months frozen); 3 to 5 days for fresh steaks, chops, and roasts (4 to 6 months for frozen chops, 6 to 12 months for frozen steaks and roasts).

## COOKING

- Start with 4 oz (125 g) of raw meat to end up with 3 oz (90 g) cooked.
- Trim all visible fat from your meat. Reduce fat further by broiling, grilling, or roasting on a rack (so fat can drip away).
- Cook ground beef until it reaches 160°F (71°C). Don't eat ground beef patties that are still pink in the middle.
- Chill soups and stews so that the congealed fat can be removed easily, and then reheat the dishes before serving.
- Layer thinly sliced cold roast beef on mini rye toast spread with horseradish and plain yogurt for an appetizer.
- Stir-fry thin strips of boneless beef top sirloin with red bell pepper, garlic, spinach, and a splash of balsamic vinegar.

# WHAT'S THE BEST CUT OF VEAL?

The following cuts all contain 10 grams or less of total fat per 3-oz (90-g) serving, and are organized first by cooking method, then from least to most fatty. Trim all visible fat before you cook.

| CUT | CALORIES & FAT PER 3-OZ (90 G) PORTION | | AVERAGE SIZE | TOTAL TIME | BEST COOKING METHOD | DONENESS GUIDELINE |
|---|---|---|---|---|---|---|
| Round steak | 179 | 5.4g | ¼ in (0.5 cm) thick | 30 min | Braise by covering with liquid, covering dish, and either simmering on stove top or baking in 325°F (160°C) oven | Cook until veal is fork-tender |
| | | | ½ in (1 cm) thick | 45 min | | |
| Shoulder (chuck, arm or blade roast) | 201 | 8.7g | ¼ in (0.5 cm) thick | 30 min | | |
| | | | ½ in (1 cm) thick | 45 min | | |
| Sirloin | 173 | 5.5g | 3-4 lb (1.5-2 kg) | 1¾-2½ hr | Roast at 325°F (160°C) | Cook until internal temperature reaches 145°F (63°C) (medium-rare) or 160°F (71°C) (medium) |
| Loin | 192 | 7.8g | | | | |
| Rib (chop) | 180 | 10g | 1 in (2.5 cm) thick | 14 min | Broil; position broiler pan so that meat is approximately 3-4 in (7.5-10 cm) from the heat | |

- Roast chunks of marinated veal round steak with cherry tomatoes and pearl onions.

## RECIPES TO TRY

- Caraway-Coated Pepper Steak with Cherry Sauce
- Pot Roast with Root Vegetables
- Beef-Fillet Salad with Mustard Vinaigrette
- Tuscan Veal Chops
- Beef in Lettuce Wraps

# BEETS

**Typical serving size:** ½ cup boiled, sliced (68 g), 29 calories

## HOW THEY HARM

Kidney stones and gout (beet greens can aggravate these conditions)
Discolored urine and stools

## WHAT THEY HEAL

Cancer
Cardiovascular disease
Dementia
High blood pressure
Constipation
Eyes and nerves

## NUTRIENTS

Beta-carotene
Calcium
Fiber
Folate
Iron
Potassium
Protein
Vitamin B6
Vitamin C
Vitamin K

## BUYING

Choose beets that:
- are small, with greens still attached
- have unblemished skin
- have sturdy, unwilted greens

Avoid beets that are:
- elongated with round, scaly areas around the top surface
- wilted, flabby, rough, or shriveled

**Best time to buy:** summer and autumn

Beets are also available canned and pre-cooked for easier preparation.

## STORING

**Where:** Refrigerator.
**How:** Trim each beet, but leave about 1 inch (2.5 cm) of the stem. Place in a plastic bag.
**For how long:** 2 weeks.

The greens (which are rich in nutrients) wilt quickly, so use them within a day or two.

## COOKING

- Boil beets unpeeled to retain nutrients and deep red color.
- Add shredded raw beets to salads.
- Stir finely chopped beet greens into vegetable soup shortly before the end of cooking.
- Stir-fry matchstick-cut beet slices with sliced red cabbage.
- Cook and serve beet greens, the most nutritious part of the vegetable, like spinach or Swiss chard.

## RECIPES TO TRY

- Raspberry-Beet Smoothie
- Balsamic Beets with Toasted Pecans
- Barley and Beet Salad
- Orange Beets

# B

# BERRIES

*See also* Cranberries, page 45

**Typical serving size:** ½ cup (62 to 76 g), 25 to 42 calories

## HOW THEY HARM

Allergies
Kidney and bladder stones
Pesticide residue
Intestinal irritation
Dark stools

## WHAT THEY HEAL

Cancer
Diabetes
Memory loss
High cholesterol
High blood pressure
Birth defects
Macular degeneration
Constipation
Skin

## NUTRIENTS

Anthocyanins (antioxidant)
Ellagic acid (cancer-fighting substance)
Fiber
Folate
Pectin (soluble fiber)
Potassium
Vitamin C

## BUYING

Choose berries that are:
- firm
- plump
- deep in color

Avoid berries that are:
- soft or watery
- mushy
- moldy
- dehydrated looking or wrinkled
- in containers with juice stains

**Best time to buy:** summer

## STORING

**Where:** Crisper drawer of refrigerator.
**How:** In original container (remove any moldy or deformed berries first).
**For how long:** 1 day to 1 week depending on ripeness (raspberries spoil faster; blueberries tend to last the longest).

## COOKING

- Wash berries just before eating or recipe preparation.
- Top strawberry halves with a dollop of part-skim ricotta cheese whipped with grated orange peel.
- Toss blueberries into a spinach salad.
- Stir raspberries into oatmeal.

## RECIPES TO TRY

- Blueberry and Cranberry Granola
- Lemony Blueberry Cheesecake Bars
- Mixed Berry and Stone Fruit Soup
- Peach and Blackberry Phyllo Pizzas
- Broccoli Salad with Almonds and Dried Cranberries

# BLACKBERRIES

*See* Berries, page 26

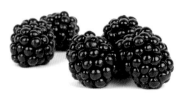

# BLUEBERRIES

*See* Berries, page 26

# BRAN

**Typical serving size:** 1 Tbsp (7 g), 14 calories

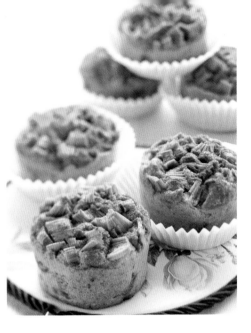

### HOW IT HARMS

Irritable bowel syndrome (can aggravate symptoms in people with this condition)

Mineral absorption (in raw bran only)

### WHAT IT HEALS

Cancer

Heart attack risk

Weight gain

Diverticulitis

Diabetes

Constipation

Hemorrhoids

### NUTRIENTS

Fiber

### BUYING

Choose bran that is:

- in a well-sealed container
- from a store that has a high product turnover because bran can go rancid

Avoid bran that:

- contains any clumps

You can find wheat and oat bran in the cereal or baking section of grocery and natural food stores.

### STORING

**Where:** Dark, dry, cool place.

**How:** In a tightly sealed container.

**For how long:** Up to 6 months in the refrigerator; up to 1 year in the freezer.

### COOKING

- Replace ¼ cup (50 mL) flour with bran in quick bread or muffin recipes.
- Coat fish fillets with bran before sautéeing.
- Add bran to a fruit smoothie.

### RECIPES TO TRY

- Pear Rhubarb Muffins
- Toasted Oat-Raisin Bread

### QUICK TIP:
**Add a little at a time**

Gradually increase your intake of bran until your body gets used to it, and drink plenty of water. This will prevent gastrointestinal problems like bloating and gas.

# B

# BREAD

*See also* Grains, page 57

**Typical serving size:** 1 slice (about 26 g), see chart on page 29 for calories

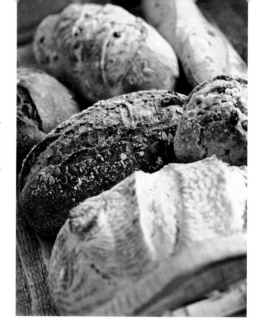

### HOW IT HARMS

Celiac disease (causes symptoms in people with this disease)

Allergies

Diabetes (white bread)

Fat storage (white bread)

High blood pressure (high-sodium bread)

### WHAT IT HEALS

Diabetes (whole grain bread)

Weight gain (whole grain bread)

Anemia (fortified or enriched bread)

### NUTRIENTS

Fiber (whole grain bread)

Folate

Iron

Niacin

Riboflavin

Thiamine

### BUYING

Choose breads that:

- are made with whole grains
- contain at least 3 g of fiber per serving
- are 100% whole wheat

Avoid breads that:

- list sugar in any form as one of the first four ingredients

### STORING

**Where:** At room temperature or in freezer, if you plan to keep it beyond its "best before" date or if you think it will become moldy. Don't store bread in the fridge. A single day in the fridge is equivalent to 3 days at room temperature.

**How:** In its wrapper.

**For how long:** You'll see the "best before" date on the plastic tie or wrapper. In the freezer, 3 months.

Eat crusty bread and rolls the day you buy them, because they become stale quickly.

### COOKING

- Make French toast with (day-old) raisin bread.
- Cut dried rye bread into croutons to garnish a red cabbage salad.
- Serve minestrone over a slice of dry whole wheat bread.

### RECIPES TO TRY

- Tomato Biscuits
- Multigrain Seeded Loaf
- Carrot-Flecked Corn Bread
- Cod with Gremolata Crust

# WHAT KIND OF BREAD IS HEALTHIEST?

Choose the highest-fiber breads that are appropriate for your dishes. Here's a guide to some of the most common types, listed in order from most to least grams of fiber per 2-oz (60-g) serving.

| TYPE | CALORIES PER 2-OZ (60 G) SERVING | GRAMS OF FIBER PER 2-OZ (60 G) SERVING | DESCRIPTION | BEST FOR |
|---|---|---|---|---|
| Multigrain | 149 | 4.2 | Made with a combination of flours and added ingredients, including sprouts and seeds; nutrition facts often comparable to whole wheat bread | All-purpose bread; use leftovers in casseroles and to make bread crumbs |
| Pita (6.5 in or 17 cm in diameter, whole wheat) | 149 | 4.1 | Flat, leavened bread that puffs up during baking and then flattens out to leave a hollow middle, or pocket | Pairing with Middle Eastern dips and salads; excellent base for personal pizzas; cut into wedges and bake until crisp as an alternative to chips |
| Tortilla (corn: 3 tortillas 6 in or 15 cm in diameter) | 120 | 4 | Unleavened Mexican bread made of corn or wheat flour, salt, and water | Mexican dishes and wrap-style sandwiches; thick flour tortillas can make a base for personal pizzas or appetizers |
| (wheat: 8 to 10 in or 20 to 25 cm in diameter) | 187 | 4 | | |
| Whole Wheat | 138 | 3.8 | Yeast bread made with whole wheat flour | All-purpose bread; use leftovers in casseroles and to make bread crumbs |
| Rye | 145 | 3.3 | Heavy and dense; may be seasoned with caraway seeds; most softer, deli-type rye breads are made with more wheat flour than rye | All-purpose sandwich bread; pairs well with Eastern European–style dishes like sauerkraut and a variety of sausages |
| Corn bread | 175 | 1.3 | Cornmeal-based quick bread; may be savory or slightly sweet depending on recipe | Stuffing, pairing with Southwestern dishes; slather with equal parts butter and honey for a decadent snack |
| Foccacia | 160 | 1.1 | Disc-shaped yeast bread made from a dough similar to pizza; traditionally flavored with olive oil, onions, garlic, and herbs | Pairing with soups and salads; toss bite-size pieces with olive oil and toast in the oven to make croutons |
| Challah | 170 | 1 | Rich, moist yeast bread usually formed into a distinct braided shape and brushed with egg white for a shiny exterior | French toast, bread pudding; pulse leftover bread in food processor for fresh bread crumbs |
| French (baguette) | 150 | 1 | A long, narrow loaf; crusty exterior | Crostini-style appetizers; use leftover slices in casseroles |
| Sourdough | 140 | 1 | White-flour bread leavened with a fermented wild yeast culture known as a starter | All-purpose bread; pairs well with strong flavors, especially assertive cheeses |

# BROCCOLI

**Typical serving size:** ½ cup cooked, chopped (78 g), 27 calories; ½ cup raw, chopped (44 g), 15 calories

## HOW IT HARMS

Bloating and flatulence

## WHAT IT HEALS

Bladder cancer
Colorectal cancer
Breast cancer
Lung cancer
Cardiovascular disease
Bone health
Colds
Skin
Weight gain

## NUTRIENTS

Antioxidants
Beta-carotene
Calcium
Fiber
Folate
Potassium
Sulforaphane (anticancer compound)
Vitamin C

## BUYING

Choose broccoli bunches with:
- florets that are dark green, purplish, or bluish green
- tightly closed buds
- stalks that are very firm and slender

Avoid bunches that have:
- pale or yellowing florets
- bendable or rubbery stalks
- open, flowering, discolored, or water-soaked bud clusters
- tough, woody stems

## STORING

**Where:** Crisper drawer of refrigerator.
**How:** Unwashed in an open plastic bag.
**For how long:** A day or two after purchasing.

## COOKING

- Steam, cook in the microwave, or stir-fry with a little broth or water to preserve vitamin and mineral content.
- Cut an X in the bottom of each stalk for more even cooking.
- Cooked broccoli should be tender enough so that it can be pierced with a sharp knife, and still remain crisp and bright green in color.
- Stir-fry broccoli chunks with garlic and teriyaki sauce.
- Roast florets coated with oil and curry powder on a baking sheet until browned.
- Simmer chopped broccoli in chicken broth until tender; puree for soup.

## RECIPES TO TRY

- One-Egg Omelet with Chopped Broccoli, Tomatoes and Cheddar
- Orange Beef with Broccoli and Jicama
- Vegetable Pot Pie
- Pasta Primavera
- Orange-Walnut Broccoli

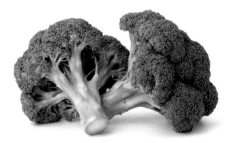

# BRUSSELS SPROUTS

**Typical serving size:** 1 cup cooked (155 g), 65 calories

## HOW THEY HARM

Bloating and flatulence

## WHAT THEY HEAL

Cancer
Cardiovascular disease
High blood pressure
Birth defects
Digestion
Cataracts
Weight gain

## NUTRIENTS

Beta-carotene
Fiber
Folate
Phytochemicals
Potassium
Vitamin C

## BUYING

Choose brussels sprouts that are:
- small, firm, compact sprouts
- bright green in color
- unblemished
- displayed in stores chilled

Avoid brussels sprouts that have:
- yellow or wilted leaves
- a strong, cabbage-like odor
- a puffy or soft feel

**Best time to buy:** autumn

## STORING

**Where:** Refrigerator.
**How:** Do not wash or trim sprouts before storing them in a plastic bag. Remove any yellow or wilted outer leaves. For sprouts packaged in a cellophane-covered container, take off the wrapping, examine them, remove any that are in bad condition, return them to container, and re-cover with cellophane.
**For how long:** 3 to 5 days.

## COOKING

- Cut an X in the bottom of the stem for even cooking when using the sprouts whole.
- Make a slaw with shaved brussels sprouts.
- Roast brussels sprouts with pork loin and carrot chunks.
- Sprinkle shredded cheddar cheese over cooked brussels sprouts.

## RECIPES TO TRY

- Braised Chicken with Winter Vegetables
- Fruity Brussels Sprouts
- Brussels Sprouts with Caraway Seeds

# BUCKWHEAT

*See* Grains, page 57

# BULGUR

*See* Grains, page 57

# BUTTERNUT SQUASH

*See* Squash, page 108

# BUTTER AND MARGARINE

Butter and margarine are both high in calories—one tablespoon has more than 100 calories—and they both contain fats that may be harmful to your heart. So it's important to use both in moderation and choose the one that will be most satisfying to you.

### KEEP IT HEALTHY

**Make it soft.** Buy soft trans fat free margarines in tubs. The softer your spread, the less you'll use.

**Combine it with other ingredients.** You can reduce the amount of butter or margarine you need to use by boosting flavor with herbs, spices, or low-fat ingredients. Top baked potatoes with chives and blended low-fat cottage cheese. When making cakes, cut the amount of butter or margarine by one-third to one-half and add about half a cup of applesauce for moisture.

**Halve it with olive oil.** Beat a soft stick of butter until it is smooth. Then slowly beat in ¼ to ½ cup olive oil. You've just significantly cut the amount of saturated fat while adding loads of healthy monounsaturated fat.

**Choose margarine with plant sterols.** Research has shown that these types of margarines actually improve cholesterol levels.

# CABBAGE

**Typical serving size:** ½ cup cooked, shredded (75 g), 17 calories; 1 cup raw, chopped (89 g), 22 calories

### HOW IT HARMS

Bloating and flatulence

High in calories (some coleslaw and sauerkraut)

Sulfites (sauerkraut and other prepared foods

### WHAT IT HEALS

Colon cancer

Breast cancer

Cancers of the uterus and ovaries

Diabetes

Weight gain

### NUTRIENTS

Beta-carotene

Fiber

Folate

Indoles (anticancer compound)

Potassium

Sulphoraphane (anticancer compound)

Vitamin C

Vitamin K

### BUYING

Choose cabbage that has:
- a tight, heavy head
- a vibrant green or red color, depending on type

Avoid cabbage that has:

- wilted, discolored, or dried outer leaves
- large blemishes
- separation of the leaves from the core

## STORING

**Where:** Refrigerator.

**How:** Unwashed and covered loosely with a plastic bag.

**For how long:** Up to 2 weeks for fresh, uncut heads; 5 to 6 days for sliced cabbage.

To prevent discoloration, rub cut surfaces with lemon juice.

## COOKING

- Cook cabbage quickly in an uncovered pan with as little water as possible to minimize odor. Overcooking can destroy the cabbage's stores of vitamin C.
- Stir-fry sliced green cabbage with scallions and grated ginger until golden.
- Use shredded savoy cabbage as a base for shrimp salad.
- Add slices of napa cabbage to beef noodle soup.

## RECIPES TO TRY

- Pork Chops and Cabbage
- Pasta with Cabbage, Apples and Leeks
- Thai-Style Beef Sandwich
- Brown Rice with Cabbage and Chickpeas
- Napa Cabbage Slaw with Peanut Dressing

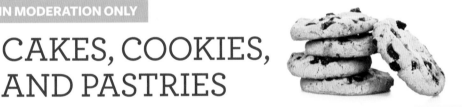

IN MODERATION ONLY

# CAKES, COOKIES, AND PASTRIES

The combination of fat and sugar in these foods makes them nearly irresistible—no wonder they're high on most people's list of favorite foods. Research has shown that this combo actually turns on pleasure sensors in the brain, making you desire more. Unfortunately these tasty treats offer little to no nutritional value, and eating too many of them can lead to weight gain (some desserts can have as many as 1,500 calories), diabetes, and high cholesterol. Additionally, most packaged baked goods are loaded with trans fats, man-made fats that contribute to heart disease. About the only upside to these foods are the mood and energy boosts they provide, However, both are short lived. But don't try to deprive yourself of these foods entirely, it will only make you crave them more. Instead, indulge wisely.

### KEEP IT HEALTHY

**Go for small portions.** You'll still enjoy the pleasures of these foods without all the fat and calories.

**Make your own.** Cut down on sugar and find healthy substitutes for unhealthy fat with the Healthy Baking tips on page 11.

# CANTALOUPE

*See* Melons, page 34

# CARROTS

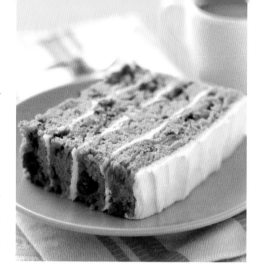

**Typical serving size:** ½ cup raw, chopped (64 g), 26 calories; ½ cup cooked, sliced (78 g), 27 calories

## HOW THEY HARM

Skin yellowing

## WHAT THEY HEAL

High cholesterol

Diabetes

Cancer

Macular degeneration

Cataracts

Night blindness

## NUTRIENTS

Beta-carotene

Fiber

Potassium

## BUYING

Choose carrots that have:

- bright green tops
- firm bodies, small to medium size
- smooth, even color without cracks

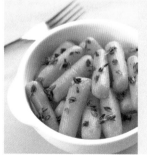

### QUICK TIP:

### Cook for more nutrition

Cooking increases carrots' nutritional value because it breaks down the tough cellular walls that encase the beta-carotene.

Avoid carrots that have:

- large green areas at the top
- soft spots
- wilted leaves

## STORING

**Where:** Crisper drawer of refrigerator.

**How:** In perforated plastic bags without green tops; keep carrots away from apples and pears.

**For how long:** Up to 2 weeks.

## COOKING

- Add a pat of butter or a tablespoon of olive oil to cooked carrots for better beta-carotene absorption.
- Stir ½ cup shredded carrot into oatmeal raisin cookie dough.
- Roast carrots tossed in soy sauce and honey until golden brown.
- Add shredded carrots and minced chives to scrambled eggs.

## RECIPES TO TRY

- Carrot Cake with Cream Cheese Glaze
- Flank Steak with Carrots and Red Pepper
- Tuna and Carrot Sandwich on Rye
- Braised Carrot, Celery, and Fennel

# CANDIES

While chocolate (especially dark chocolate) provides some health benefits (see page 42) and sugarless gum may help prevent cavities, the only thing other types of candy have to offer is sugar. While you may enjoy a quick energy burst, the jolt can have an equally negative effect. The rapid rise in blood sugar from eating candy causes insulin levels to spike. And when your blood sugar crashes after a high, you're likely to feel hungry and tired. Sweets and sugary foods also form an acid bath that is corrosive to tooth enamel and create an environment where destructive, cavity-causing bacteria flourish. The one group that actually benefits from candy in small amounts is people who have hypoglycemia, when they experience severe drops in blood glucose. It's unlikely that anyone can swear off candy forever, so enjoy it only occasionally.

### KEEP IT HEALTHY

**Pick your favorites.** Don't waste the calories on candy that's just so-so. When you do indulge, make sure it's a type you really love and then savor it.

**Have sugarless gum.** It's calorie-free and may help stimulate saliva flow to flush food particles out of your mouth.

**Chew, don't suck.** Candies that linger in the mouth longer are more damaging to teeth than those quickly swallowed. However, be careful of chewy caramels and other candies that leave sticky particles behind.

**Go nuts.** You can minimize blood sugar spikes by choosing candy with nuts in it.

# CAULIFLOWER

**Typical serving size:** ½ cup cooked (62 g), 14 calories; ½ cup raw (50 g), 13 calories

### HOW IT HARMS
Bloating and flatulence

### WHAT IT HEALS
Cancer
Weight gain

### NUTRIENTS
Bioflavonoids (anticancer compounds)
Fiber
Folate
Indoles (anticancer compounds)
Potassium
Vitamin B6
Vitamin C

### BUYING
Choose cauliflower that has:
- a firm head
- compact florets
- a snowy, white color
- crisp, green leaves

Avoid cauliflower that has:
- brown spots
- loose sections

**Best time to buy:** autumn

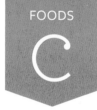

### STORING

**Where:** Crisper drawer of refrigerator.
**How:** In a plastic bag.
**For how long:** Up to 5 days.

### COOKING

- Boil or steam cauliflower in a minimum amount of water to retain flavor and nutrients.
- Stir-fry cauliflower florets with smoked paprika and garlic.
- Simmer cauliflower in some chicken broth until tender; puree.
- Sauté cauliflower florets and garlic in olive oil until golden; toss with whole-wheat pasta and slivered green olives.

### RECIPES TO TRY

- Spiced Cauliflower with Peas
- Cauliflower and Spinach Casserole
- Vegetable Pot Pie
- Cauliflower Salad with Cashews
- Broccoli and Cauliflower with Cream Sauce

# CELERIAC

(also known as Celery Root)

**Typical serving size:** ½ cup cooked (78 g), 21 calories

### WHAT IT HEALS

Weight gain
Cardiovascular disease

### NUTRIENTS

Fiber
Phosphorous
Potassium
Vitamin B6
Vitamin C
Vitamin K

### BUYING

Choose celeriacs that are:
- small- to medium-size
- firm
- heavy for their size
- smooth

Avoid celeriacs that:
- have soft spots

**Best time to buy:** autumn and winter

### STORING

**Where:** Refrigerator.
**How:** In an unsealed plastic bag.
**For how long:** Up to 1 week. If it turns soft, do not eat.

### COOKING

- Place peeled celeriac in some water with a squeeze of lemon juice immediately after cutting, to prevent it from changing color.
- Add shredded celeriac in place of celery in potato salad.
- Cook shredded celeriac with a wild rice pilaf.
- Layer sliced celeriac with potatoes in a gratin.

### RECIPES TO TRY

- Ham and Celeriac Pitas
- Sweet Potato and Celery Root Puree
- Pot Roast with Root Vegetables

# CEREALS

Not all cereals are created equally. While more than 90% of all commercial cereals are enriched or fortified with various vitamins and minerals—especially iron, niacin, thiamine, vitamin B6, and folic acid—many are high in sugar, and some are also high in salt. Even if you choose whole grain varieties, they can have too much sugar and salt. Granola types can also be high in fat from added oils. In addition, it's very easy to pour out much larger portions than recommended, so you could end up consuming more calories than you think. But if you take the time to read labels and keep portion size in check, cereal can be a healthy way to start your day.

### KEEP IT HEALTHY

**Read carefully.** Some cereals are low in calories and sugar when consumed in small servings. Pay extra attention to the serving size, which often varies from one box to the next.

**Start with whole grain varieties or ones with bran added.** Check the ingredient list. Whole grain or bran should be at the top.

**Look for high-fiber cereals.** Aim for at least 4 g per serving.

**Keep salt and sugar in check.** A serving should have no more than 240 mg of sodium and 13 g of sugar.

# CELERY

**Typical serving size:** ½ cup raw, diced (60 g), 9 calories

## WHAT IT HEALS

Weight gain

High blood pressure

Inflammation

Cancer

## NUTRIENTS

Beta-carotene

Fiber

Folate

Phthalides (compounds that may lower blood pressure)

Phytochemicals

Potassium

## BUYING

Look for celery stalks that are:

- light green
- crisp
- firm
- uniform in color
- have dark leaves

Avoid celery stalks that are:

- bruised
- browning
- hollow

## STORING

**Where:** Refrigerator.

**How:** Wrap the stalks loosely in plastic wrap.

**For how long:** 1 week.

QUICK TIP:
## Re-crisp your celery

To perk up celery that's gone limp, place stalks in ice water in the refrigerator for a few hours.

### COOKING

- Fill ribs with cashew butter and sprinkle dried cranberries on top.
- Scatter thinly sliced celery over tacos.
- Add minced celery to meat loaf.
- Add the leaves to soups, salads, and other dishes enhanced by the flavor of celery.

### RECIPES TO TRY

- Spicy Vegetable Cocktail
- Honey-Roasted Rack of Lamb
- Three-Bean Salad with Manchego Cheese
- Shellfish Salad with Herbed Lemon Dressing

**WARNING!**
**FOOD-DRUG INTERACTION**

Tyramine—found in aged cheeses such as cheddar, blue cheese, and camembert—also interacts with monoamine oxidase (MAO) inhibitors, drugs sometimes used to treat depression, and can cause a life-threatening rise in blood pressure.

# CHEESE

*See also* Milk and Dairy Products, page 39

**Typical serving size:** Varies; see chart on page 50

### HOW IT HARMS

High in saturated fat and sodium
Migraines
Allergies
Bacterial infection
Drug interaction

### WHAT IT HEALS

Diabetes
Metabolic syndrome
Bones
Muscles
Tooth decay

### NUTRIENTS

Calcium
Phosphorous
Potassium
Protein
Vitamin B12

### BUYING

Choose cheese that:
- contains the words "pasteurized milk" in the ingredient list
- has uniformity in color and texture
- is within the "use-by" date noted on the packaging

Avoid cheese that:
- is missing or has an incomplete label, or does not contain a factory seal

Take advantage of the broad range of low-fat cheeses on the market. Production methods have improved to allow for smoother texture and better taste.

### STORING

**Where:** Crisper drawer of refrigerator.
**How:** Wrap hard cheese such as parmesan or gouda in waxed paper, then in plastic wrap; wrap blue cheeses and semihard cheeses in plastic wrap; and keep fresh cheeses (like mozzarella or feta) in their packaging in water and change the water every couple of days.
**For how long:** Hard cheeses up to several months; softer cheeses from 1 to 3 weeks after opening; large pieces of cheese tend to keep longer than shredded cheese.

### COOKING

- Puree low-fat cottage cheese in a blender, then season to taste with salt-free herb blend.

# WHICH CHEESE SHOULD YOU CHOOSE?

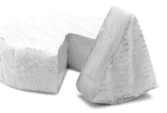

Keep calories and fat in check while selecting the best type of cheese for the dishes you're creating. The cheeses here are organized from least to most fatty.

| TYPE | CALORIES PER 1-OZ (30 G) SERVING | FAT PER 1-OZ (30 G) SERVING | DESCRIPTION | BEST FOR |
|---|---|---|---|---|
| Cottage cheese (low-fat) | 81 per 4 oz (125 g) serving | 1.2 g per 4 oz (125 g) serving | Technically a mild-flavored cheese curd that is not pressed or cured | Lasagna, jello salads, and desserts, as well as pairing with fresh fruit |
| Mozzarella (part-skim) | 72 | 4.5 g | Mild, semisoft unripened white cheese; fresh mozzarella is sold in a brine solution; low-moisture mozzarella can be refrigerated for up to a month | Italian-style dishes and salads |
| Feta (sheep milk) | 75 | 6 g | Compressed curds are cut into blocks and soaked in a brine solution; crumbles easily; salty, tangy flavor | Mediterranean-style dishes, salads |
| Brie | 95 | 7.8 g | Pale, creamy cheese under a rind of edible white mold; soft texture; flavor becomes stronger with age | Appetizers and cheese plates |
| Gouda | 101 | 7.8 g | Yellow semihard cheese that develops a nutty sweetness as it ages; young cheeses (aged less than 6 months) are noticeably softer and creamier | Appetizers and cheese plates |
| Swiss | 106 | 7.8 g | Pale yellow to off-white cheese that may or may not have holes depending on the variety; in general, flavors become more pronounced with age; most young cheeses (aged less than 6 months) are noticeably softer and creamier | Sandwiches and fondue (gruyere and emmental) |
| Blue | 100 | 8 g | Creamy white and streaked with blue-green ribbons of mold; soft and often crumbly texture; flavor can be strong or mild depending on variety | Fruit, salads, pasta dishes |
| Monterey jack | 100 | 8 g | Mild, semihard white cheese sometimes marbled with colby (sold as colby jack) or hot peppers (pepper jack); excellent melting cheese | Fruit, Mexican-style dishes, dips |
| Parmesan | 122 | 8.1 g | Hard, dry, and sharply flavored cheese sold in wedges or already grated | Italian-style dishes |
| Havarti | 110 | 9 g | Buttery semisoft cheese, similar to swiss, that can be flavored with dill or caraway seeds | Grilled cheese sandwiches |
| Cheddar | 113 | 9.3 g | Pale yellow to off-white; hard texture; sharp flavor becomes stronger with age | Macaroni and cheese; sandwiches with other strong flavors |

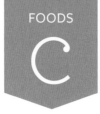

- Replace grated parmesan with half the amount of intensely flavored grated romano for pastas and salads.
- Scatter crumbled reduced-fat feta cheese on veggie pita pizzas.

### RECIPES TO TRY

- Huevos Rancheros
- Pumpkin Maple Cheesecake
- Turkey Braciole Stuffed with Provolone and Spinach
- Baked Pasta with Garlic and Greens
- Mediterranean Salad with Edamame

# CHERRIES

**Typical serving size:** ½ cup fresh with pits (59 g), 37 calories; ¼ cup dried (40 g), 140 calories

### HOW THEY HARM

**Allergies**

### WHAT THEY HEAL

**Inflammation**

**Cancer**

**High cholesterol**

**Gout**

**Arthritis**

### NUTRIENTS

**Anthocyanins (antioxidant)**

**Beta-carotene**

**Pectin (soluble fiber)**

**Potassium**

**Quercetin (flavonoid)**

**Vitamin C**

### BUYING

Look for cherries that are:
- plump
- firm
- green stemmed

Avoid cherries that are:
- bruised

**Best time to buy:** early summer

### STORING

**Where:** Refrigerator.

**How:** Unwashed, with stems attached in an open bag or container.

**For how long:** About 3 to 5 days; cherries spoil quickly, so eat them as soon as possible.

### COOKING

- Stir quartered cherries into a wild rice pilaf just before serving.
- Fold pitted cherries into a Waldorf salad.
- Puree cherries and combine them with ice and cold seltzer for a refreshing drink.

### RECIPES TO TRY

- Caraway-Coated Pepper Steak with Cherry Sauce
- Fruit Salad with Spiced Coconut
- Savory Cranberry Chutney
- Fruity Granola Mix

# CHIA

*See* Nuts and Seeds, page 77

# CHICKEN

*See* Poultry, page 96

# CHICKPEAS

*See* Beans and Other Legumes, page 20

# CHILES

**Typical serving size:** ½ cup raw, chopped (75 g), 30 calories; 2 Tbsp dried (4 g), 30 calories

## HOW THEY HARM
Hemorrhoids
Gastric discomfort

## WHAT THEY HEAL
Cancer
Blood clots
Nasal congestion
Weight gain

## NUTRIENTS
Beta-carotene
Bioflavonoids (anticancer compounds)
Capsaicin (may prevent blood clots)
Vitamin C

## BUYING
Choose chile peppers that have:
- smooth skin
- deep color

Avoid chiles that are:
- bruised or wrinkled
- mushy or have soft spots

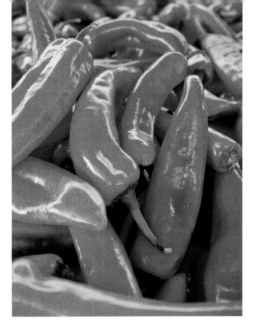

Red varieties generally have a higher nutritional content than the green ones.

## STORING
**Where:** Fresh, in the refrigerator; dried, in a cool dry place away from sunlight.
**How:** Fresh, in a plastic bag; dried, in an airtight container.
**For how long:** Fresh, up to 2 weeks; dried, up to 4 months.

## COOKING
- Remove the white ribs and seeds from chiles for a milder flavor.
- Blend three or four tomatoes, cilantro, chopped onion, a couple of chiles, and a pinch of salt for instant fresh salsa.
- Mix some minced jalapeño chiles into hamburger patties.
- Add a pinch of dried red chiles to pasta salad.
- Include some minced serrano chiles in a marinade for flank steak.

## RECIPES TO TRY
- Quinoa with Chiles and Cilantro
- Green Pork Chili

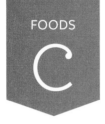

FOODS

# CHIPS AND CRACKERS

*See* Convenience and Processed Foods, page 47

# CHOCOLATE

**Typical serving size:** Varies; in general, 1 oz (28 g), 150 calories

### HOW IT HARMS
High in sugar and fat
Migraines

### WHAT IT HEALS
High blood pressure
Cardiovascular disease
Mood disorders

### NUTRIENTS
Epicatechin (disease-fighting flavonoids)
Procyanidins (disease-fighting flavonoids)

### BUYING
Choose chocolate that:
- is dark, with at least 60% cocoa for the most antioxidants
- has a smooth shiny surface, if visible

Avoid chocolate that has:
- a whitish or gray coating (which indicates blooming)
- milk or white chocolate
- a long ingredient list

White chocolate is a mixture of cocoa butter, milk solids, and sugar. It has no cocoa solids and does not keep well. The darker the chocolate, the less fat and sugar it has.

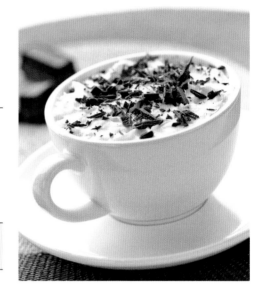

### STORING
**Where:** In a cool, dry place. Do not store in the refrigerator because this causes "blooming," or separation of cocoa butter from the chocolate.
**How:** In a tightly sealed container or bag.
**For how long:** Up to 1 year.

### COOKING
- Use crunchy, unsweetened cocoa nibs in place of chocolate chips in baked goods.
- Substitute ½ cup unsweetened cocoa powder for the flour in pancake recipes.
- Dip slices of crystallized ginger into melted bittersweet chocolate.

### RECIPES TO TRY
- Nutty Chocolate Chip Cookies
- Chocolate-Almond Biscotti
- Chocolate Banana Soufflés

# CLAMS

*See* Shellfish, page 103

# COFFEE

Drinking more than 400 to 500 mg a day of caffeine can pose a number of health problems. Some may just be annoying, like feeling jittery or making frequent trips to the bathroom. But others can be more serious. Caffeine prompts a temporary rise in blood pressure, increases calcium excretion, may interfere with conception, and may raise the risk of miscarriage. If you are susceptible to cardiac arrhythmias, have high blood pressure, suffer from migraines or headaches, are at risk for osteoporosis, are trying to conceive, or are pregnant, you should talk to your doctor about the effect that caffeine may have on you.

If you're not at risk for any of these serious health problems, go ahead and enjoy your cup of joe. Research shows that a moderate intake can reduce your risk of diabetes, Alzheimer's disease, colon cancer, Parkinson's disease, and skin cancer.

### KEEP IT HEALTHY

**Limit caffeine to less than 500 mg a day.** That's the amount in about four 6-oz (180 mL) cups. Most coffee cups today are much bigger, so you may only get to have one or two cups a day. And don't forget to include other sources of caffeine, such as tea or soft drinks, in your tally.

**Watch out for specialty coffee drinks.** While a 6-oz (180 mL) cup of sugar-free black coffee has only 4 calories, coffee drinks with syrups and whipped cream often have more fat and calories than a rich dessert.

# COCONUTS

**Typical serving size:** 1 cup raw, shredded (80 g), 283 calories

### HOW THEY HARM

High cholesterol

### WHAT THEY HEAL

Cravings

Digestion

Weight gain

### NUTRIENTS

Fiber

Potassium

### BUYING

Choose coconuts that have:

- a firm shell

Avoid coconuts with:

- dark or soft spots

### STORING

**Where:** Refrigerator once it's cut.

**How:** Wrapped tightly in plastic.

**For how long:** Up to 5 days; whole coconuts can be kept at room temperature for up to a month.

### COOKING

- Use reduced-fat coconut milk in place of cow's milk for french toast.
- Toss shredded fresh coconut in a

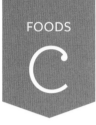

shrimp salad with lime dressing.
- Sprinkle shredded coconut on high-fiber breakfast cereal.
- Blend shredded raw coconut into smoothies.

## RECIPES TO TRY

- Thai Roasted Shrimp
- Fruit Salad with Spiced Coconut
- Thai Coconut Rice

# COLLARD GREENS

*See* Kale and Other Cooking Greens, page 65

# CORN

**Typical serving size:** 1 medium ear (90 g), 77 calories; ½ cup kernels (82 g), 67 calories

## HOW IT HARMS

Pellagra (a niacin or tryptophan deficiency)

## WHAT IT HEALS

Cardiovascular disease
Cancer
Macular degeneration

## NUTRIENTS

Ferulic acid (anticancer compound)
Fiber
Folate
Lutein (antioxidant)
Potassium
Thiamine

## BUYING

Choose corn that has:
- moist, green husks
- shiny silks
- plump and healthy kernels all the way to the tip
- some heft for its size
- been frozen rather than canned
- no salt added, if you must buy canned

To check the condition of the kernels, don't strip the husk—it dries out the corn and leaves it susceptible to fungus. Instead, feel around the silk end for firm, plump kernels.

Avoid corn that:
- feels wrinkled, mushy, or dry

**Best time to buy:** summer

## STORING

**Where:** Crisper drawer of refrigerator.
**How:** With husks attached.
**For how long:** Within 1 to 2 days.

## COOKING

- Use plain popcorn in place of bread for a poultry stuffing recipe.
- Stir corn kernels into a vegetable casserole.
- Toss corn kernels into a salad made with cooked red quinoa, minced onion, cilantro, and some salsa.

## RECIPES TO TRY

- Carrot-Flecked Corn Bread
- Sweet and Spicy Snack Mix
- Cod and Vegetable Stew
- Bulgur with Dried Cherries and Corn

# CONDIMENTS

While condiments certainly add zest to food, they generally contribute little nutrition and sometimes add a lot of sugar, fat, sodium, cholesterol, or nitrites. Too much of those can lead to weight gain, high blood pressure, diabetes, heart disease, and even cancer. Used judiciously, though, condiments add variety and make food tastier.

### KEEP IT HEALTHY

**Stick to the good guys.** Salsas, chutney, mustards, and hummus tend to be the lowest in fat and calories, although commercially prepared versions may still contain excess sugar or fat. Those made with cream, butter, egg yolk, and cheese tend to be the most unhealthy. Read labels carefully or make your own.

**Buy modified versions.** Many condiments are available in low-fat, nonfat, no-added-sugar, or other healthier options.

**Check ingredients.** If you have allergies or food intolerances, the culprits may be in these products, so read the labels carefully.

# CRANBERRIES

*See also* Berries, page 26

**Typical serving size:** ½ cup whole (48 g), 22 calories; ¼ cup dried (30 g), 90 calories

### HOW THEY HARM
Blood sugar spikes
Drug interaction

### WHAT THEY HEAL
Urinary tract infections
Cardiovascular disease
Cancer

### NUTRIENTS
Anthocyanins (antioxidants)
Fiber
Flavonols (plant chemical that prevents heart disease)
Proanthocyanidins (plant chemical that prevents heart disease)
Vitamin C

## BUYING

Choose cranberries that are:
- firm
- brightly colored
- unsweetened
- bouncy when dropped
- fresh or frozen

Avoid cranberries that are:
- bruised or mushy
- dry or shriveled
- canned or sweetened

**Best time to buy:** autumn

## STORING

**Where:** Fresh, in the refrigerator; dried, in a cool dark place or in the refrigerator.

**How:** In their original plastic packaging or tightly wrapped.

**For how long:** Fresh, up to 4 weeks; frozen, up to a year; dried, 6 months on a shelf or up to a year in the refrigerator.

## WARNING!
**FOOD-DRUG INTERACTION**

Do not drink cranberry juice if you are on the medication warfarin. The interaction between the juice and the drug may lead to bleeding.

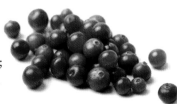

### COOKING

- Add dried cranberries to walnut biscotti dough.
- Stir some fresh cranberries into braised chicken about 10 minutes before cooking time is finished.
- Add some fresh cranberries to an apple cobbler or pie filling.

### RECIPES TO TRY

- Rice-Stuffed Squash
- Savory Cranberry Chutney
- Cranberry-Peanut Cereal Bars
- Broccoli Salad with Almonds and Dried Cranberries

# CUCUMBERS

**Typical serving size:** ½ cup sliced (52 g), 7 calories

### WHAT THEY HEAL

Weight gain

### NUTRIENTS

Folate

Potassium

### BUYING

Choose cucumbers that are:
- firm
- brightly colored

Avoid cucumbers that have:
- soft spots, blemishes, or bruises
- wrinkled or dry looking skin

**QUICK TIP: Snack on cucumbers in hot weather**

The interior flesh of cucumbers is about 20 degrees cooler than the outside temperature even if they aren't chilled. And their high water content—about 95%—will keep you hydrated.

**Best time to buy:** summer

### STORING

**Where:** Crisper drawer of refrigerator.

**How:** Unwashed and unpeeled; if peeled, wrap tightly in plastic wrap.

**For how long:** 1 to 2 days for unwaxed or peeled; up to 1 week for waxed.

### COOKING

- If cucumber skin is waxed, peel before using.
- Layer thinly sliced cucumbers on cheese, ham, or turkey sandwiches.
- Puree peeled, seeded cucumber with plain yogurt, garlic, chopped dill, and a bit of ice water for a refreshing summer soup.
- Dip cucumber sticks in baba ghanoush.

### RECIPES TO TRY

- Chunky Gazpacho with Garlicky Croutons
- Greek Lamb Kebabs
- Poached Salmon with Cucumber-Dill Sauce
- Minty Melon Cups
- Japanese Sushi Rolls

# CONVENIENCE AND PROCESSED FOODS

Convenience foods that require little or no preparation—from ready-to-eat breakfast cereals and canned, dried, or frozen fruits and vegetables, to prepackaged heat-and-serve meals—are practically a necessity in our busy lifestyles. Unfortunately, many are much less healthy than home-cooked versions because of extra sugar, salt, and fat, all of which can have adverse health effects. They also tend to be loaded with artificial flavorings, emulsifiers, fillers, preservatives, and trans fats that can increase your risk for heart disease. And processing often strips vitamins and minerals from foods. But nutritious picks that help busy cooks put meals together quickly do exist; you just have to be a savvy shopper.

### KEEP IT HEALTHY

**Go for fresh options.** Precut veggies and fruit and rotisserie chicken are quick healthy options. Just don't eat the skin on the chicken.

**Boost nutrition.** Add a fresh side salad to a meal consisting of processed food, like frozen lasagna, to provide a wide assortment of valuable nutrients.

**Watch out for sauces.** Vegetables and many fruits harvested and quick-frozen at their peak often have more vitamins than those picked before maturity, shipped long distances, and then placed on shelves. But you can undo those benefits if you choose varieties in high-calorie, high-fat sauces and syrups. Stick to plain varieties for the healthiest option.

**Limit salt.** Scan the nutrition panel carefully, and keep your daily intake under 2,300 mg of sodium.

**Watch out for red-flag ingredients.** Be wary of ingredient lists with the words "corn sweetener," "corn syrup," "corn syrup solids," "high-fructose corn syrup," "hydrogenated fats," or "vegetable shortening."

**Choose whole grains.** Look for packaged rice or noodle products made with brown rice or whole wheat pasta whenever possible. If you can't find prepackaged foods with whole wheat pasta or brown rice, cook some up separately and then add it to the dish. Along with more fiber, it will increase the amount of food you have, so the sodium, sugar, and fat per serving will be less.

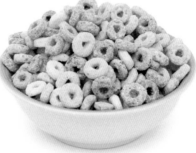

# D

Dates contain tyramine, an organic compound found in aged cheese, certain processed meats, red wine, and other products. Anyone taking monoamine oxidase (MAO) inhibitors to treat depression should avoid dates, because tyramine can interact with these drugs to produce a life-threatening rise in blood pressure. In some people, tyramine can also trigger migraine headaches.

# DATES

**Typical serving size:** 5 to 6 dates (40 g), 126 calories

## HOW THEY HARM

Weight gain
Tooth decay
Drug interaction

## WHAT THEY HEAL

Cancer
Bone loss
Cardiovascular disease
High blood pressure

## NUTRIENTS

Calcium
Fiber
Iron
Magnesium
Manganese
Niacin
Polyphenols (anticancer compounds)
Potassium
Vitamin B6

## BUYING

Choose dates that are:
- shiny
- uniformly colored

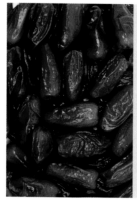

**QUICK TIP:**
### Refresh your dates

If they've been stored for an extended period of time, immerse them in hot water (about 80°F or 30°C) for about 20 to 30 minutes, allowing water to absorb to improve texture and taste. Remove, pat dry with a paper towel.

Avoid dates that are:
- cracked
- discolored or have yellow or brown blemishes

Fresh dates are classified according to their moisture content, falling into three categories: soft, semisoft, and dry. Most varieties in North America are semisoft, which are marketed fresh, as well as dried after part of their moisture has been evaporated.

**Best time to buy:** autumn

## STORING

**Where:** At room temperature.
**How:** In an airtight container.
**For how long:** Several months. Refrigerated dates last up to 1 year.

## COOKING

- Blend a couple of dates into a smoothie in place of other sweeteners and for added fiber.
- Stuff dates with whole blanched almonds and drizzle with melted white chocolate.
- Stir some chopped dates into tabbouleh salad.
- Create a sweet and sour sauce for sautéed chicken breasts by deglazing the skillet with sherry vinegar and chopped dates.

## RECIPES TO TRY

- Hot Cereal with Apples and Dates
- Fruity Brussels Sprouts
- Chewy Date-Walnut Bars

# DUCK

*See* Poultry, page 96

# EDAMAME

*See* Soy, page 105

# EGGPLANTS

**Typical serving size:** ½ cup cooked (50 g), 18 calories (with no fat added)

### HOW THEY HARM

Fat and calorie magnet

### WHAT THEY HEAL

Weight gain

### NUTRIENTS

Fiber

Anthocyanins (antioxidants)

## BUYING

Choose eggplants that are:
- firm with thin skin
- smaller
- heavy for their size
- deep purple to light violet or white

Avoid eggplants that are:
- cracked or discolored
- bruised or shriveled
- yellowish or have blue or brown streaks

## STORING

**Where:** Crisper drawer of refrigerator.
**How:** Whole, no container or bag needed.
**For how long:** 5 to 7 days.

## COOKING

- Eggplants' spongy texture causes them to soak up more fat and calories than potatoes. For healthier cook-ing, use a preparation that requires minimal fat, such as broiling, baking, roasting, or stewing. If sautéing, use a nonstick pan and little oil.
- Grill baby eggplant slices, then spread with ricotta cheese, pesto, and finely chopped tomato. Roll into tubes.
- Grill eggplant wedges, then toss in a bowl with hoisin sauce and chile paste just to coat.
- Stir-fry eggplant cubes in olive oil with chopped onion, zucchini, and tomato.
- Slice eggplant into thin slivers and use in place of noodles in lasagna.
- Cut eggplant in half and roast until soft. Scoop out the insides and mix with a bit of olive oil, salt, pepper, a crushed garlic clove, and a squeeze of lemon for a quick baba ghanoush.
- Use it in place of meat in stews, cas-seroles, and sandwiches.

## RECIPES TO TRY

- Penne with Fresh Tomato Sauce and Grilled Eggplant
- Rustic Grilled Vegetable and Rigatoni Salad
- Grilled Eggplant Sandwiches with Red Pepper–Walnut Sauce

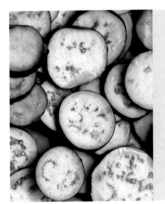

**QUICK TIP:**
**Sprinkle with salt**

To eliminate bitterness in some eggplants, sprinkle cubed or sliced eggplant with salt. Let it stand for half an hour, then drain it and blot it dry. The salt draws out excess moisture and reduces bitterness.

# E

# EGGS

**Typical serving size:** 1 large (50 g), 75 Calories

## HOW THEY HARM
Allergies
Bacterial infection

## WHAT THEY HEAL
Cardiovascular disease
Cancer
Cataracts and macular degeneration
Memory

## NUTRIENTS
Beta-carotene
Choline
Iron
Lutein
Protein
Vitamin B12
Vitamin D
Vitamin E
Zeaxanthin (antioxidant)
Zinc

## BUYING

Choose eggs that are:
- enhanced with omega-3s (they're lower in saturated fat and higher in vitamin E than regular eggs)
- brown or white—they're equally nutritious (free-range eggs may have slightly higher levels of carotenoids)

Avoid eggs that are:
- cracked or stuck to the bottom
- past the "use-by" date

## STORING

**Where:** In the main part of the refrigerator, not on the inside of the door.

## QUICK TIP:
### Limit eggs if indicated
Doctors recommend that people with high cholesterol eat no more than three yolks a week. People with diabetes should limit consumption, too.

**How:** In its carton with the pointed end of the egg down.
**For how long:** Up to 3 weeks. (Eggs age more in 1 day at room temperature than in 1 week in the refrigerator.)

## COOKING

- To be certain that eggs have been cooked long enough, boil them for at least 4 minutes, poach them for 5 minutes, or fry them for 3 minutes. Both the yolk and the white should be firm. Omelets and scrambled eggs should be cooked until firm and not runny.
- Refrigerate hard-cooked eggs for up to a week for quick, easy snacks or sandwich fillings.
- Stir-fry leftover cooked noodles or rice with leftover veggies and a beaten egg for a quick meal.
- Top steamed asparagus with a poached egg and a sprinkling of parmesan cheese.

## RECIPES TO TRY

- Asparagus, Egg, and Ham Sandwiches
- Mushroom and Bell Pepper Frittata
- Zucchini-Carrot Crustless Quiche Squares
- Fried Rice with Tofu and Vegetables

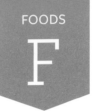

# FENNEL

**Typical serving size:** 1 cup sliced (87 g), 25 calories

## HOW IT HARMS

Skin irritation

## WHAT IT HEALS

Weight gain
High blood pressure
High cholesterol
High blood sugar
Cancer

## NUTRIENTS

Beta-carotene
Calcium
Fiber
Folate
Iron
Potassium
Vitamin C

## BUYING

Choose fennel that has:
- firm bulbs
- bright green stalks and leaves

Avoid fennel that is:
- blemished
- soft or has mushy spots

**Best time to buy:** autumn to early spring

## STORING

**Where:** Crisper drawer of refrigerator.
**How:** Unwashed in a sealed plastic bag.
**For how long:** Up to 5 days.

## COOKING

- All parts of the plant are edible. It can be prepared raw in salads, or braised or sautéed as a side dish.
- Marinate shrimp in cracked fennel seeds, lemon juice, and olive oil before grilling.
- Dip fennel wedges into hummus.
- Sauté fennel and sweet onion wedges until browned, then season with balsamic vinegar.
- Use in place of celery in stews and soups.

## RECIPES TO TRY

- Braised Carrot, Celery, and Fennel
- Grilled Oysters with Fennel and Spinach
- Warm Kasha and Seafood Salad
- Sicilian Pasta Salad

# FIGS

**Typical serving size:** 2 small (80 g), 60 calories; ¼ cup dried (50 g), 124 calories

## HOW THEY HARM

Diarrhea
Tooth decay
Canker sores

## WHAT THEY HEAL

Cardiovascular disease
High cholesterol
Diabetes
Cancer
Bone loss
Constipation

## NUTRIENTS

Calcium
Fiber
Iron
Manganese
Pectin (soluble fiber)
Potassium
Vitamin B6

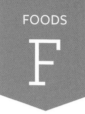
## BUYING

Choose figs that are:
- ripe and unblemished
- a deep purple
- soft, but not mushy

Avoid figs that are:
- moldy or smell fermented
- mushy or blemished

**Best time to buy:** late summer to early autumn

## STORING

**Where:** Refrigerator.
**How:** In a paper towel–lined container.
**For how long:** Within 2 days.

## COOKING

- Macerate quartered dried figs in orange juice.
- Use chopped dried figs in place of raisins.
- Bake halved fresh figs with fresh pineapple wedges sprinkled with cinnamon.

## RECIPES TO TRY

- Sesame Fig Bars
- Nutty Muesli
- Fresh Figs with Raspberries and Rose Cream
- Grilled Fruit en Brochette

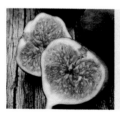

### QUICK TIP: Pick the sweetest

Fig connoisseurs say to look for a drip of moisture at the hole on the bottom of the fruit.

# FISH

*See also* Shellfish, page 103

**Typical serving size:** About the size of a deck of cards, or 3 oz (85 g); calories vary depending on variety (see chart on page 53)

## HOW IT HARMS

Pollutants
Parasites
Bacteria and viruses

## WHAT IT HEALS

Cardiovascular disease
Stroke
Inflammation
Memory loss
Macular degeneration

## NUTRIENTS

Calcium (canned salmon and
  sardines with bones)
Magnesium
Niacin
Omega-3 fatty acids
Protein
Vitamin A (oily fish such as salmon)
Vitamin D (oily fish such as salmon)
Vitamin B12
Zinc

## BUYING

Shop at a busy fish counter—it means faster turnover and fresher fish. Or look for markets that keep fish covered (both top and bottom) with ice. The best sources of omega-3 fats are oily cold-water fish such as salmon, mackerel, trout, sardines, herring, and anchovies. You'll also find them in halibut, bluefish, ocean perch, bass, red snapper, and smelts. Limit your intake of large bottom-feeders such as tuna, shark, king mackerel, tilefish, and

# WHICH TYPE OF FISH OR SHELLFISH TO CHOOSE?

In general, cook fish for 10 minutes for every inch of thickness, or until it flakes easily with a fork. Before cooking clams, oysters, and mussels, discard any that don't close with a light tap on the shell; cook until the shells open, and avoid eating any that do not open during cooking. When preparing lobster, scallops, shrimp and squid, cook just until firm; longer cooking times can result in a tough, chewy texture. Octopus traditionally requires a longer cooking time, usually at least an hour, to become tender. Because most of the fat in fish is healthy (as noted on the chart below), don't shy away from fatty types.

| TYPE | CALORIES PER 3 OZ (90 G) COOKED PORTION | FAT PER 3 OZ (90 G) COOKED PORTION | BEST FOR |
|---|---|---|---|
| Anchovies | 162 | 9*g | Pizza and pasta dishes; due to their intense flavor, smaller portions are more typical |
| Bass | 124 | 4g | Fillets and paired with a wide variety of dishes; excellent grilled, pan-seared, or roasted |
| Catfish | 115 | 6.5g | Fillets and paired with Southern foods; excellent when pan-seared or baked |
| Clams | 126 | 1.7g | Steaming and eating right out of the shell; also great in soups and pasta dishes |
| Cod (Pacific) | 89 | 0.7g | Fillets; excellent when pan-seared or baked with a topping to prevent dryness |
| Crab (blue) | 87 | 1.5g | Crab cakes, pasta dishes, salads |
| Halibut | 119 | 2.5g | Fillets or fish tacos; excellent either grilled or broiled |
| Herring | 173 | 9.9*g | Appetizers; if pickled, choose herring in wine sauce versus cream sauce for less fat and fewer calories (calories listed do not include any sauce) |
| Lobster | 76 | 0.7g | Steaming and eating right out of the shell; also great in soups, risottos, salads, and pasta dishes |
| Mackerel | 223 | 15.1*g | Fillets and paired with other strong flavors, such as garlic and olives; great when grilled (whole), pan-seared, or roasted |
| Mussels | 146 | 3.8g | Steaming and eating right out of the shell; also great in pasta dishes |
| Octopus | 139 | 1.8g | Mediterranean and Asian dishes; to save time, look for chopped, frozen octopus |
| Oysters | 139 | 3.9g | Eating raw right out of the shell; also great in soups and stuffing |
| Red snapper | 109 | 1.5g | Fillets and paired with Caribbean dishes; best grilled, pan-seared, or roasted |
| Salmon | 155 | 6.9*g | Fillets and paired with a wide variety of dishes; excellent grilled, pan-seared, or smoked; choose wild salmon when feasible |
| Sardines | 136 | 7.9*g | Appetizers; typically sold in smaller cans |
| Scallops | 150 | 1g | Main dishes and appetizers; best pan-seared or broiled |
| Shrimp | 84 | 0.9g | Main dishes and appetizers; excellent in most cooking methods, including pan-seared, baked, grilled, steamed, and boiled |
| Squid | 60 | 1.5g | Main dishes and appetizers; best when cooked very briefly |
| Tilapia | 109 | 2.2g | Fillets and when well-seasoned to compensate for its mild flavor; excellent pan-seared or baked |
| Trout | 162 | 7.2*g | Main dishes and appetizers; excellent pan-seared, baked, or smoked |
| Tuna (chunk, light) | 99 | 0.7g | Casserole and pasta dishes; opt for tuna packed in water |

* High in omega-3 fatty acids

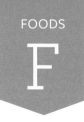

swordfish because they tend to be high in mercury.

Choose fish that has:
- bright, bulging, and clear eyes (whole fish)
- bright red gills (whole fish)
- bright, glossy skin with tight scales (whole fish)
- moist, resilient skin (fillets)
- firm flesh
- a fresh, briny odor

Avoid fish that has:
- gray or cloudy eyes (whole fish)
- grayish or pink gills (whole fish)
- any discoloration (fillets)
- gaps in the flesh (fillets)
- a fishy odor

When buying canned fish, choose those packed in water rather than oil. For tuna, go with the light or albacore variety.

### STORING

**Where:** In the coldest part of the refrigerator, or in the freezer.
**How:** Wrapped in plastic wrap.
**For how long:** Fresh, 1 to 2 days; frozen, within 3 months for fatty fish, and 6 months for lean fish.

### COOKING

- Serve slivers of smoked whitefish with a spinach salad.
- Brush grilled halibut with teriyaki sauce.
- Crumble drained canned salmon into a pasta salad.

### RECIPES TO TRY

- Roasted Mackerel with Cherry Tomatoes and Potatoes
- Monkfish and Mussel Kebabs
- Snapper and Snaps in a Packet
- Grilled Salmon Salad
- Tossed Tuna Salad Niçoise

# FLAX

*See also* Nuts and Seeds, page 77

**Typical serving size:** 1 to 2 Tbsp, ground (7 to 14 g), 33 to 66 calories

### HOW IT HARMS

Fetus and nursing infants (check with doctor if pregnant or nursing)
Bleeding problems (avoid if you have a bleeding disorder)
Drug interaction

### WHAT IT HEALS

Cardiovascular disease
High cholesterol
Menopause symptoms
Cancer
Constipation

### NUTRIENTS

Alpha linolenic acid (ALA—a heart healthy omega-3 fatty acid)
Fiber
Lignans (phytoestrogens)

### BUYING

In the grocery, you can find flaxseeds and flaxmeal in the same aisle as flour. Flaxseed oil is often found in the pharmacy section.

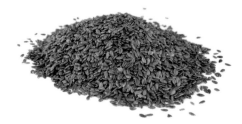

**WARNING!**
**FOOD-DRUG INTERACTION**
Because the lignans in flax are phytoestrogens, it may affect drugs such as Tamoxifen that are used to treat hormone-sensitive conditions. While some research suggests that it helps these conditions, more studies are needed. Talk to your doctor before eating flax while on Tamoxifen, or if you have hormone-sensitive ailments such as breast or uterine cancer, endometriosis, or fibroids.

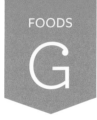
Choose flaxseeds that are:
- whole (grind them in a blender or coffee grinder as needed)
- from a store with a high turnover, if ground
- refrigerated, if ground
- vacuum-packed, if ground

Avoid flaxseeds that:
- are not in an opaque container
- don't come with a "use-by" date

## STORING

**Where:** In the refrigerator or freezer, especially if ground.

**How:** In an airtight, opaque container in the fridge if whole or in oil form; in the freezer if ground.

**For how long:** Up to 1 year if whole; if ground, a few weeks in the freezer or until the best-before date on the package.

If flaxseed tastes bitter or smells sharp or fishy, throw it away.

## COOKING

- Replace 2 Tbsp of flour in cookie recipes with an equal amount of flaxmeal.
- Use flaxmeal to bread fish or chicken cutlets to be baked or sautéed.
- Spread corn on the cob with a blend of flaxseed oil and Cajun seasoning.
- Add ground flax to muffin or pancake batter.
- Sprinkle ground flax onto oatmeal.

## RECIPES TO TRY

- Broccoli Salad with Almonds and Dried Cranberries
- Berry-Flaxseed Smoothie
- Chicken-Kale Soup with Roasted Pepper Puree
- Cranberry-Peanut Cereal Bar
- Whole Wheat Flaxseed Bread

# FLOUR

*See* Grains, page 57

# GARLIC

*See also* Herbs and Spices, page 61

**Typical serving size:** 3 cloves (9 g), 12 calories

## HOW IT HARMS

Bleeding problems

Stomach irritation

Drug interaction

## WHAT IT HEALS

High blood pressure

Atherosclerosis

Cardiovascular disease

Diabetes

Colon and rectal cancer

Infections

Tick bites

## NUTRIENTS

Allicin

Antibacterial, antifungal, and antiviral compounds

## BUYING

Choose garlic that:
- is dry
- has lots of papery sheath covering it
- looks and feels plump and firm
- is white or off-white

Avoid garlic that is:
- shriveled
- moldy
- mushy
- sprouting

**WARNING!**
**FOOD-DRUG INTERACTION**
Garlic may interfere with the effectiveness of saquinavir, a drug used to treat HIV infection.

**Best time to buy:** late summer

## STORING

**Where:** In a cool, dark, and dry place with plenty of circulation or a clay garlic holder; not in the refrigerator.
**How:** In its papery covering.
**For how long:** Several weeks.

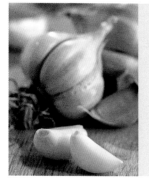

### QUICK TIP:
**Prepare before cooking**

To activate garlic's full nutritional power, it should be chopped or crushed and then left to stand for 10 minutes before cooking. This allows allicin and its potent derivatives to be activated.

## COOKING

- Boil peeled garlic cloves with potatoes to season the mash.
- Stir-fry spinach with extra-virgin olive oil and plenty of minced garlic.
- Wrap a whole head of garlic in foil and bake in the oven for 30 minutes for a soft spread for breads or potatoes.
- Sauté garlic and add it to tomato sauce, or mince it and add it raw.

## RECIPES TO TRY

- Braised Mixed Greens with Dried Currants
- Roasted Tomatoes with Garlic and Herbs
- Turkey, Spinach, and Rice in Roasted Garlic Broth
- Bok Choy, Tofu, and Mushroom Stir-Fry
- Romaine Lettuce with Chunky Tomato Vinaigrette

# GINGER

**Typical serving size:** 1 tsp or 1-in (2.5-cm) diameter slice, raw (2 g), 2 calories; 1 tsp ground (2 g), 6 calories

## HOW IT HARMS

Bleeding problems
Miscarriage
Inflamed mouth and mucous membranes
Drug interaction

## WHAT IT HEALS

Motion sickness and nausea
Pain
Cancer
Flatulence

## NUTRIENTS

Beta ionone (cancer-fighting compound)
Gingerols (phenol compound)
Shogaols (phenol compound)

## BUYING

Fresh ginger can be found at any supermarket, but dried and powdered forms are readily available, as are ginger juices and teas.

Choose ginger that:
- is plump and firm
- has smooth skin
- has a spicy fragrance

Avoid ginger that is:
- withered
- cracked
- moldy
- blemished

Here's a comforting way to relieve congestion: Make ginger tea by simmering one or two slices of fresh ginger root in water for 10 minutes; add a pinch of cinnamon for extra flavor.

## STORING

**Where:** In the refrigerator or freezer.
**How:** Unpeeled and dry, in a sealed plastic bag with all the air pressed out.
**For how long:** 2 weeks in the refrigerator; up to 2 months in the freezer.

## COOKING

- Sauté minced ginger with broccoli and a little olive oil for an antioxidant feast.
- Add grated fresh ginger to butternut squash soup.
- Top baked tilapia with grated ginger, soy sauce, and a few drops of canola oil.
- Whisk grated ginger into a salad dressing of canola oil and rice wine vinegar.

## RECIPES TO TRY

- Chicken Breast with Peaches and Ginger
- Jerk Turkey Breast with Ginger Barbecue Sauce
- Shrimp and Vegetable Stir-Fry
- Pork, Pear, and Potato Salad
- Fruit Parfait with Ginger Tea Cream

# GRAINS

*See also* Barley, page 20; Bran, page 27; Oats, page 78; Quinoa, page 98; Rice, page 101; Wheat and Wheat Germ, page 115

**Typical serving size:** ½ cup cooked whole grains, 73 to 151 calories

## HOW THEY HARM

**Cardiovascular disease (refined grains)**
**Atherosclerosis (refined grains)**
**Diabetes (refined grains)**
**Celiac disease**

## WHAT THEY HEAL

**Diabetes (whole grains)**
**Cardiovascular disease (whole grains)**
**Cancer (whole grains)**
**Digestive health (whole grains)**
**Diverticular disease (whole grains)**
**Anemia (whole grain and enriched flours)**

## NUTRIENTS

**B vitamins (whole grains and enriched)**
**Complex carbohydrates (whole grains)**
**Fiber (whole grains)**
**Folate (enriched)**
**Iron (whole grains and enriched)**
**Magnesium (whole grains)**
**Vitamin E (whole grains)**
**Zinc (whole grains)**

## BUYING

Choose grains that:
- are unrefined; look for the words "whole wheat flour" as the first ingredient on breads and cereals
- have a "100% Whole Grains" label

**WARNING!**
**FOOD-DRUG INTERACTION**

Consuming ginger while on medications that slow bleeding such as warfarin may cause bleeding and bruises. If you are on these medications, do not eat ginger.

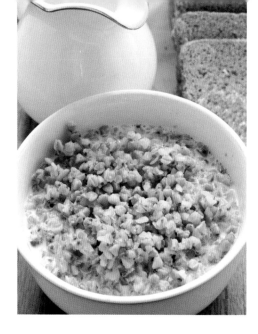

**FOOD-DRUG
INTERACTION**
Grapefruit juice
can enhance the
effects of certain
medications,
possibly resulting
in adverse
effects. Drugs to
watch out for
include those for
high blood
pressure, anxiety,
depression,
elevated lipids,
and more. As a
precaution, it is
best to avoid
taking any drug
with grapefruit
juice until you
have asked your
doctor or
pharmacist if it is
safe to do so.

If you have a gluten sensitivity, you can
find flours made from all sorts of grains,
nuts, and other foods, including potato, almonds, rice, chickpeas, and buckwheat.

Avoid grains that are:
- refined
- labeled wheat flour

## STORING

**Where:** In a cool, dry place, in the refrigerator, or in the freezer.
**How:** In an airtight container or in bags
with the air pressed out.
**For how long:** 2 to 6 months.

## COOKING

- Add some cooked roasted buckwheat
  groats (kasha) to a bean or lentil
  salad.
- Replace ½ cup of the flour in muffin
  recipes with rolled oats.
- Serve grits as a side dish instead of
  mashed potatoes.
- Stuff bell peppers with seasoned
  cooked millet.

## RECIPES TO TRY

- Warm Kasha and Seafood Salad
- Multigrain Seeded Loaf
- Buckwheat Pancakes with Fruit Sauce
- Whole Wheat Pasta with Sausage and
  Greens
- Wheat Berry Salad with Dried
  Apricots

# GRAPEFRUITS

**Typical serving size:** ½ grapefruit
(123 g), 52 calories; or ¾ cup (177 mL)
juice, 70 calories

## HOW THEY HARM

Allergies
Canker sores
Drug interaction

## WHAT THEY HEAL

High cholesterol
Cancer
Weight gain
Inflammation

## NUTRIENTS

Beta-carotene (pink and red
  varieties)
Bioflavonoids
Fiber
Limonoids (cancer fighters)
Lycopene (antioxidant)
Monoterpenes (cancer fighters)
Pectin (soluble fiber)
Phenolic acid (cancer fighter)
Potassium
Terpenes (cancer fighters)
Vitamin C

## BUYING

Choose grapefruits that are:
- firm
- heavy for their size
- bright and colorful

Avoid grapefruits that are:
- wrinkled
- bruised
- have blemishes

**Best time to buy:** winter

## STORING

**Where:** At room temperature or in the crisper drawer of the refrigerator.
**How:** Unpeeled or cut.
**For how long:** Up to 1 week at room temperature; 2 to 3 weeks in the fridge.

## COOKING

- Add grapefruit wedges to a smoothie.
- Dip wedges into melted bittersweet chocolate.
- Stir-fry boneless chicken breast cubes with garlic and cumin, add grapefruit chunks and toss until heated.

## RECIPES TO TRY

- Tropical Fruit Salad
- Roast Pork and Quinoa Salad
- Chicken Salad with Citrus

### QUICK TIP: Serve it warm

Turn this typical warm weather breakfast fruit into a toasty treat. Cut a grapefruit in half and discard the center membrane and seeds. Sprinkle with sugar and cinnamon and broil until browned.

# GRAPES AND RAISINS

**Typical serving size:** ½ cup or about 15 grapes (46 g), 31 calories; 1 oz or about 55 raisins (28 g), 85 calories

## HOW THEY HARM

Asthma attacks in sulfur-sensitive people

Allergies in people with aspirin allergies

## WHAT THEY HEAL

Cardiovascular disease

Cancer

Muscle cramps

Anemia

## NUTRIENTS

Anthocyanins (antioxidants)

Ellagic acid (anticancer compound)

Iron

Potassium

Quercetin (antioxidant)

Resveratrol (anticancer compound)

Vitamin C

European table grapes have more nutrients, such as vitamin C, than American varieties. Red and purple varieties have more nutrients, such as anthocyanins and resveratrol, than green.

## BUYING

Choose grapes that are:
- plump
- without blemishes
- uniform in color

Avoid grapes that are:
- wrinkled or brownish
- white where the stem meets the fruit

Buy raisins in single-serving boxes to limit portion size and keep calories reasonable.

**Best time to buy:** summer

### STORING

**Where:** Refrigerator.
**How:** Unwashed, in a ventilated plastic bag.
**For how long:** Up to 1 week.

### COOKING

- Sauté red grapes with chard or kale.
- Freeze grapes on a tray, then store in a freezer-proof container for quick snacks.
- Add dark raisins to a tossed green salad.
- Add golden raisins to braised pork.

### RECIPES TO TRY

- Fruit Salad with Spiced Coconut
- Rice Salad with Chicken and Grapes
- Turkey Braciole Stuffed with Provolone and Spinach
- Brown Rice with Cabbage and Chickpeas

# GREEN BEANS

*See* Beans and Other Legumes, page 20; Peas and Pea Pods, page 89

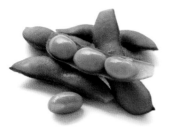

# GUAVAS

| **Typical serving size:** 1 medium (90 g), 45 calories |
| --- |

### HOW THEY HARM

Allergies

### WHAT THEY HEAL

Cancer
Cardiovascular disease
Constipation
Weight gain

### NUTRIENTS

Vitamin C
Pectin (soluble fiber)
Potassium

### BUYING

Choose guavas that:
- are firm but not hard (skin yields slightly when pressed)
- have a fragrant, musky aroma

Avoid guavas that:
- are wrinkled
- are bruised
- smell fermented

**Best time to buy:** late autumn and early winter

### STORING

**Where:** Counter, if unripe; crisper drawer of refrigerator, if ripe.
**How:** Unwrapped.
**For how long:** Up to 4 days when ripe.

To hasten ripening, place the guava in a brown paper bag with a banana or an apple.

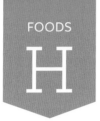

## COOKING

- Toss chopped guavas into an arugula salad.
- Simmer chopped guavas with brown sugar and cinnamon.
- Add guava chunks to a smoothie.

## RECIPES TO TRY

- Guavas and Plums with Vanilla Syrup
- Fresh Fruit Soup

# HERBS AND SPICES

*See also* Garlic, page 54; Ginger, page 56

**Typical serving size:** varies according to recipe, negligible calories

### HOW THEY HARM
Allergies
Pesticides

### WHAT THEY HEAL
Digestion
Bloating and flatulence
Inflammation
High blood pressure
Colds and flus
Cancer
Nausea and motion sickness
Fainting
Stomach cramps

### NUTRIENTS
See chart on page 62

## BUYING
Choose:
- whole spices to grind at home for the freshest, most pungent flavor
- organic herbs to avoid pesticides
- herbs that smell robust

Avoid:
- herbs with brown spots
- herbs that smell moldy
- herbs that are limp

Spices are sold bottled in supermarkets and, less expensively, in bulk-food stores and ethnic markets.

### STORING
**Where:** Dark, dry cupboard for spices and dried herbs; refrigerator for fresh herbs.
**How:** In airtight containers for spices and dried herbs. For fresh herbs, snip ends and stand them in a glass of water; change water daily.
**For how long:** About 1 year for spices and dried herbs; up to 1 week for fresh herbs.

### COOKING
- Add chopped fresh mint to cucumber salad.
- Stir chopped fresh cilantro into hummus.
- Add a handful of chopped fresh parsley to tossed salad.
- Create a Moroccan spice blend with equal parts of ground cinnamon, coriander, and cumin.
- Sprinkle oregano on grilled zucchini slices brushed with olive oil.
- Season stir-fried shrimp with crushed fennel seeds and garlic.

### RECIPES TO TRY
- Roasted Pork with Pomegranate Sauce
- Fruit Salad with Spiced Coconut
- Fruity Granola Mix
- Minty Melon Cups
- Herb-Buttered Turnips

# WHICH HERBS AND SPICES SHOULD YOU USE?

Both fresh and dried herbs provide a wide variety of active phytochemicals that promote health and protect against chronic disease. Discover the healing power of nine popular herbs and spices and how to get more of them into your diet.

| TYPE | HOW THEY HEAL | HOW TO USE IN COOKING |
| --- | --- | --- |
| Cayenne | Helps break up nasal and sinus congestion | Add a dash of ground cayenne to any dish that needs a little heat. For an extra kick, try a light dusting on popcorn or party mix. Excellent as part of a spice rub mix. |
| Cinnamon | Aids digestion and may help fight infection due to anti-inflammatory and antimicrobial properties | Use cinnamon's distinct warm flavor as a complement to sweet desserts and drinks, including mulled cider and Mexican hot chocolate. Also used in Greek and Moroccan cooking to add balance to savory dishes. |
| Clove | Contains eugenol, which may help curb toothache pain | Add a dash of ground cloves alongside other warming spices, including cinnamon, nutmeg, ginger, and allspice in cookies, pies, and other baked goods. |
| Cumin | May protect eyes and cardiovascular system against diabetes-related damage | Use ground cumin alongside dried coriander in Mexican and Indian cooking; also pairs nicely with sautéed onions and canned beans (add a squirt of fresh lime to balance cumin's earthy notes); for maximum flavor, toast lightly just before using to release fragrant oils. |
| Mint | Aids digestion by calming upset stomach; relieves gas | Brew as a tea by steeping fresh or dried leaves in hot water; chop fresh mint and add to fruit salads, beverages and desserts, as well as traditional Mediterranean and Middle Eastern dishes such as tabbouleh and cucumber-laced tzatziki sauce. |
| Oregano | A member of the mint family, oregano may help improve symptoms of a sinus infection as part of a steam inhalation therapy | Add fresh or dried oregano to Italian and Mediterranean dishes; pairs well with tomatoes and garlic (add a splash of lemon or vinegar to the combination to highlight oregano's herbal qualities). One teaspoon dried oregano is roughly equal to 1 Tbsp fresh; reserve fresh oregano for dishes that are seasoned just before serving, as heat quickly dissipates the flavor. |
| Rosemary | Distinct piney scent was once thought to aid memory; today research indicates it may help relieve asthma and allergy symptoms | Use chopped fresh rosemary along with garlic in marinades, dressings and side dishes for a classic Mediterranean combination; especially good tucked inside roasted fish or poultry, or chopped and scattered over roasted potatoes. The herb's tough, woody stems are excellent to use as skewers when grilling fish and other delicate proteins. |
| Thyme | Reduces inflammation and helps fight infection; excellent in mouthwashes and natural cough drops | Keep this versatile herb in your pantry for dressing up a wide variety of sauces and sides; complements poultry, seafood, potato, and egg dishes. |
| Turmeric | A relative of ginger; has anti-inflammatory compounds that may fight pain and swelling associated with arthritis | Use a teaspoon when cooking curry sauces and rice dishes; add a dash when assembling potato salads or mixing up egg recipes to impart a distinct yellow hue to the finished dish. |

# HONEY

*See* Sugar and Other Sweeteners, page 62

# HONEYDEW

*See* Melons, page 73

# HUMMUS

*See* Condiments, page 45

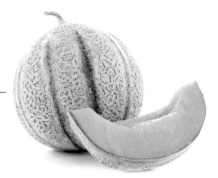

# ICE CREAM

This creamy frozen treat is another one of those fat-sugar combos—like cakes, cookies, and pastries—that's just so hard to say no to, especially during summer months. Along with loads of calories, ice cream contains big helpings of saturated fat, which is bad for your heart and your waistline. Its redeeming qualities are a healthy dose of calcium and protein. To enjoy the good while limiting the bad, keep portions small, indulge only occasionally, and follow these guidelines.

### KEEP IT HEALTHY

**Opt for alternatives, such as fruit sorbets or low-fat frozen yogurt.** Just be sure to read labels carefully—some of these products may have more sugar and calories.

**Look for slow-churned or double-churned.** These types of light or reduced-fat ice cream contain up to half the fat and two-thirds the calories of original and have a creamier texture.

**Choose cones wisely.** A sugar cone contains 60 calories, while a chocolate-dipped waffle cone has more than 200. And avoid high-calorie toppings like candy.

**Top it with fruit.** The fiber will fill you up so you'll be satisfied with less. Nuts are another option; just watch the portion size since they're high in calories.

# JICAMA

**Typical serving size:** ½ cup sliced (60 g), 23 calories

## HOW IT HARMS

Allergies

## WHAT IT HEALS

Cardiovascular disease

Stroke

Weight gain

High blood sugar

Constipation

Skin

Cataracts

## NUTRIENTS

Fiber

Potassium

Vitamin C

### BUYING

Choose jicama:
- between 1 and 2 lb (500 g and 1 kg); larger ones may be less sweet
- with firm, smooth, slightly shiny skin
- that is heavy for its size

Avoid jicama that is:
- blemished or cracked
- moldy
- discolored

**Best time to buy:** late autumn through spring

### STORING

**Where:** Refrigerator.

**How:** Uncut, in a plastic bag; cut, wrapped in plastic.

**For how long:** Uncut, 2 to 3 weeks; cut, up to 1 week.

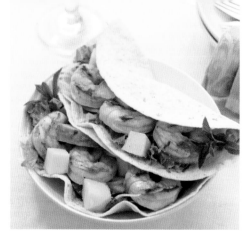

- Season jicama sticks with lime juice and chili powder.
- Eat it with a dip, diced in a salad, or added to stir-fries.
- Top jicama slices with tapenade for an appetizer.
- Shred jicama and add it to slaws. It's a great topping for fish tacos.

### COOKING

- Peel jicama and remove the fibrous white area just beneath the skin.

### RECIPES TO TRY

- Orange Beef with Broccoli and Jicama
- Avocado, Jicama, and Orange Salad
- Jamaican Jerked Chicken Salad

**IN MODERATION ONLY**

# JAMS, JELLIES, AND OTHER SPREADS

High in sugar, jams and jellies are no substitute for the abundant nutrition found naturally in fruits. In fact, most of the vitamin C and other key nutrients are destroyed during the intense cooking process involved in producing them. Low-calorie, reduced-sugar jams aren't much better because they're often sweetened with concentrated fruit juice, fructose, and corn syrup and thickened with starches, giving you only empty calories. Soft spread-cheese-based products contain only trace amounts of vitamin A and calcium and are high in sodium, fat, and cholesterol. Chocolate and marshmallow spreads are just spreadable sugar. About the only upside to these products is the quick boost of energy they provide. But that's really only helpful for people prone to hypoglycemia. So whenever possible, choose the real thing—sliced strawberries with peanut butter for a sandwich, cheese slices on crackers, or melted dark chocolate—instead of the processed stuff. But when you can't, follow these guidelines.

### KEEP IT HEALTHY

**Go for all-fruit.** Choose preserves made of 100% fruit.

**Skip additives.** That includes added oils, salt, sugar, and preservatives.

**Measure how much you use.** And use the least amount possible. A tablespoon (15 mL) of regular jelly has about 60 calories and 11 g of sugar.

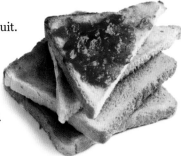

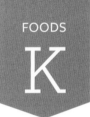
# JUICES

Even if you choose the healthiest juices, they still contain a lot of calories because of the natural fruit sugar. Canned or bottled vegetable juices tend to have less sugar than fruit juices but more salt, which can increase blood pressure. Fruit juice should not be given to infants under 6 months old because it can cause diarrhea, poor weight gain or delayed development, and tooth decay. If consumed in moderation, drinking juice can be an easy way to get more of the recommended 5 to 10 servings of fruits and vegetables. About 4 oz (125 mL) of juice is equal to 1 serving. Since juice lacks fiber and other compounds found in whole pieces of fruit and vegetables, it's best to make only 2 or 3 of your fruit servings from juice. And when you do, choose wisely.

### KEEP IT HEALTHY

**Strive for 100%.** Look for juices labeled "100% juice" for the most nutrients.

**Go unsweetened.** Choose juices that do not have added sugars.

**Look for plant sterols.** These cholesterol-lowering compounds that have been used in margarine are now showing up in orange juice.

**Step away from "fruit drinks" and "fruit punch."** They contain extra sugar (usually corn syrup) and other additives with less actual fruit juice.

# KALE AND OTHER COOKING GREENS

*See* also Spinach, page 107

**Typical serving size:** ½ cup cooked, chopped (65 g), 18 calories

### HOW THEY HARM

Bloating and flatulence

### WHAT THEY HEAL

Cardiovascular disease

Cancer

Eye conditions

Bone health

### NUTRIENTS

Beta-carotene

Bioflavonoids

Calcium

Carotenoids

Fiber

Folate

Indoles (anticancer compounds)

Iron

Lutein (antioxidant)

Magnesium

Potassium

Vitamin C

### BUYING

Choose kale that has:

- crisp edges
- deep color
- small to medium size leaves

Avoid kale that has:
- wilted leaves
- yellowed or brown leaves

### STORING

**Where:** Refrigerator.
**How:** Rinsed, slightly damp, wrapped in a paper towel, and in a plastic bag.
**For how long:** Within 3 days.

### COOKING

- Simmer finely chopped mustard greens in vegetable soup.
- Add some chopped Italian lacinato kale to marinara sauce for pasta.
- Stuff blanched collard green leaves instead of cabbage leaves.

### RECIPES TO TRY

- Summer Greens Scramble
- Baked Pasta with Garlic and Greens
- Chicken-Kale Soup with Roasted Pepper Puree

# KETCHUP

*See* Condiments, page 45

# KIWI

**Typical serving size:** 1 large kiwi or ½ cup sliced (90 g), 56 calories

### WHAT THEY HEAL

High blood pressure
High cholesterol
Cancer
Macular degeneration
Weight gain

### NUTRIENTS

Lutein (antioxidant)
Pectin (soluble fiber)
Phytochemicals
Potassium
Vitamin C
Vitamin E
Zeaxanthin (antioxidant)

### BUYING

Choose kiwis that:
- are firm, but give to slight pressure
- have rough, fuzzy skin

Avoid kiwis that are:
- blemished
- wrinkled

### STORING

**Where:** Room temperature, or in the refrigerator.
**How:** Unpeeled and uncut.
**For how long:** About 1 week at room temperature; up to 4 weeks in the fridge.

### COOKING

- Kiwi skin is edible if it is de-fuzzed.
- Toss chunks with strawberries and chopped fresh mint.
- Grill unpeeled halved kiwi to serve with grilled pork chops.
- Serve kiwi slices over lemon yogurt.

### RECIPES TO TRY

- Tropical Fruit Salad
- Jamaican Jerked Chicken Salad

QUICK TIP:
**Tenderize meat with kiwis**
Rub meat with a cut kiwi and wait 30 to 60 minutes before cooking to tenderize.

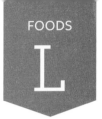

# KOHLRABI

**Typical serving size:** 1 cup raw, chopped (135 g), 36 calories

### HOW IT HARMS

Bloating and flatulence

### WHAT IT HEALS

Cancer
Cardiovascular disease

### NUTRIENTS

Bioflavonoids
Fiber
Indoles (anticancer compounds)
Iron
Isothiocyanates (anticancer compounds)
Potassium
Vitamin C

## BUYING

Choose kohlrabi with:

- a diameter of less than 3 in (7.5 cm) (larger ones can be tough and woody)
- thin rinds
- fresh tops

Avoid kohlrabi with:

- blemishes
- cracks

## STORING

**Where:** Crisper drawer of refrigerator.
**How:** Remove leaf stems and place in a sealed plastic bag.
**For how long:** Several weeks.

## COOKING

- Simmer chunks of kohlrabi with green split peas to puree for soup.
- Stir-fry chopped kohlrabi with a slice of diced bacon until crisp-tender.
- Serve raw kohlrabi sticks on a veggie platter with dip.

## RECIPES TO TRY

- Maple-Glazed Chicken with Root Vegetables

# LAMB

**Typical serving size:** 3 oz (85 g), 160-200 calories, depending on cut

### HOW IT HARMS

Weight gain

### WHAT IT HEALS

Muscles
Anemia
Immunity

### NUTRIENTS

Conjugated linoleic acid (fatty acids that improve cholesterol levels)
Iron
Phosphorous
Potassium
Protein
Vitamin B12
Zinc

## BUYING

Look for lamb that is:

- firm
- red colored with some white marbling

Avoid lamb that:

- has holes in its packaging
- is past the "use-by" date

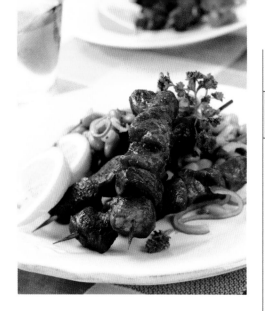

## STORING

**Where:** In the refrigerator at 40°F (4°C) or below, or in the freezer.

**How:** In its original packaging and covered to prevent cross-contamination (overwrap tightly when freezing).

**For how long:** 1 to 2 days for ground lamb or stew meat in the fridge (3 to 4 months in the freezer); 3 to 5 days for lamb chops, roasts, and steaks in the fridge (6 to 9 months in the freezer).

## COOKING

- Sauté thinly sliced lamb with slivered onions and curry powder.
- Stuff a pita bread half with sliced roast lamb, cucumber, plain yogurt, and fresh dill.
- Marinate skewered chunks of lamb, onion, and bell pepper in lemon-garlic salad dressing before grilling.

## RECIPES TO TRY

- Skillet Okra and Lamb
- Lamb Burgers with Fruit Relish
- Savory Lamb Stew with Sweet Potatoes
- Greek Lamb Kebabs

# LEEKS

**Typical serving size:** 1 raw (89 g), 50 calories

## HOW THEY HARM

Flatulence

## WHAT THEY HEAL

Cancer
High cholesterol
High blood pressure

## NUTRIENTS

Beta-carotene
Kaempferol (anticancer compound)

## BUYING

Choose leeks that have:

- firm, crisp stalks
- as much white and light green regions as possible

Avoid leeks that have:

- yellow or withered tops

## STORING

**Where:** Refrigerator.
**How:** Unwashed, in a plastic bag.
**For how long:** Up to 2 weeks.

## COOKING

- Serve steamed whole leeks with cheddar cheese sauce.
- Roast chunks of leeks with brussels sprouts tossed in canola oil and sprinkled with sesame seeds.
- Toss sliced raw leeks with beets in reduced-fat ranch dressing.
- Chop green tops of leeks and add to soups and stocks.

## RECIPES TO TRY

- Lentil and Rice Paella with Clams
- Pasta with Cabbage, Apples, and Leeks
- Vegetable Stock

# LEGUMES

*See* Beans and Legumes, page 20

# LEMONS AND LIMES

**Typical serving size:** ½ cup sectioned and peeled (106 g), 31 calories

## HOW THEY HARM

Skin irritation

Fungicides and pesticides

Sun sensitivity

Canker sores

Tooth enamel damage

## WHAT THEY HEAL

High cholesterol

Cancer

Cardiovascular disease

Kidney stones

Varicose vein pain

Dry mouth

## NUTRIENTS

Bioflavonoids (anticancer compound)

Limonene (in the zest; cholesterol-lowering compound)

Rutin (flavonoid)

Vitamin C

## BUYING

Look for lemons and limes that are:
- not waxed
- heavy for their size
- bright skinned

Avoid lemons and limes that have:
- bruises or wrinkles
- large blemishes or discoloration
- soft spots

## STORING

**Where:** At room temperature or in the crisper drawer of refrigerator.

**How:** In a plastic bag in the refrigerator.

**For how long:** Several days at room temperature; about 2 weeks in the refrigerator.

## COOKING

- Macerate sliced strawberries in lemon juice and a sprinkling of sugar.
- Stuff a halved lemon and bouquet garni into the chicken cavity before roasting.
- Toss grated lime peel and juice with hot cooked quinoa.
- Freeze lemon or lime juice mixed with the grated peel in small resealable freezer bags for convenience.
- Use lime juice as a salt substitute for meat and fish dishes.

## RECIPES TO TRY

- Scallops Florentine
- Trout with Lemon-Mushroom Stuffing
- Shellfish Salad with Herbed Lemon Dressing
- Grilled Chicken Sandwiches with Basil Mayonnaise
- Angel Food Cake with Strawberries

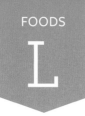

# LENTILS

*See also* Beans and Other Legumes, page 20

**Typical serving size:** ½ cup cooked (99 g), 115 calories

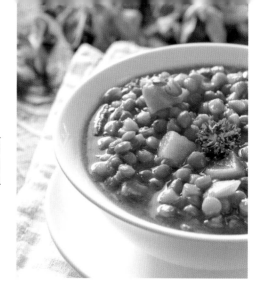

## HOW THEY HARM

Bloating and flatulence

## WHAT THEY HEAL

High cholesterol
Blood sugar spikes
Weight gain
Constipation
Anemia
Cardiovascular disease
Reproductive health
Cancer

## NUTRIENTS

B vitamins
Fiber
Folate
Iron
Magnesium
Niacin
Potassium
Protein

## BUYING

Choose lentils that are:
- uniform size
- brightly colored

Avoid lentils that are:
- not in clear packaging
- cracked, shriveled, or have holes

The common khaki-colored lentils are widely available in supermarkets; the more delicate green and red lentils may be harder to find.

## STORING

**Where:** A cool, dry place.
**How:** In an airtight container.
**For how long:** Up to 6 months. Cooked lentils may be stored in a sealed container in the refrigerator for up to 1 week.

## COOKING

- Sort through lentils before cooking and discard any that are shriveled.
- Don't mix new lentils with older ones, because older lentils will take longer to cook.
- Red lentils cook faster than the khaki ones.
- Coarsely grind cooked seasoned lentils in a food processor, then shape into patties for frying or grilling.
- Use lentils in place of beans in minestrone.
- Toss cooked lentils with cooked rotini pasta and shredded provolone cheese.

## RECIPES TO TRY

- Lentil and Rice Paella with Clams
- Artichokes with Lentils and Lima Beans
- Lentil Soup with Canadian Bacon

# LETTUCE AND OTHER SALAD GREENS

*See also* Spinach, page 107

**Typical serving size:** 1 cup (20 to 55 g depending on variety), 4 to 10 calories

## HOW THEY HARM

Food poisoning

## WHAT THEY HEAL

Cancer
Cardiovascular disease
Weight gain

## NUTRIENTS

Antioxidants
Beta-carotene
Calcium
Folate
Iron
Potassium
Vitamin C

Amounts vary from one variety to another, with dark green or other deeply colored leaves being more nutritious than paler varieties. Arugula, watercress, escarole, and mache are some of the most nutritious varieties.

## BUYING

Look for lettuce with:
- fresh, crisp leaves
- good, bright color

Avoid lettuce with:
- decay like wilting or sliminess
- blemishes
- tip burn, a tan or brown area around the margins of the leaves
- very hard or irregular shaped heads
- insect damage

## STORING

**Where:** Crisper drawer of the refrigerator.

**How:** Discard brown and wilted leaves, separate leaves and rinse, spin them dry, and layer between sheets of paper towel.

**For how long:** Up to 1 week; if using within 3 days, you can store greens in a plastic bag in the refrigerator.

## COOKING

- Pair romaine lettuce with apples, pecans, blue cheese and cider vinaigrette.
- Try arugula with beets, walnuts, feta cheese, and red wine vinaigrette.
- Stir-fry sliced romaine lettuce with some Chinese black beans and grated ginger as a side dish.
- Make a pureed soup by blending simmered lettuce, garlic, thyme, and chicken broth; garnish with grated parmesan.
- Braise sliced escarole with raisins, garlic, balsamic vinegar, and a pinch of ground red pepper.

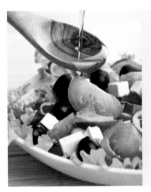

**QUICK TIP: Dress your salad with a little oil**

Oil enhances the absorption of beta-carotene, which is plentiful in arugula and romaine varieties of lettuce. Beta-carotene plays an important role in preventing cancer and vision loss.

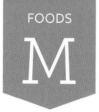
**RECIPES TO TRY**

- Watermelon and Feta Salad
- Asian Chicken Salad
- Buckwheat Noodles with Tofu and Green Vegetables
- Endive, Apple, and Watercress Salad
- Salmon and Fennel Lettuce Wraps

# LIMES

*See* Lemons and Limes, page 69

# LIVER

*See* Organ Meats, page 83

# LOBSTER

*See* Shellfish, page 103

# MANGOES

**Typical serving size:** ½ cup sliced (83 g), 54 calories

## WHAT THEY HEAL

Cancer

High blood pressure

High cholesterol

Weight gain

## NUTRIENTS

Beta-carotene

Pectin (soluble fiber)

Potassium

Vitamin C

**BUYING**

Look for mangoes that:
- yield slightly when gently pressed
- emit a fruity aroma
- have a green or yellow-green color with a red blush

Avoid mangoes that:
- have large dark spots
- are completely green
- have shriveled skin

**Best time to buy:** summer

**STORING**

**Where:** At room temperature and out of the sun until ripened; in refrigerator, once ripe.

**How:** In a plastic bag if cut.

**For how long:** 1 to 2 weeks uncut; no more than 3 days once cut.

**COOKING**

- Use mangoes in any recipe that calls for peaches.
- Sprinkle mango chunks with toasted coconut.
- Add mango chunks to a pork stir-fry.

**RECIPES TO TRY**

- Broiled Salmon with Avocado-Mango Salsa
- Fruit Salad with Spiced Coconut
- Indian-Style Turkey Burger
- Fish Tacos
- Yogurt Parfait

# MARGARINE

*See* Butter and Margarine, page 32

# MELONS

**Typical serving size:** ½ cup diced (78 to 85 g), 23 to 31 calories, depending on type

## HOW THEY HARM
Bacterial infection

## WHAT THEY HEAL
Cancer
Cardiovascular disease
High blood cholesterol
Weight gain

## NUTRIENTS
Beta-carotene
Bioflavonoids and carotenoids (anticancer compounds)
Fiber
Lycopene (antioxidant in watermelons)
Potassium
Vitamin C

## BUYING
Look for melons that:
- are whole to preserve nutritional content
- have a smooth, slightly sunken scar near where the stem was
- have a deep, intense fragrance

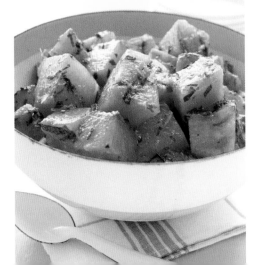

- rattle when shaken or produce a slightly hollow sound when thumped

Avoid melons that:
- are lopsided or have a flat side
- have cracks, soft spots, or dark bruises
- have stems on the scar

**Best time to buy:** summer to early autumn

## STORING
**Where:** Crisper drawer of refrigerator.
**How:** Whole and unwashed; in a sealed container if cut.
**For how long:** 5 to 7 days; the riper they are, the shorter they will keep. Toss cut melons that have been left at room temperature for more than 4 hours.

## COOKING
- Before cutting, scrub the skin with a clean vegetable brush under running water and blot it dry.
- Add finely chopped watermelon to barbecue sauce.
- Grill sliced honeydew melon with Cajun seasoned catfish fillets.
- Stir cantaloupe cubes into chicken salad.

## RECIPES TO TRY
- Crab Cakes with Melon Relish
- Chicken-Melon Salad
- Cantaloupe and Orange Soup
- Fruit Parfait with Ginger Tea Cream

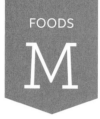
# MILK AND DAIRY PRODUCTS

*See also* Butter and Margarine, page 32; Cheese, page 38; Ice Cream, page 63; Yogurt, page 116

**Typical serving size:** 1 cup (236 mL), calories vary (see chart below)

## HOW THEY HARM

High cholesterol (whole milk and milk products)
Lactose intolerance
Allergies
Acne

## WHAT THEY HEAL

Bone loss
Insulin resistance
High blood pressure

## NUTRIENTS

Calcium
Magnesium
Potassium
Protein
Riboflavin
Vitamin B12
Vitamin D

## BUYING

Choose milk:

- dated several days in the future (the date on the carton indicates the last day on which the milk can be sold)
- in a cardboard or opaque container

Avoid milk:

- on or past its "use-by" date
- in a clear or translucent container

## STORING

**Where:** Toward the back of the refrigerator.
**How:** A temperature just above freezing is ideal, but milk should not be frozen.

## WHICH MILK SHOULD YOU DRINK?

In recent years, some new milk options have popped up in grocery stores, and they're not all created equally. Here's what you need to know to find the best milk for you.

| | | PER FLUID 8-OZ SERVING | | | | | |
|---|---|---|---|---|---|---|---|
| | | CALORIES | TOTAL FAT (G) | SAT FAT (G) | CALCIUM (MG) | PROTEIN (G) | VITAMIN D (IU) |
| | Whole (3.25% milk fat) | 149 | 7.9 | 4.6 | 276 | 7.7 | 124* |
| | Reduced-fat (2% milk fat) | 122 | 4.8 | 3.1 | 293 | 8 | 120* |
| | Low-fat (1% milk fat) | 102 | 2.4 | 1.5 | 305 | 8.2 | 117* |
| | Skim (0% milk fat) | 83 | 0 | 0 | 299 | 8.3 | 115* |
| | Buttermilk (low-fat) | 98 | 2.2 | 1.3 | 284 | 8.1 | 0 |
| LACTOSE–FREE | Almond milk (unsweetened) | 40 | 3 | 0 | 450* | 1 | 100* |
| | Soymilk (original and vanilla) | 104 | 3.6 | 0.5 | 299* | 6.3 | 104* |
| | Rice milk (unsweetened) | 113 | 2.3 | 0 | 283* | 0.7 | 101* |
| | Coconut milk (unsweetened) | 80 | 5 | 5 | 300* | 1 | 120* |

*Indicates nutrient added to the milk during processing; may vary according to brand

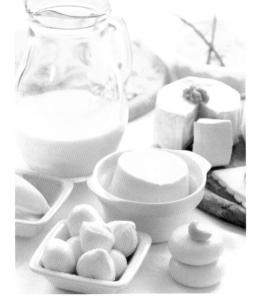

**For how long:** 1 to 5 days beyond "use-by" date.

## COOKING

- Freeze cubes of milk mixed with an equal amount of orange juice; process cubes in a food processor to make sherbet.
- Cook rice in milk instead of water for a creamy side dish.
- Simmer sliced red potatoes and onions in milk for a quick soup; season with dill and black pepper.

## RECIPES TO TRY

- Chai
- Macaroni and Cheese with Spinach
- Potato Salad with Sun-Dried Tomatoes, Scallions, and Basil

### QUICK TIP: Try dry milk

To boost calcium, add nonfat dry milk (from a sprinkling up to ¼ cup) when baking or to soups, casseroles, stews, egg dishes, meatloaf, and mashed potatoes. A ¼ cup (125 g) of dry milk has 210 mg of calcium.

# MUSHROOMS AND TRUFFLES

**Typical serving size:** ½ cup raw, sliced (35 g), 8 calories; ½ cup cooked (78 g), 22 calories

## HOW THEY HARM

May be poisonous

## WHAT THEY HEAL

Cardiovascular disease
High blood pressure
High cholesterol
Prostate and breast cancer
Immunity
Weight gain

## NUTRIENTS

Chitin (cholesterol-lowering fiber)
Lentinan (phytochemical that may help boost immunity)
Niacin
Potassium
Selenium

## BUYING

Choose mushrooms that are:
- firm buttons
- large; the largest of any variety have the most flavor

Avoid mushrooms with:
- bruises

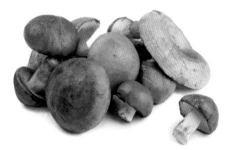

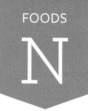
**STORING**

**Where:** Crisper drawer of refrigerator.
**How:** In a paper bag.
**For how long:** 5 days.

**COOKING**

- Rinse mushrooms only before using them. Do not peel them or remove the stalks.
- Squeeze a little lemon juice on mushrooms to retain their color.
- Mix sautéed chopped mushrooms into turkey meat loaf.
- Grill portobello mushroom caps mounded with wild rice stuffing.
- Sprinkle truffle oil over sautéed mushrooms as a bruschetta topping.

**RECIPES TO TRY**

- Mushroom and Bell Pepper Frittata
- Trout with Lemon-Mushroom Stuffing
- Bok Choy, Tofu, and Mushroom Stir-Fry
- Baked Rice with Wild Mushrooms and Cheese
- Vegetable-Stuffed Mushrooms

# MUSTARD GREENS

*See* Kale and Other Cooking Greens, page 65

# NECTARINES

*See* Peaches and Nectarines, page 87

# NUTS AND SEEDS

*See also* Flax, page 54; Peanuts and Peanut Butter, page 88

**Typical serving size:** 1 oz (28g), calories vary (see chart on page 77)

**HOW THEY HARM**

**High in fat and calories**
**Allergies**
**Dehydration (chia seeds)**

**WHAT THEY HEAL**

**Diabetes**
**Cardiovascular disease**
**High cholesterol**
**Cancer**
**Low energy**
**Constipation**
**Anemia**
**Weight gain**

**NUTRIENTS**

**Calcium**
**Fiber**
**Flavonoids**
**Folate**
**Iron**
**Magnesium**
**Manganese**
**Monounsaturated fats**
**Omega-3 fatty acids**
**Potassium**
**Protein**
**Selenium**
**Vitamin E**
**Zinc**

**BUYING**

Choose nuts or seeds that are:
- plump
- uniform in color and size

# WHICH NUT AND SEED IS BEST?

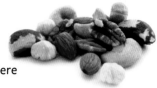

While these little gems are high in fat and calories, most of it is healthy poly-unsaturated and monounsaturated fat. To keep your waistline from expanding as you enjoy all the good nutrition in nuts and seeds, keep an eye on your portions. Here are guidelines for serving sizes and how many calories they pack.

| TYPE | AVERAGE NUMBER OR AMOUNT PER OUNCE | CALORIES PER 1-OZ (30 G) SERVING | FAT PER 1-OZ (30 G) SERVING | BEST FOR |
|---|---|---|---|---|
| Almond | 24 | 163 | 14 g | Use sliced or chopped to add light crunch to salads, baked goods; whirl smoked almonds with roasted peppers and a splash of vinegar for a quick and easy vegetable dip. |
| Brazil nut | 9 | 192 | 19 g | General snacking and pesto; try tossing toasted, chopped nuts with roasted asparagus. |
| Cashew | 16-18 | 156 | 12.4 g | Curries and stir-fries; use as an alternative to peanuts; to make a dairy-free "cream sauce" that you can season countless ways, soak raw cashews overnight in enough water to cover them and then puree until smooth. |
| Hazelnut | 20 | 178 | 17.2 g | Italian dishes and desserts; for an easy and elegant side dish, toss green beans with a little cooked chopped bacon and toasted hazelnuts. |
| Macadamia | 10-12 | 200 | 21 g | Desserts; toast with sweetened coconut and sprinkle over fresh pineapple. |
| Pecan | 20 halves | 196 | 20.4 g | Desserts and breakfast dishes; chop and mix with raisins and chopped dried apples for an easy addition to your oatmeal routine. |
| Pine nut | 3 Tbsp | 190 | 19.3 g | Pesto and pasta dishes; use sparingly as they are more expensive than many nuts; store in freezer to extend freshness. |
| Pistachio | 47 | 158 | 12.6 g | Italian dishes and salads; try dried apricots dipped in melted dark chocolate and then chopped pistachios. |
| Pumpkin seed | 3 Tbsp | 160 | 12.6 g | Trail mixes and Mexican dishes (including mole sauce); scatter a small handful over rice pilaf for an attractive (and flavorful) garnish. Also sold as pepitas. |
| Sesame seed | 3 Tbsp | 162 | 14 g | Asian dishes and general baking; make an easy gourmet crust by pressing sesame seeds into salmon or tuna fillets before pan searing. |
| Sunflower seed (shelled) | ¼ cup | 150 | 11 g | General snacking; use as a coating for cheese balls or add to granola mix for a classic combination. |
| Walnut | 14 halves | 185 | 18.5 g | General baking and salads; chop finely and use to coat boneless, skinless chicken breasts before oven roasting. |

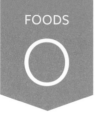

Avoid nuts or seeds that are:

- moldy
- close to or past their "use-by" date

## STORING

**Where:** Cool, dry place when unopened, in the refrigerator once opened.
**How:** In an airtight container or sealed plastic bag.
**For how long:** Up to 6 months.

## COOKING

- Sprinkle lemon-pepper seasoning over hot roasted sunflower seeds.
- Scatter chopped walnuts over a chicken stir-fry.
- Scatter pistachios over a salad of watercress, sliced orange, and red onion.
- Sprinkle sesame seeds into tuna salad.
- Puree raw almonds, roasted red peppers, and garlic as a sandwich spread.

## RECIPES TO TRY

- Pasta with Walnut Cream Sauce
- Spiced Almonds
- Blueberry and Cranberry Granola
- Cauliflower Salad with Cashews
- Balsamic Beets with Toasted Pecans

# OATS

*See also* Grains, page 57

**Typical serving size:** ½ cup cooked with water (117 g), 83 calories

## HOW THEY HARM

Blood sugar spikes (instant oatmeal)

## WHAT THEY HEAL

Cardiovascular disease
High cholesterol

High blood pressure
Diabetes
Constipation
Weight gain

## NUTRIENTS

Beta-glucan (soluble fiber that can help lower cholesterol)
Calcium
Folate
Iron
Manganese
Polyphenols and saponins (antioxidants)
Protein
Thiamine
Vitamin E

## BUYING

Choose:

- steel-cut or whole oat products

Avoid:

- flavored or instant oatmeal

## STORING

**Where:** A cool, dry place or freezer.
**How:** In an airtight container; in a plastic bag with the air squeezed out if freezing.
**For how long:** About a year.

## COOKING

- Stir ¼ cup steel-cut oats into a beef stew to thicken.
- Sprinkle rolled oats atop quick bread loaves before baking.
- Serve cooked oats topped with a poached egg.
- Use rolled oats instead of breadcrumbs in meat loaf, or to coat chicken or fish patties before cooking.

**RECIPES TO TRY**

- Hot Cereal with Apples and Dates
- Multigrain Pancakes or Waffles
- Spinach Stuffed Meat loaf
- Chewy Oatmeal Raisin Cookies
- Cherry Crisp

# OILS

*See also* Olives and Olive Oil, page 80

**Typical serving size:** 1 Tbsp (15 mL), 120 calories

### HOW THEY HARM

High in saturated fat (coconut, palm kernel, and palm oil)

Bacterial infection

### WHAT THEY HEAL

High cholesterol

Hormone production

Nutrient absorption

### NUTRIENTS

Monosaturated and omega-3 fats

### BUYING

Choose:

- single-source oils, such as pure canola or pure olive

Avoid:

- blended oils

### STORING

**Where:** A cool, dark place.

**How:** In original container.

**For how long:** About 6 months.

### COOKING

- Choose canola oil for sautéeing or stir-frying.

- Use olive oil in a carrot muffin recipe.
- Drizzle roasted sesame oil over zucchini wedges after they're grilled.

**RECIPES TO TRY**

- Romaine Lettuce with Chunky Tomato Vinaigrette
- Buckwheat Noodles with Tofu and Green Vegetables
- Walnut Shortbread

# OKRA

**Typical serving size:** ½ cup cooked (80 g), 18 calories

### WHAT IT HEALS

High cholesterol

Constipation

Weight gain

### NUTRIENTS

Beta-carotene

Fiber

Folate

Magnesium

Pectin (soluble fiber)

Potassium

Thiamine

Vitamin C

### BUYING

Choose okra with:

- firm pods
- bright green color
- shallow ridges in pods

Avoid okra with:

- yellow or black discoloration
- shriveling
- any bruising, pitting, or decay

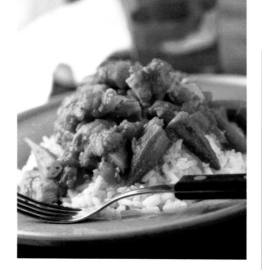

## STORING

**Where:** Crisper drawer of refrigerator.
**How:** Unwashed and loosely wrapped in a perforated plastic bag.
**For how long:** 3 days.

## COOKING

- Sauté baby okra in canola oil and garlic until crisp-tender, toss with teriyaki sauce.
- Bake whole baby okra flavored with olive oil, fine bread crumbs, garlic, and parmesan cheese.
- Use sliced okra in a chicken potpie filling.

## RECIPES TO TRY

- Savory Lamb Stew with Sweet Potatoes
- Skillet Okra and Lamb

### QUICK TIP:
### Use as a thickener

Okra is high in starch, pectin, and soluble fiber, which help thicken soups and stews when it is cooked. As okra cooks, its fats are released and naturally thicken the soups and stews.

# OLIVES AND OLIVE OIL

*See also* Oils, page 79

**Typical serving size:** 4 small olives (13 g), 16 calories; 1 Tbsp oil (15 mL), 120 calories

### HOW THEY HARM

Blood pressure (olives)

### WHAT THEY HEAL

High blood cholesterol
Cancer
Inflammation
Immunity
Weight gain

### NUTRIENTS

Lignans (compounds that may protect against cancer)
Monounsaturated fats
Phytochemicals
Vitamin E

### BUYING

Choose:
- oils that are minimally processed, such as extra-virgin or cold-pressed
- low-sodium varieties of canned olives

Avoid:
- olives that are soft or mushy

### STORING

**Where:** Refrigerator for olives; dark, cool place for oil.
**How:** In an airtight container.
**For how long:** Up to 2 months for olives; several years for oil (if the oil turns cloudy, toss it).

## COOKING

- Stir slivered ripe olives into risotto.
- Toss hot spaghetti with extra-virgin olive oil and garlic.
- Add minced green olives to egg salad.

## RECIPES TO TRY

- Green Beans with Tomatoes and Olives
- Penne with Fresh Tomato Sauce and Grilled Eggplant
- Grilled Salmon with Sautéed Greens
- Linguine with Clams
- Tuna and Cannellini Salad with Lemon

# ONIONS

**Typical serving size:** ½ cup raw (80 g), 32 calories

### HOW THEY HARM

Bloating and flatulence

### WHAT THEY HEAL

Lung cancer and other cancers
Heart attacks
High cholesterol
High blood sugar
Bacterial infections

### NUTRIENTS

Beta-carotene
Chromium
Flavonoids
Potassium
Vitamin C

## BUYING

Choose onions that:
- are firm
- have crackly, dry skin
- have a mild odor

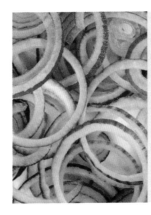

**QUICK TIP: Go raw**

Cooking onions at a high heat significantly reduces the benefits of diallyl sulfide, their cancer-protective phytochemical. For the biggest health boost, enjoy fresh raw onions. Mincing (or even chewing) the onion helps to release its phytochemical power.

- have fresh, crisp, green tops that extend 2 to 3 in (5 to 7.5 cm) up from the root (spring onions/scallions)

Avoid onions that:
- feel soft
- have black spots
- have green sprouts showing at the top
- have a strong, oniony smell
- have yellowing, wilted, discolored, or decayed tops (spring onions/scallions)

## STORING

**Where:** A cool, dry place away from direct light and away from potatoes. Store scallions and cut onions in the refrigerator.

**How:** With skin on for whole onions; tightly wrapped in plastic if cut; in a plastic bag for scallions.

**For how long:** 3 to 4 weeks uncut; 2 to 3 days cut; 3 days for scallions (use them before they begin to soften).

## COOKING

- Broil pita bread topped with sautéed onions and grated swiss cheese until bubbly.
- Stir sliced scallions into scrambled eggs.
- Marinate slivers of sweet onion in cider vinegar in the refrigerator for several hours to make quick pickled onions.

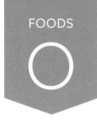
## RECIPES TO TRY

- Pineapple-Chipotle Chicken
- Herbed Turkey Meatballs and Fusilli
- Spinach Salad with Chickpeas
- Tuscan Bean Soup
- Sloppy Joes

# ORANGES AND TANGERINES

**Typical serving size:** 1 medium orange (131 g), 63 calories; 1 medium tangerine (109 g), 50 calories; ½ cup juice (4 fl oz, 120 mL), 52 calories

## HOW THEY HARM

Allergies

Tooth enamel erosion

Drug interaction

Canker sores

## WHAT THEY HEAL

Cancer, including thyroid cancer

High blood pressure

High cholesterol

Inflammation

Weight gain

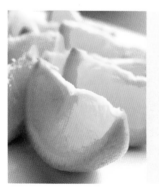

### QUICK TIP:
**Don't be a perfect peeler**

Eat the orange with the pith, the spongy white layer between the zest and the pulp. Although bitter, the pith stores a good amount of the fruit's fiber and antioxidant plant chemicals.

## NUTRIENTS

Beta-carotene

Bioflavonoids

Fiber

Folate

Nobiletin (flavonoid that may have anti-inflammatory actions)

Potassium

Thiamine

Vitamin C

## BUYING

Choose oranges that:

- are firm
- are heavy for their size
- have bright orange skin

Avoid oranges that:

- have bruised, wrinkled skin
- are discolored
- are canned

**Best time to buy:** winter and spring

## STORING

**Where:** At room temperature, or crisper drawer of refrigerator (preferred spot for tangerines).
**How:** Unpeeled.
**For how long:** Up to 2 weeks.

## COOKING

- Mix orange chunks with cottage cheese and mint.
- Quickly sauté orange slices as a topping for vanilla ice cream.
- Simmer tangerine sections, sliced pears, brown sugar, and a pinch of cloves in a saucepan to make a compote to serve with yogurt or on toast.
- Grill tangerine sections with sea scallops threaded on skewers.

## RECIPES TO TRY

- Orange Beef with Broccoli and Jicama
- Cantaloupe and Orange Soup
- Orange and Pomegranate Compote
- Asian Chicken Salad
- Orange Beets

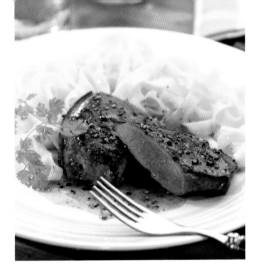

# ORGAN MEATS

**Typical serving size:** 3 to 4 oz (85 to 115 g), 165 to 216 calories

### HOW THEY HARM

Toxins

Gout

High cholesterol

Vitamin A toxicity

Creutzfeldt-Jakob disease risk

### WHAT THEY HEAL

Anemia

Vitamin B12 deficiency

Protein deficiency

### NUTRIENTS

Folate

Iron

Niacin

Potassium

Protein

Vitamin B12

Zinc

## BUYING

Choose organ meat that:

- is from a local butcher
- has the Safe Food Handling label on the package when buying at a supermarket
- is tightly wrapped and cold to the touch
- is shiny
- has a pleasant smell

Avoid organ meat that is:

- soaking in a large amount of liquid

## STORING

**Where:** In the coldest part of the refrigerator or the meat drawer or bin.

**How:** Loosely wrapped.

**For how long:** 1 to 2 days (3 to 4 months if frozen).

## COOKING

- Sauté chicken livers and minced onion, mash, and use as a sandwich spread.
- Add some finely chopped beef tripe to chili.
- Sauté veal sweetbread with chopped bacon.

## RECIPES TO TRY

- Calf's Liver with Rigatoni

# OYSTERS

*See* Shellfish, page 103

# PAPAYAS

**Typical serving size:** 1 medium (304 g), 119 calories

### HOW THEY HARM

Allergies

### WHAT THEY HEAL

Cardiovascular disease

Colon cancer

Inflammation

Arthritis

Macular degeneration

### NUTRIENTS

Beta-carotene

Fiber

Folate

Potassium

Vitamin C

Vitamin E

### BUYING

Choose papaya that:
- have reddish-orange skin
- are slightly soft to the touch or yield to gentle pressure

Avoid papayas with:
- blemished skin
- large dark spots
- mold or are soft
- leaking at the stem end

### STORING

**Where:** At room temperature to ripen; in the refrigerator when ripe.

**How:** Uncut in a plastic bag.

**For how long:** Up to 3 days.

### COOKING

- Prepare a salad with shredded green papaya and ginger vinaigrette.
- Add papaya chunks to chicken curry.
- Top 2% Greek yogurt with papaya chunks and finely chopped roasted peanuts.

### RECIPES TO TRY

- Papaya and Avocado Salad

# PARSNIPS

**Typical serving size:** 1 cup cooked (156 g), 111 calories

### HOW THEY HARM

Allergies

### WHAT THEY HEAL

High cholesterol

Weight gain

Constipation

Cancer

Birth defects

### NUTRIENTS

Fiber

Folate

Potassium

Vitamin C

Vitamin K

### BUYING

Choose parsnips that are:
- firm and dry without pits
- about the size of a medium carrot

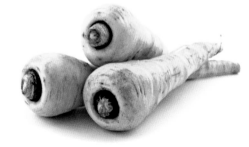

Avoid parsnips that are:
- very large
- covered with roots
- soft and shrunken or have moist spots

**Best time to buy:** autumn and winter

## STORING

**Where:** In the refrigerator.
**How:** Unwashed with tops removed and in an unsealed bag.
**For how long:** 3 weeks or more.

## COOKING

- Don't peel them. The most nutritious part of a parsnip is just below the surface of the skin.
- To bring out their sweetness, accent parsnips with nutmeg, ginger, mace, or cinnamon.
- Boil parsnip and carrot chunks until tender, drain and mash.
- Add chunks of parsnip to shepherd's pie.
- Make latkes from grated parsnip instead of potato.

## RECIPES TO TRY

- Honey-Roasted Rack of Lamb
- Braised Chicken with Winter Vegetables
- Carrot and Parsnip Puree
- Roasted Root Vegetables

**QUICK TIP: Beware of allergies**

You might want to avoid parsnips if you have a history of allergies to birch pollen as well as foods like walnuts, figs, carrots, and parsley. Symptoms in sensitive people usually include a slight swelling and itching of the lips and mouth.

# PASSION FRUIT

**Typical serving size:** 1 medium (18 g), 17 calories

## HOW IT HARMS

Bloating and flatulence

## WHAT IT HEALS

Vision
Immunity
Constipation
Weight gain

## NUTRIENTS

Fiber
Vitamin A
Vitamin C

## BUYING

Choose passion fruit that are:
- heavy and firm
- red, purple, or yellow
- wrinkled
- fragrant

Avoid passion fruit that is:
- lightweight or feels hollow

**Best time to buy:** winter and spring

## STORING

**Where:** In the refrigerator when ripe (ripen smooth-skinned passion fruit at room temperature).
**How:** In a plastic bag.
**For how long:** Up to 7 days.

## COOKING

- Seeds are edible, but if you'd like to remove them, strain the pulp and juice

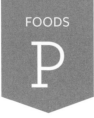

through a cheesecloth or another non-aluminum sieve.

- Spoon passion fruit over grilled bananas.
- Dollop passion fruit over sautéed chicken breasts.
- Add some passion fruit to an apple crumble.

### RECIPES TO TRY

- Berry Salad with Passion Fruit
- Kiwi-Passion Fruit Salad

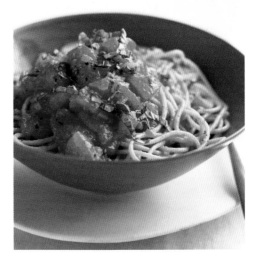

# PASTA

**Typical serving size:** ½ cup (70 g), about 110 calories

### HOW IT HARMS

Weight gain (white pasta)

Diabetes (white pasta)

### WHAT IT HEALS

Mood

Diabetes (whole grain pasta)

Cardiovascular disease (whole grain pasta)

Colon cancer

### NUTRIENTS

Fiber

Iron

Niacin

Thiamine

### BUYING

Choose pasta that is:

- whole wheat
- high fiber

Avoid pasta that is:

- white

### STORING TIPS

**Where:** A cool, dry place for dried pasta; refrigerator for fresh pasta.

**How:** Sealed container for dried; airtight container for fresh.

**For how long:** Indefinitely for dried; within a few days of purchase for fresh.

### COOKING

- Simmer orzo pasta in chicken broth and Italian herb seasoning for a side dish.
- Fill an omelet with some leftover sauced pasta.
- Toss cooked whole grain spaghetti with bottled Thai peanut sauce and cilantro.

### QUICK TIP:
#### Pick diabetes-friendly pasta

If you have diabetes, you'll minimize blood sugar spikes if you choose whole grain pasta, which contains three times the fiber of white pasta. Other options are the new higher protein pastas that are enriched with soy flour and milk solids and have a lower glycemic index (see page 354).

## RECIPES TO TRY

- Whole Wheat Pasta with Sausage and Greens
- Linguine with Clams
- Farfalle with Winter Squash Sauce
- Penne with Fresh Tomato Sauce and Grilled Eggplant
- Sicilian Pasta Salad

# PEACHES AND NECTARINES

**Typical serving size:** 1 medium peach (98 g), 38 calories; 1 medium nectarine (142 g), 62 calories

### HOW THEY HARM

Allergies
Cyanide poisoning (pit only)

### WHAT THEY HEAL

High cholesterol
Cancer
Weight gain
Constipation

### NUTRIENTS

Beta-carotene
Carotenoids (antioxidants)
Fiber
Pectin (soluble fiber)
Potassium

## BUYING

Choose peaches or nectarines that are:
- yellow or creamy with a rosy blush
- moderately firm
- fragrant

Avoid peaches or nectarines with:
- green undertones
- wrinkled skin or bruises, or ones that are rock hard
- tan circles on their skin

**Best time to buy:** spring, summer, early autumn

## STORING

**Where:** Refrigerator when ripe; at room temperature if unripe.
**How:** Uncut if ripe; in a paper bag to ripen.
**For how long:** 3 or 4 days when ripe; 2 or 3 days to ripen.

## COOKING

- Make salsa with peaches or nectarines in place of tomatoes.
- Stir chunks of peaches or nectarines into pancake batter.
- Top grilled peach or nectarine halves with a dollop of whipped ricotta cheese and honey.

## RECIPES TO TRY

- Chicken Breast with Peaches and Ginger
- Peach and Blackberry Phyllo Pizzas
- Wheat Germ Smoothie
- Mixed Berry and Stone Fruit Soup
- Watermelon and Feta Salad

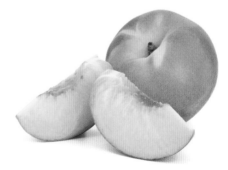

## P

# PEANUTS AND PEANUT BUTTER

*See also* Other Beans and Legumes, page 20

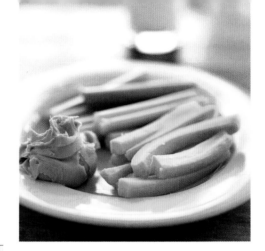

**Typical serving size:** 1 oz (28 g) peanuts, 166 calories; 2 Tbsp peanut butter (32 g), 188 calories

## HOW THEY HARM

High in trans fats (peanut butter)

Allergies

## WHAT THEY HEAL

Diabetes

High blood pressure

Cardiovascular disease

Low energy

Weight control

## NUTRIENTS

Fiber

Folate

Magnesium

Monosaturated fats

Potassium

Sterols (plant compounds that improve cholesterol)

Vitamin E

## BUYING

Choose:
- unsalted peanuts
- fresh-ground peanut butter

Avoid:
- peanuts that are moldy or have an "off" taste
- peanut butter with added sugar, salt, or trans fats (hydrogenated ingredients)

## STORING

**Where:** Refrigerator or freezer (nuts only).
**How:** Tightly sealed container.
**For how long:** Up to 1 year for peanut butter in the fridge, up to 2 weeks if it's fresh ground; about 3 months for shelled nuts in the fridge, up to 6 in the freezer.

Nuts still in their shells can be kept in a cool, dry place, but keeping them in the fridge will help them last up to 9 months.

## COOKING

- Scatter chopped roasted peanuts over roasted sweet potato sticks.
- Toss chopped roasted peanuts with corn kernels, bell pepper, and onion for a salad.
- Spread peanut butter over a pork tenderloin before roasting.

## RECIPES TO TRY

- Whole Wheat Noodles with Peanut Sauce and Chicken
- Bulgur with Dried Cherries and Corn
- Banana-Peanut Bread
- Asian Peanut Dip
- No-Bake Flaxseed-Nut Bars

# PEARS

**Typical serving size:** 1 medium (166 g), 96 calories

## HOW THEY HARM

Allergies

Tooth decay (dried pears)

## WHAT THEY HEAL

High cholesterol

Constipation

High blood pressure

Diabetes

## NUTRIENTS

Antioxidants

Fiber

Pectin (soluble fiber)

Potassium

Vitamin C

## BUYING

Choose pears that:
- have a smooth skin
- yield slightly to the touch at the stem
- have a slight fragrance

Avoid pears that:
- are dark or bruised

## STORING

**Where:** Room temperature until ripe, then refrigerator.
**How:** Uncut.
**For how long:** A few days.

## COOKING

- Make a salsa with chopped pears, basil, and orange juice.
- Use pears instead of apples in pastry recipes.
- Grill pear halves with agave nectar and nutmeg.

## RECIPES TO TRY

- Pear Rhubarb Muffins
- Buckwheat Pancakes with Fruit Sauce
- Grilled Fruit en Brochette
- Minty Melon Cups
- Pork, Pear, and Potato Salad

# PEAS AND PEA PODS

*See also* Beans and Other Legumes, page 20

**Typical serving size:** ½ cup green peas (49 g), 73 calories; 10 pea pods (34 g), 14 calories

## HOW THEY HARM

Gout

## WHAT THEY HEAL

Cancer

Constipation

High cholesterol

Macular degeneration

## NUTRIENTS

Coumestrol (anticancer compound)

Fiber

Iron

Lutein (antioxidant)

Pectin (soluble fiber)

Protein

Vitamin C

## BUYING

Choose fresh peas that are:
- less developed and have flatter pods
- firm
- bright green

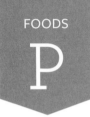
Avoid peas that are:
- decaying
- wilted

If you can't get fresh peas, choose frozen over canned.

### STORING

**Where:** Refrigerator.
**How:** Unwashed in a perforated plastic bag or unsealed container.
**For how long:** 3 to 5 days.

### COOKING

- Cook peas in as little water as possible until just tender to minimize the loss of vitamins.
- Stir fresh or frozen baby peas and basil into a cheese risotto.
- Simmer fresh or frozen baby peas and chopped onion in chicken broth until tender; puree for soup.
- Serve pea pods with hummus for dipping.
- Add pods with the peas to soup stock for added flavor and nutrition.

### RECIPES TO TRY

- Asparagus and Chicken Stir-Fry
- Snapper and Snaps in a Packet Spanish Rice
- Scallops Florentine
- Bulgur with Spring Vegetables
- Spiced Cauliflower with Peas

# PECANS

*See* Nuts and Seeds, page 77

# PEPPER, GROUND

*See* Herbs and Spices, page 61

# PEPPERS

**Typical serving size:** ½ cup chopped (75 g), 20 calories

### HOW THEY HARM

Digestion
Joint function
Pesticides
Canker sores

### WHAT THEY HEAL

Cancer
Cardiovascular disease
Macular degeneration
Immunity

### NUTRIENTS

Antioxidants
Beta-carotene
Bioflavonoids (anticancer compounds)
Folate
Lutein (antioxidant)
Phenolic acid (anticancer compound)
Sterols (cholesterol-lowering compound)
Vitamin B6
Vitamin C
Zeaxanthin (antioxidant)

## BUYING

Choose peppers that:
- feel heavy for their size
- have smooth, unwrinkled skin

Avoid peppers that:
- have soft or dark spots
- are dull, shriveled, or pitted

**Best time to buy:** summer and early autumn

## STORING

**Where:** Refrigerator.
**How:** In a plastic bag.
**For how long:** About 5 days.

## COOKING

- Mix chopped green bell peppers into turkey meat loaf.
- Stuff Anaheim peppers with seasoned ground beef, then braise in marinara sauce.
- Stir some minced fresh cayenne pepper into a pasta salad.

## RECIPES TO TRY

- Flank Steak Roll with Carrots and Red Peppers
- Grilled Eggplant Sandwiches with Red Pepper–Walnut Sauce
- Beef, Onion, and Pepper Fajitas
- Couscous-Stuffed Peppers
- Basil-Scented Sautéed Vegetables

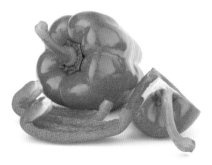

# PERSIMMONS

**Typical serving size:** 1 medium (5 to 6 cm) (168 g), 118 calories

## HOW THEY HARM
Bloating and flatulence

## WHAT THEY HEAL
Cancer
Immunity
High blood pressure
Digestion
Weight gain

## NUTRIENTS
Fiber
Potassium
Vitamin A
Vitamin C

## BUYING

Choose:
- Hachiya varieties that are very soft
- Fuyu varieties that are crisper
- plump, well-rounded fruit with leaf still attached
- deeply colored fruit with glossy skin

Avoid persimmons with:
- blemishes
- cracks
- bruises
- yellow patches (which indicate unripe fruit)

## STORING

**Where:** Refrigerator if ripe; room temperature if unripe.
**How:** Inside a plastic bag if ripe; in a paper bag with an apple to ripen.
**For how long:** Up to 3 days in the fridge; 1 to 3 days to ripen.

Store puréed persimmon flesh in the freezer for up to 6 months.

### COOKING

- Toss slices of ripe persimmon into an escarole and walnut salad.
- Add chopped persimmon to a bread pudding.
- Stir persimmon chunks into oatmeal with maple syrup.

### RECIPES TO TRY

- Nutty Muesli
- Cauliflower Salad with Cashews

# PINEAPPLES

**Typical serving size:** 1 cup diced (155g), 78 calories

### HOW THEY HARM

Allergies

Canker sores

### WHAT THEY HEAL

Cancer

Blood clots

Inflammation

Metabolism

### NUTRIENTS

Bromelain (anti-inflammatory)

Ferulic acid (plant chemical that protects against cancer)

Fiber

Manganese

Potassium

Vitamin C

### BUYING

Choose pineapples that:

- exude a fragrant odor
- have light yellow or white flesh
- are dense and heavy for their size
- have green, fresh-looking leaves
- make a dull, solid sound when thumped

Avoid pineapples with:

- brown patches
- bruises and soft spots on the base

When buying canned pineapple, choose 100% fruit juice over pineapple in heavy syrup.

**Best time to buy:** summer

### STORING

**Where:** Refrigerator if cut; on the counter if whole.

**How:** In an airtight container when cut.

**For how long:** 3 days in the fridge if cut; a few days at room temperature if whole.

### COOKING

- Blend crushed pineapple with part-skim ricotta cheese for a spread.
- Freeze the juice from no-sugar-added canned pineapple in ice pop trays for snacks.
- Stir some pineapple chunks into a three-bean salad.
- Add pineapple to stews or marinades for a natural tenderizer.

### RECIPES TO TRY

- Jamaican Jerked Chicken Salad
- Pineapple-Chipotle Chicken
- Twice-Baked Stuffed Sweet Potatoes
- Grilled Fruit en Brochette

# PLUMS AND PRUNES

**Typical serving size:** 1 medium plum (66 g), 40 calories; ¼ cup prunes (40 g), 122 calories

## HOW THEY HARM
Allergies
Cyanide poisoning (pit only)
Tooth decay (prunes)

## WHAT THEY HEAL
Cancer
Weight gain
Constipation
Bone loss

## NUTRIENTS
Anthocyanins (antioxidant)
Fiber
Iron
Isatin (a natural laxative)
Potassium
Riboflavin
Vitamin C
Vitamin K

## BUYING
Choose plums that:
- are brightly colored
- yield slightly to the touch

Avoid plums that are:
- too soft or too hard
- bruised or discolored
- shriveled or have skin breaks
- leaky

**Best time to buy:** late spring to early autumn

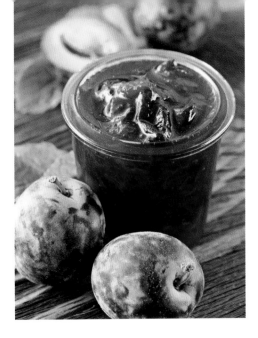

## STORING
**Where:** At room temperature to ripen; in refrigerator when ripe.

**How:** In a paper bag to ripen for plums; in an airtight container in a cool, dark place for prunes.

**For how long:** 2 to 3 days for plums; up to 6 months for prunes.

## COOKING
- Blend a plum and yogurt smoothie.
- Add plum slices to a skillet of sautéed chicken.
- Simmer prunes in spiced red wine until tender.

## RECIPES TO TRY
- Buckwheat Pancakes with Fruit Sauce
- Mixed Berry and Stone Fruit Soup
- Guavas and Plums with Vanilla Syrup

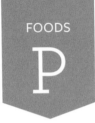
# POME-GRANATES

**Typical serving size:** ½ cup arils (seeds) (87 g), 59 calories

## HOW THEY HARM

Drug interaction

## WHAT THEY HEAL

Prostate cancer
High cholesterol
High blood pressure
Erectile dysfunction

## NUTRIENTS

Anthocyanins (antioxidant)
Copper
Ellagic acid (antioxidant)
Fiber
Folate
Potassium
Vitamin C

## BUYING

Choose pomegranates that:
- are heavy for their size
- have a bright, fresh color
- have thin, yet tough skin

Avoid pomegranates with:
- blemishes or broken skin
- mold around the crown

**Best time to buy:** autumn and early winter

## STORING

**Where:** A cool, dark place or in the refrigerator.
**How:** Unpeeled.
**For how long:** 2 weeks in a cool place; up to 2 months in the fridge. Seeds can be frozen for up to 1 year.

## COOKING

- Make a spritzer with pomegranate juice and sparkling apple cider.
- Add pomegranate seeds to poultry stuffing.
- Scatter pomegranate seeds over roasted brussels sprouts.

## RECIPES TO TRY

- Bulgur with Dried Cherries and Corn
- Creamy Citrus and Vanilla Rice Pudding
- Roasted Pork with Pomegranate Sauce
- Orange and Pomegranate Compote

# PORK

*See also* Smoked and Cured Meats, page 104

**Typical serving size:** 3 oz (85 g), 105 to 180 calories, depending on cut

## HOW IT HARMS

High blood pressure (cured or smoked products)
Parasites

## WHAT IT HEALS

Bones
Muscles
Heart and nervous system function
Anemia
Immunity

## NUTRIENTS

Iron
Protein
Selenium
Thiamin
Vitamin B12
Zinc

Choose pork that is:
- smooth and pink
- lean
- fresh (check date stamp on packages, which reflects the last date of sale)

Avoid pork that is:
- gray or damp looking

## STORING

**Where:** Refrigerator.

**How:** In original package and wrapped if uncooked; in a sealed container if cooked.

**For how long:** Up to 3 days uncooked (1 week for bacon), 5 days cooked. Freeze bacon for up to 1 month.

## COOKING

- Braise pork shoulder in dark beer, tomato puree, sliced onion, and Cajun seasoning.
- Stir-fry thin slices of pork tenderloin with Granny Smith apples and sage.
- Add some crumbled bacon to navy bean soup.

## RECIPES TO TRY

- Pork Chops and Cabbage
- Ham and Celeriac Pitas
- Green Pork Chili
- Spinach-Stuffed Meat Loaf
- Roast Pork and Quinoa Salad

### QUICK TIP: Cook to perfection

Cook pork tenderloin, chops, and roasts to an internal temperature of 145°F (63°C). When using ground pork to make meatballs or patties, cook them until they reach 160°F (71°C).

# POTATOES

**Typical serving size:** 1 medium (154 g), 140 calories

## HOW THEY HARM

Toxic risk (green and sprouted potatoes)

Digestion (if sensitive to night shade)

Joint function (if sensitive to night shade)

Diabetes (depending on preparation)

## WHAT THEY HEAL

Cancer

Hypertension

## NUTRIENTS

Chlorogenic acid (anticancer compound)

Fiber

Kukoamines (compounds that may lower blood pressure)

Magnesium

Potassium

Vitamin B6

Vitamin C

## BUYING

Choose potatoes that:
- are firm and blemish free

Avoid potatoes that have:
- bald spots (except new potatoes)
- wrinkles or cracks
- sprouted
- a green tinge

## STORING

**Where:** In a cool, dark place, but not in the refrigerator or near onions.

**How:** Uncut and unpeeled.

**For how long:** Up to 2 weeks.

### COOKING

- Don't remove the skin. Fiber is in the skin, and many of the nutrients are near the surface.
- Scrub them under water with a vegetable brush.
- Baking, steaming, or microwaving preserves the maximum amount of nutrients.
- Roast cubed potatoes in extra-virgin olive oil, garlic, and rosemary until crisp.
- Toss cooked marble-size red potatoes in Greek yogurt and chopped dill for a quick salad.
- Simmer cubed potatoes with Mexican seasoning, canned diced tomatoes and enough water to cover until tender.

### RECIPES TO TRY

- Pot Roast with Root Vegetables
- Braised Chicken with Winter Vegetables
- Potato Salad with Sun-Dried Tomatoes, Scallions, and Basil
- New Potatoes with Nori
- Mashed Turnips with Carrots and Potatoes

# POULTRY

*See also* Smoked and Cured Meats, page 104

**Typical serving size:** 3 oz (85 g), calories vary (see chart on page 97)

### HOW IT HARMS

Bacterial contamination

### WHAT IT HEALS

Anemia
Cardiovascular disease
Immunity
Bones and muscles

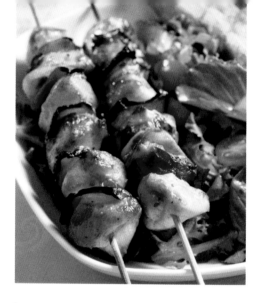

### NUTRIENTS

Iron
Niacin
Phosphorous
Potassium
Protein
Vitamin B6
Vitamin B12
Zinc

### BUYING

Choose poultry that:

- has a current date stamp (for rotisserie chicken, check time stamps to see when it was prepared, and purchase within 2 to 4 hours after)
- has white to deep yellow colored fat
- is skinless for less fat

Avoid poultry with:

- rough, dry, or bruised skin
- gray or pasty-colored fat

### STORING

**Where:** Coldest part of the refrigerator or freezer.
**How:** Securely wrapped.
**For how long:** Up to 3 days in fridge if cooked or raw; 2 months if frozen raw, 1 month if frozen cooked.

# WHICH TYPE OF POULTRY IS HEALTHIEST?

Choose the leanest cuts and cook your poultry to perfection with this guide, organized from least to most fatty.

| CUT | CALORIES & FAT PER 3-OZ (90-G) COOKED PORTION | | AVERAGE SIZE | TOTAL TIME | BEST COOKING METHOD | DONENESS GUIDELINE |
|---|---|---|---|---|---|---|
| Turkey breast | 110 | 0.5 g | 4-6 lb (2-3 kg) | 1 ½ - 2 ¼ hr | Roast at 325°F (160°C) | Until internal temperature is 165°F (74°C) |
| Ground turkey, extra-lean | 120 | 1.5 g | Varies | Varies with amount and size of skillet | Brown in skillet over medium-high heat | |
| Chicken tenders | 139 | 3.0 g | 2 oz (60 g) each | 15-20 min | Roast at 350°F (180°C) | |
| | | | | 4-6 min per side | Grill | |
| Chicken breast (boneless, skinless) | | | 4-6 oz (125-175 g) | 20-30 min | Roast at 350°F (180°C) | |
| | | | | 6-8 min per side | Grill | |
| Chicken breast (bone-in, skinless) | | | 6-8 oz (175-250 g) oz each | 30-40 min | Roast at 350°F (180°C) | |
| | | | | 10-15 min per side | Grill | |
| Duck, breast (boneless skinless) | 144 | 6 g | 8-10 oz (250-300g) | 12 min | Roast at 425°F (220°C) | |
| Chicken thigh (boneless, skinless) | 176 | 9.2 g | 3-5 oz (90-150 g) | 20-30 min | Roast at 350°F (180°C) | |
| | | | | 6-8 min per side | Roast at 350°F (180°C) | |

## COOKING

- Remove the skin after cooking to reduce fat and calories while maximizing flavor.
- Dip boneless chicken breast strips into buttermilk, then coat in crushed bran cereal and bake.
- Stir-fry chicken chunks with peanuts and Chinese pea pods.
- Slow-cook turkey drumsticks with chunks of onion, carrot, and celery in chicken broth.

## RECIPES TO TRY

- Curried Chicken Salad Sandwiches
- Turkey, Spinach, and Rice in Roasted Garlic Broth
- Pesto Chicken Spirals with Roasted Peppers
- Herbed Turkey Meatballs and Fusilli
- Grilled Duck Breast with Polenta

# PRUNES

*See* Plums and Prunes, page 93

# PUMPKINS

**Typical serving size:** 1 cup cooked, mashed (245 g), 49 calories

### HOW THEY HARM
Choking hazard (seeds)

### WHAT THEY HEAL
Cancer

High blood pressure

Crohn's disease

### NUTRIENTS
Beta-carotene

B vitamins (seeds)

Fiber

Iron

Potassium

Vitamin C

Vitamin E (seeds)

### BUYING
Choose pumpkins that:
- have a hard, tough rind with the stem attached
- are heavy for their size
- are free of decay

Avoid pumpkins that:
- are used for jack-o-lanterns
- have cuts or punctures
- have sunken or moldy spots

### STORING
**Where:** In a cool, dry place.

**How:** Uncut.

**For how long:** About 1 month.

### COOKING
- Bake pumpkin pie filling in oiled custard cups for individual puddings.
- Roast pumpkin seeds and add them to trail mix.

QUICK TIP:

## Try it for Crohn's disease

There's no one diet that seems to work for people living with the inflammatory problems associated with Crohn's disease. However, pumpkins and pumpkin seeds tend to be well tolerated by most.

- Simmer a quick soup with canned pumpkin, evaporated fat-free milk, cumin, and garlic.

### RECIPES TO TRY
- Shrimp Seviche with Avocado and Pumpkin Seeds
- Broccoli and Pearl Barley Salad
- Whole Wheat Pumpkin Rolls
- Sweet and Spicy Snack Mix

# QUINOA

*See also* Grains, p 57

**Typical serving size:** ½ cup cooked (93 g), 111 calories

### HOW IT HARMS
Kidney stones

### WHAT IT HEALS
Celiac disease

Cancer

Cardiovascular disease

Diabetes

Weight gain

### NUTRIENTS
B vitamins

Complex carbohydrates

Fiber

Folate
Iron
Lysine (amino acid)
Magnesium
Niacin
Phosphorous
Potassium
Protein
Quercetin (antioxidant)
Saponins (phytochemicals that help
   prevent heart disease and cancer)
Thiamine
Zinc
Vitamin E

## BUYING

Look for quinoa:
- in white, red, and black varieties
  (darker colors tend to have a stronger,
  earthy flavor while lighter colors are
  more mild)
- in health food stores and supermarkets, next to rice

## STORING

**Where:** In a cool, dark place.
**How:** In an airtight package.
**For how long:** Up to 6 months, or freeze
   indefinitely.

## COOKING

- Rinse thoroughly in a mesh strainer
  before cooking.
- Flavor cooked quinoa with a spoonful
  of pesto.
- Stir some cooked quinoa into a sweet
  potato salad.
- Use quinoa instead of rice to stuff bell
  peppers.

## RECIPES TO TRY

- Roast Pork and Quinoa Salad
- Springtime Quinoa
- Quinoa with Chiles and Cilantro

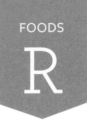

# RADISHES

**Typical serving size:** 5 medium raw
(23 g), 5 calories

## HOW THEY HARM

Bloating and flatulence
Allergies

## WHAT THEY HEAL

Weight gain
Cancer

## NUTRIENTS

Folate
Iron
Potassium
Vitamin C

## BUYING

Choose radishes that:
- are brightly colored
- feel solid
- have crisp greens, if attached

Avoid radishes that are:
- really big (red globe radishes)
- blemished

**Best time to buy:** spring to early summer

## STORING

**Where:** Refrigerator.
**How:** Remove any attached greens and
   place in plastic bags.
**For how long:** About 2 weeks.

## COOKING

- Dip radishes into baba
  ghanoush.
- Add sliced radishes to
  a vegetable stir-fry.

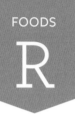
- Dip raw radishes into extra-virgin olive oil, coarsely ground black pepper, and sea salt.

### RECIPES TO TRY

- Warm Kasha and Seafood Salad
- Pork, Pear, and Potato Salad

# RAISINS

*See* Grapes and Raisins, page 59

# RASPBERRIES

*See* Berries, page 26

# RHUBARB

**Typical serving size:** ½ cup diced (122 g), 26 calories

### HOW IT HARMS

Poisonous (leaves)
Mineral absorption
Kidney stones
Gallstones

### WHAT IT HEALS

Cancer
High blood pressure

### NUTRIENTS

Fiber
Polyphenols (anticancer compounds)
Potassium
Vitamin C

### BUYING

Choose rhubarb with:
- firm stalks
- no blemishes
- red flesh

Avoid rhubarb that is:
- green-fleshed
- discolored or scarred
- wilted, flabby, or mushy

**Best time to buy:** spring

### STORING

**Where:** Crisper drawer of refrigerator or in the freezer.
**How:** Cut off the leaves, if any, and discard. Wash stalks in cold water, pat dry, and place them in a plastic bag. Cut into ½-in (1 cm) pieces if freezing.
**For how long:** One week in the fridge; up to 1 year in the freezer. Do not use if the stalks become mushy or discolored.

### COOKING

- Baking rhubarb for 20 minutes releases high levels of polyphenols.
- Simmer sliced rhubarb, raisins, honey, vinegar, and ginger to make a chutney.
- Cook a chopped stalk of rhubarb with curried lentils.
- Roast chunks of rhubarb sprinkled with brown sugar just until crisp-tender.
- Stew to make a sauce to complement poultry, meats, pork, and desserts.

### RECIPES TO TRY

- Pear Rhubarb Muffins
- Rhubarb-Blackberry Crumble

# RICE

*See also* Grains, page 57

**Typical serving size:** ½ cup cooked (93g), 85 to 120 calories

### HOW IT HARMS

Blood sugar spikes (white rice)

### WHAT IT HEALS

Colon cancer (brown rice)
Diarrhea
Diabetes (brown rice)
Celiac disease

### NUTRIENTS

B vitamins
Fiber (brown rice)
Lysine (especially wild rice)
Magnesium
Phytochemicals
Protein (especially wild rice)
Vitamin E (brown rice)

## BUYING

Choose rice that is:
- brown
- short, medium, or long varieties
- covered and dry, if buying in bulk

Avoid rice that is:
- white

## STORING

**Where:** Refrigerator or freezer for brown rice; a cool, dry cupboard for white rice.
**How:** In an airtight container.
**For how long:** Up to 6 months for brown rice; 1 year for white. To store cooked rice, let it cool, then place it in an airtight container in the coldest part of the refrigerator for no more than 5 days or in the freezer for up to 6 months.

## COOKING

- Scatter leftover cooked brown rice over a vegetable frittata.
- Cook wild rice in apple juice.
- Toss cooled cooked rice with chopped tomatoes and basil in Italian dressing.

## RECIPES TO TRY

- Snapper and Snaps in a Packet
- Rice Salad with Chicken and Grapes
- Japanese Sushi Rolls
- Creamy Citrus and Vanilla Rice Pudding

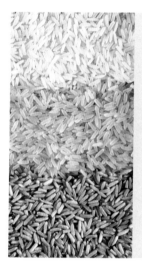

**QUICK TIP: Get the right rice**
Long-grain rice such as basmati is fragrant and delicate, making it a nice complement to curries and other spicy dishes. Instant rice is good for quick meals and works well in casseroles, side dishes, and soups. Wild rice, a very distant cousin of rice, is technically a water grass. It works well in pilafs, soups, and stuffings. Choose arborio rice for risotto because of its creamy texture.

# RYE

*See* Grains, page 57

# SAUSAGES

*See* Smoked and Cured Meats, page 104

**IN MODERATION ONLY**

# SALT AND SODIUM

You need 1,300 to 1,500 mg of sodium per day for your body to function. North Americans typically consume 4,000 to 7,000 mg per day. Some people are more salt-sensitive than others, and they will get the biggest payoff from cutting back on salt. Everyone can benefit, though. Along with contributing to high blood pressure in sensitive individuals, a high-salt diet may increase your risk of kidney stones by stealing calcium from your body. Here's how to cut your intake down to only the essential amount.

### KEEP IT HEALTHY

**Hide your salt shaker.** Don't add salt at the table. Taste your food first instead of salting out of habit. Cut the amount of salt in recipes by half—you probably won't even notice the difference. One teaspoon provides more than 2,000 mg of sodium.

**Limit processed and preserved foods.** Everyday food items like cereals, cold cuts, canned soups, canned vegetables, prepackaged meals, and baked goods are bursting with sodium. It's also found in MSG (monosodium glutamate); meat tenderizers; sauces and condiments such as ketchup, soy sauce, salad dressings, chili sauce, and steak sauce; soups; cured or smoked foods; olives; and pickles.

**Choose low-sodium or no-salt-added canned foods.** Whenever possible, rinse canned foods with water before cooking to remove more sodium. This works well with canned beans.

**Season with sodium-free herbs and spices.** Good choices include garlic powder or fresh garlic, onion flakes, dry mustard, coriander, lemon, mint, cumin, chili powder, curry, rosemary, thyme, basil, bay leaves, ginger, hot peppers, black pepper, chives, and parsley.

**Use kosher salt.** The grains are larger so it tastes saltier and you can use it more sparingly.

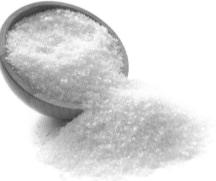

**Opt for the least processed option.** Eat fresh or frozen fish instead of canned or dried varieties. Choose sliced roast beef or chicken over bologna, salami, or other processed meat.

# SEAWEED

## HOW IT HARMS
High in sodium

## WHAT IT HEALS
Thyroid function
Muscles
Immunity
Metabolism

## NUTRIENTS
Beta-carotene
Folate
Iodine
Protein
Vitamin A

## BUYING
Look:
- in Asian markets and natural food stores

## STORING
**Where:** Cool cupboard, if dried; refrigerator, if fresh.
**How:** Well wrapped in an airtight container.
**For how long:** Up to 1 year, if dried; up to 1 to 2 days, if fresh.

## COOKING
- Sprinkle snipped dried dulse over Manhattan clam chowder.
- Toss sliced fresh wakame with thinly sliced cucumbers, rice wine vinegar and a sprinkling of sugar for a salad.
- Add some ready-to-eat dried wakame to the filling of a vegetable omelet.

## RECIPES TO TRY
- Warm Kasha and Seafood Salad
- Japanese Sushi Rolls
- New Potatoes with Nori
- Miso Soup with Tofu

# SHELLFISH

**Typical serving size:** 2 to 3 oz shelled (56 g to 85 g), calories vary (see chart on page 53)

## HOW IT HARMS
Allergies

## WHAT IT HEALS
Cancer
Weight gain
Cardiovascular disease
Anemia
Thyroid function

## NUTRIENTS
Iodine
Iron
Omega-3 fatty acids
Protein
Selenium
Vitamin B12

## BUYING
Buy shellfish that:
- is well covered with ice, or for lobsters, in aerated tanks with circulating water
- smells briny

## QUICK TIP:
**Try lemon instead of butter**

A simple squeeze of lemon juice can be enough to flavor shellfish as long as it hasn't been overcooked.

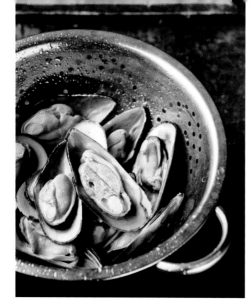

Avoid shellfish that:
- smells like iodine
- smells fishy

Most shrimp are trimmed and frozen in bulk at sea, then thawed for sale. Shrimp processed in this way should be labeled "previously frozen."

### STORING

**Where:** On the bottom shelf in the back of the refrigerator.
**How:** In a shallow pan on a bed of ice.
**For how long:** 24 hours from purchase. Purchased frozen shellfish can be kept frozen for up to 6 months.

### COOKING

- Make a salad with slices of grilled squid, tomatoes, red onions, and ripe olives.
- Season stir-fried shrimp with Thai peanut sauce.
- Marinate soft-shell crabs in Italian dressing for one 1 hour before grilling.

### RECIPES TO TRY

- Pan-Seared Scallops with Oranges and Sun-Dried Tomatoes
- Thai Roasted Shrimp
- Shellfish Salad with Herbed Lemon Dressing
- Crab Cakes with Melon Relish
- Oysters with Tomato Salsa

**IN MODERATION ONLY**

# SMOKED AND CURED MEATS

You might want to skip the deli line the next time you go food shopping. The reddish-pink color of cured meats, including cold cuts, is due to the presence of nitrites, chemicals that may cause cancer. These types of meat also tend to have a high sodium content that can increase blood pressure. Aside from some protein, these foods offer little nutritionally so they're best consumed infrequently.

### KEEP IT HEALTHY

**Look for lower-sodium options.** Even these will be high in sodium; some brands still top 460 g per serving. So limit the quantity and frequency that you eat these types of food.

**Select the least processed meats.** Choose sliced roast beef or chicken over bologna, salami, or other processed meat.

**Go color free.** Lean cuts of white meat such as turkey breast have less fat and are a healthier option to most cold cuts.

# SHRIMP

*See* Shellfish, page 103

---

# SOY

*See also* Beans and Other Legumes, page 20

**Typical serving size:** Varies (see chart on page 106)

### HOW IT HARMS
Cancer risk
Thyroid function

### WHAT IT HEALS
Cardiovascular disease
Breast and prostate cancers
Osteoporosis
Menopause

### NUTRIENTS
Calcium
Essential amino acids (only plant product to contain all of them)
Isoflavones (potential anticancer compounds)
Protein

### BUYING
Look for:
- edamame (green soy beans) in the pod in the produce section, if fresh, or shelled in the frozen food section, if frozen
- tofu in the produce or refrigerated (dairy) section
- soy flour with other flours
- soymilk in the dairy section

Avoid soy products with:
- lots of salt, sugar, or other additives

### STORING
**Where:** Edamame and tofu, in the refrigerator or freezer; low-fat soy flour, and shelf-stable soymilk in a cupboard; full-fat soy flour, in the freezer; regular soymilk, in the refrigerator.
**How:** In airtight packages or containers.
**For how long:** Edamame, up to 5 days; tofu, before "use-by" date; low-fat soy flour, up to 1 year; full-fat soy flour, up to 1 year; soymilk, 7 to 10 days after opening or as indicated on the label.

### COOKING
- Simmer rice in miso broth in place of water.
- Use thinly sliced soft tofu to replace half of the cheese in a lasagna recipe.
- Add some steamed edamame to a three-bean salad.

### RECIPES TO TRY
- Mediterranean Salad with Edamame
- Edamame Hummus with Pita Crisps
- Miso Soup with Tofu
- Bok Choy, Tofu, and Mushroom Stir-Fry

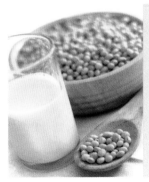

### QUICK TIP:
**Pair it with vitamin C**

The iron in soy products is not well absorbed. To improve absorption, add foods high in vitamin C—such as orange juice, tomatoes, peppers, strawberries, or melons—to your meal.

# WHAT'S THE DIFFERENCE BETWEEN SOY PRODUCTS?

Most soy foods contain some amount of isoflavones, which are plant-based, estrogen-like nutrients that may play a role in fighting heart disease and osteoporosis. However, ingesting high amounts of isoflavones may be problematic for people with some types of cancer and other hormone-sensitive conditions. Talk with your doctor about including soy foods in your diet. This chart lists products from highest to lowest isoflavone content.

| TYPE | WHAT IT IS | HOW IT'S USED | TYPICAL SERVING SIZE | ISOFLAVONE CONTENT (MG PER SERVING) |
|---|---|---|---|---|
| Edamame | Japanese name for young soybeans | Steamed and served in the pod, sometimes sprinkled with salt and a squirt of fresh lemon | ½ cup | 160 |
| Soy flour, full-fat | Made from roasted soybeans that have been finely ground; rich in protein | Substitute up to ¼ all-purpose flour with soy flour in recipes; makes baked goods brown faster, so adjust baking time accordingly. | ¼ cup | 107 |
| Soy flour, low-fat | | As an egg substitute in baking, mix 1 Tbsp soy flour with 1 Tbsp cold water; can be used to make homemade soymilk (mix with water, heat, and strain it) | ¼ cup | 79 |
| Tempeh | Made from cooked soybeans that have been pressed into a cake; firm texture and subtle, nutty flavor | Use in salads, sandwiches, burgers, chili-style dishes, and stir-fries as an alternative to chicken, pork, or beef | 4 oz (125 g) | 54 |
| Tofu, soft | Versatile, high-protein pressed soymilk curds; moisture content determines softness; good source of calcium when made with calcium sulfate; virtually flavorless | May be grilled, baked, or fried in a variety of sweet and savory dishes; for best results, always drain regular tofu by pressing the blocks between paper towels before slicing | 4 oz (125 g) | 37 |
| Tofu, firm | | | 4 oz (125 g) | 28 |
| Soymilk | Processed beverage; available sweetened or flavored | Use as you would regular milk in most recipes; scalds easily so always stir when heating; doesn't set as easily in pudding and pie recipes, so experiment by adding small amount of cornstarch to soymilk before heating | 8 oz (250 g) | 24 |
| Miso | Rich, salty Japanese condiment made from fermented soybeans and grains (usually rice or barley); it comes in a paste, concentrated broth, or freeze-dried; darker-colored miso indicates stronger flavors | Use in soups, marinades, and salad dressings; to preserve nutrients, do not boil | 1 tsp | 2 |
| Soy cheese | Processed soymilk product designed to resemble dairy-based cheeses | Use in recipes as you would regular cheese; melting times and consistency may vary by brand | 1 oz (30 g) | 2 |
| Meat analogues | Term used to describe processed meatless foods that are often made from soy and designed to resemble common meats | Use tofu hot dogs and sausages, meatless crumbles and burgers, as well as soy-based chicken chunks and strips in place of animal protein, especially in saucy dishes where spices are the dominant flavor | Varies | Varies* |
| Non-dairy soy frozen desserts | Term used to describe processed soymilk product designed to resemble ice cream | Use in frozen dessert recipes as you would regular ice cream; variety of brands and flavors are available | ½ cup | Varies |
| Soy sauce | Salty brown liquid made from fermented soybeans and grains (usually rice or barley) | Traditionally used throughout Asia as an all-purpose seasoning; salt-sensitive people should use lower-sodium soy sauce when available | 1 Tbsp | None |

*These processed products have proprietary blends so isoflavone content isn't standard.

# SOFT DRINKS

Apart from a quick energy boost from the caffeine or sugar, soft drinks and soda pop offer little to no nutritional value. The extra sugar in sodas can lead to weight gain and tooth decay, and many contain acids that erode tooth enamel. Research suggests that one soda a day increases a child's chances of becoming obese by 60%. Colas also contain large amounts of phosphates, which may impair calcium absorption. Even worse is that kids are likely to drink less milk if they're consuming soda. While diet soft drinks have fewer calories, they may still contribute to weight gain by tricking your taste buds into craving more sugar, and they contain artificial sweeteners and caffeine. The one time when soda can actually benefit you is if you have an upset stomach. Ginger ale or cola can help to quell nausea and provide energy for people unable to take solid food.

### KEEP IT HEALTHY

**Choose a healthier fizz.** Carbonated drinks are refreshing, so try sparkling water, club soda, or sodium-free seltzer.

**Mix your own soft drink.** Combine 100% fruit juice with one of the carbonated beverages above for an energy boost with less sugar and no caffeine.

**Shrink the serving size.** Choose the smallest portion or share with a friend.

# SPICES

*See* Herbs and Spices, page 61

# SPINACH

*See also* Kale and Other Cooking Greens, page 65; Lettuce and Other Salad Greens, page 71

**Typical serving size:** 1 cup raw (30 g), 7 calories; ½ cup cooked (90 g), 21 calories

## HOW IT HARMS

Mineral absorption
Kidney and bladder stones
Drug interaction

## WHAT IT HEALS

Macular degeneration
Cancer
Congenital neurological birth defects
Anemia
Bone health

## NUTRIENTS

Bioflavonoids
Folate
Lutein (antioxidant)
Potassium
Riboflavin
Vitamin A
Vitamin B6
Vitamin C
Vitamin K
Zeaxanthin (antioxidant)

**WARNING! FOOD-DRUG INTERACTION**

Spinach may interfere with blood-thinning drugs. If your physician has prescribed blood-thinning medication such as heparin and warfarin (Coumadin), it is wise to moderate your intake of vitamin K–rich foods, such as spinach. Excess vitamin K can counteract the effects of these drugs.

## BUYING

Choose spinach that:
- has dark green leaves
- is crisp and fresh
- has no added sauce, if frozen

Avoid spinach that:
- is wilted or yellowing
- has signs of insect damage, holes in leaves

## STORING

**Where:** Crisper drawer of refrigerator.
**How:** In a plastic bag.
**For how long:** Up to 5 days.

## COOKING

- To maximize nutrients in spinach, don't overcook it. Instead, lightly steam or stir-fry to preserve vitamin content, texture, and flavor.
- Scatter chopped cooked spinach over cheese pizza.
- Season cooked spinach with soy sauce and grated ginger.
- Drain cooked pasta in a colander filled with baby spinach leaves, return the pasta and spinach to the pot, and toss with olive oil, grated romano cheese and dried red chile.

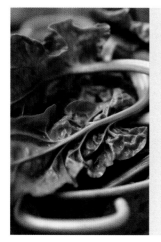

### QUICK TIP: Ditch the dirt

To effectively remove dirt and sand from spinach, submerge it in a bowl of cold water. Let the sand fall to the bottom, then remove and rinse the leaves. Dry them if making a salad. If you are cooking the spinach, the water left on the leaves may be just about the right amount with which to steam it.

## RECIPES TO TRY

- Flank Steak Roll with Carrots and Red Peppers
- Turkey Braciola Stuffed with Provolone and Spinach
- Scallops Florentine
- Cauliflower and Spinach Casserole
- Spinach, Sweet Potato, and Shiitake Salad

# SQUASH

(includes summer squash, such as chayote, patty pan, yellow crooknecks and straightnecks, and zucchini, and winter squash, such as acorn, banana, butternut, delicata, dumpling, hubbard, spaghetti, and turban)

*See also* Zucchini, page 117

**Typical serving size:** ½ cup slices, cooked (90 g), 18 calories

## WHAT IT HEALS

Vision
Bone growth
Cell functions
Immunity
Constipation
High cholesterol
Weight gain

## NUTRIENTS

Beta-carotene (especially winter varieties)
B vitamins
Fiber
Folate
Iron
Potassium
Vitamin C

## BUYING

Choose squash with:

- firm, unblemished skin or rind
- dull, brown stems (winter variety)
- long necks and smaller bottoms (butternut squash)
- shiny skin (summer variety)

Avoid:

- summer squash with pitted skin or spongy texture
- winter squash that gives when pressed hard
- winter squash with shiny green stems

## STORING

**Where:** Crisper drawer of refrigerator for summer varieties; in a cool, dark place for winter ones.

**How:** Uncut.

**For how long:** Up to 1 week for summer squash; several months for winter ones. If any soft or discolored spots develop on the squash, cut them away and discard before eating.

## COOKING

- Summer squash can be eaten raw. If it is cooked, stir-frying or steaming minimizes nutrient loss and keeps the vegetable from becoming too mushy.
- To avoid making dishes watery because of its high water content, lightly salt summer squash slices or pieces and place them on absorbent paper towels; rinse before adding them to the recipe.

> **QUICK TIP: Baked is better**
> You'll retain more nutrients if you bake or steam winter squash instead of boiling it.

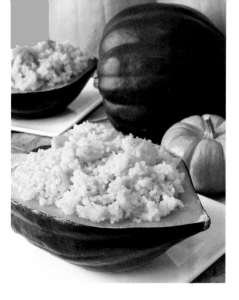

- Microwave small hard-shell squash, pierced several times with a knife, for 10 minutes on high power for easy peeling.
- Simmer chopped acorn or hubbard squash in a marinara sauce.
- Stir-fry slices of delicata squash with chopped leeks.

## RECIPES TO TRY

- Broccoli and Pearl Barley Salad
- Roasted Pork with Pomegranate Sauce
- Cider-Baked Acorn Squash with Apple Stuffing
- Fruity Butternut Squash Casserole with Papaya
- Ginger Butternut Squash Soup

# STRAWBERRIES

*See* Berries, page 26

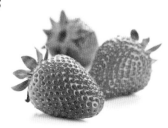

# SUGAR AND OTHER SWEETENERS

One healthy change every American should make is eating less sugar. We consume about 22 teaspoons of added sugar a day (that is, sugar added during preparation, not sugar that occurs naturally in fruit and other foods)—about 355 empty calories that can show up on your waistline and can increase your risk for diabetes and heart disease. This is sugars—that has been added during processing or preparation or at the table, not sugar that occurs naturally in foods like fruit. Despite some claims, brown sugar, honey, and molasses aren't any healthier than white sugar. Even some agave products, which have been hailed as more healthful alternatives because of their low glycemic index, actually cause blood sugar swings. And all of these sweeteners encourage the growth of oral bacteria that can lead to cavities. While it's unrealistic to think you can eliminate sugar entirely, you can make smarter choices.

### KEEP IT HEALTHY

**Monitor your intake.** It's amazing how quickly it adds up. Aim to consume under 40 g (about 10 tsp) of added sugar a day. That's about one can of Coke.

**Satisfy your sweet tooth with whole foods.** Natural sugars found in fruits and some vegetables make them a good option.

**Consider calorie-free alternatives.** Artificial sweeteners such as aspartame and sucralose (Splenda) have virtually no calories. While they may sound like a perfect choice if you're trying to lose weight, some research suggests that they may not be as helpful as expected and could contribute to weight gain, so use them wisely. They may be a good alternative for people with diabetes because they generally don't raise blood sugar. They also don't promote tooth decay.

**Be cautious with sugar alcohols.** Used in chewing gums, candies, ice cream, and many baked goods, sweeteners such as sorbitol, xylitol, maltitol, and lactitol provide fewer calories than sugar, do not promote tooth decay, and do not cause sudden jumps in blood glucose. However, they can produce a laxative effect in some people.

**Brush afterward.** More dangerous than the amount of sugar is the length of time the sugar remains in contact with the teeth.

# SWEET POTATOES AND YAMS

**Typical serving size:** ½ cup baked (2.4 oz or 68 g); 80 to 90 calories

## WHAT IT HEALS

High blood pressure
Eyes and skin
Immunity
Cardiovascular disease
Diabetes
Prostate and breast cancer
High blood sugar
High cholesterol
Insulin resistance

## NUTRIENTS

Beta-carotene
Carotenoids
Chlorogenic acid (anticancer compound)
Fiber
Potassium
Vitamin C

## BUYING

Choose yams and sweet potatoes that are:
- firm and smooth

Avoid yams and sweet potatoes that have:
- wrinkles or bruises
- sprouts or decay

## STORING

**Where:** In a dry, cool place such as a cellar, pantry, or garage.
**How:** Unwashed, uncut.
**For how long:** 1 month; stored at room temperature, 1 week.

## COOKING

- Scrub the potatoes but don't peel them, to retain more fiber and nutrients.
- Mash cooked yams or sweet potatoes with grated ginger and roasted sesame oil.
- Top roasted, split yams or sweet potatoes with chili.
- Make a soup with chunks of yam or sweet potato, chicken chunks, and chopped kale in broth.

## RECIPES TO TRY

- Savory Lamb Stew with Sweet Potatoes
- Cod and Vegetable Stew
- Black Bean and Sweet Potato Burritos
- Twice-Baked Stuffed Sweet Potatoes

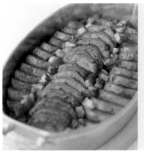

**QUICK TIP:**
**Lighten up traditional recipes**

For candied sweet potatoes, use thickened apple juice as a glaze, instead of sugar, and substitute pineapples for marshmallows.

# TANGERINES

*See* Oranges and Tangerines, page 82

# TEA

**Typical serving size:** 6 fl oz (177 mL), 2 calories

## HOW IT HARMS

Iron absorption

Increased urination

Insomnia

Migraines

## WHAT IT HEALS

Weight gain

Stroke

Diabetes

Cardiovascular disease

Cancer

Asthma

Dental health

Diarrhea

## NUTRIENTS

Antioxidants

Catechins (especially green and white varieties; compounds that may help with weight loss)

Epigallocatechin gallate (compounds that may protect against diabetes, heart disease, and cancer)

Flavonoids

Flouride

L-theanine (chemical that boosts immunity)

Phenols

Tannins (compounds that protect teeth)

Theophyllines (compounds that may help with respiratory problems)

## BUYING

Choose tea:

- in whole leaf form, when available, for best flavor and healing properties
- in bags that are made from unbleached natural fiber
- that's unsweetened

Avoid tea:

- flavored with fruit syrups and sweetened with sugar, including commercial iced teas

## STORING

**Where:** In a cool spot.

**How:** In a metal container.

**For how long:** Up to 1 year.

## COOKING

- Stir a spoonful of matcha, powdered green tea, into scrambled eggs.
- Add some cold brewed red rooibos tea to a berry smoothie.
- Use cold brewed black tea to replace water or milk in muffin recipes.

## RECIPES TO TRY

- Earl Grey Chicken
- Napa Cabbage Slaw with Peanut Dressing
- Melon Berry Compote with Green Tea and Lime
- Chai

# TOFU

*See* Soy, page 105

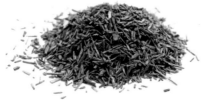

# TOMATOES

**Typical serving size:** 1 tomato (123 g), 22 calories

### HOW THEY HARM

Indigestion and heartburn
Allergies
Headaches
Canker sores

### WHAT THEY HEAL

Cancer
Cardiovascular disease

### NUTRIENTS

Chlorogenic acid (anticancer compound)
Folate
Lycopene (antioxidant)
Potassium
Salicylates (anticlotting effects)
Vitamin C

## BUYING

Choose tomatoes that:
- have deep red color and shiny, firm skin
- are vine ripened
- have reduced or no sodium added, for canned or jarred tomatoes

Avoid tomatoes that are:
- wrinkled or blemished
- pale colored
- have signs of insect or worm damage

## STORING

**Where:** At room temperature for fresh tomatoes; in a cool cupboard if canned or jarred.
**How:** Out of direct sunlight.
**For how long:** 1 week if fresh; 1 year if canned or jarred.

## COOKING

- Top a pizza with sliced tomatoes.
- Add some finely chopped tomatoes to corn bread batter before baking.
- Use sliced tomatoes instead of pineapple in an upside-down cake recipe.

## RECIPES TO TRY

- Orange Chicken with Artichokes and Sun-Dried Tomatoes
- Roasted Mackerel with Cherry Tomatoes and Potatoes
- Fusilli with Pan-Roasted Vegetables
- Tomato Biscuits

# TURKEY

*See* Poultry, page 96

# TURNIPS

**Typical serving size:** ½ cup cooked (78 g), 17 calories

### HOW THEY HARM

Bloating and flatulence
Thyroid function

### WHAT THEY HEAL

Cancer
High cholesterol
Vision
Bones
Immunity

### NUTRIENTS

Beta-carotene (turnip greens)
Calcium
Fiber
Lysine (may help with cold sores)
Potassium
Vitamin C

## BUYING

Choose turnips that:
- are firm
- feel heavy for their size
- have smooth skin
- are no more than 3 in (7.5 cm) in diameter
- have brightly colored and fresh greens

Avoid turnips that:
- are mushy
- have sunken brown spots
- have wilted or yellow greens

**Best time to buy:** winter

## STORING

**Where:** Crisper drawer of refrigerator.
**How:** In a plastic bag.
**For how long:** Up to 2 weeks.

## COOKING

- Small turnips of about 2 inches (5 cm) in diameter may only need to be well scrubbed, not peeled, before cooking.
- Shred turnips and use in coleslaw.
- Add matchstick-cut turnips to a vegetable stir-fry.
- Roast turnip chunks with carrot, onion, and walnuts.
- Replace half of the potatoes in a gratin recipe with turnips.

## RECIPES TO TRY

- Herb-Buttered Turnips
- Basil-Scented Sautéed Vegetables
- Mashed Turnips with Carrots and Potatoes

# VINEGAR

**Typical serving size:** 1 Tbsp, 3 to 14 calories, depending on variety

## HOW IT HARMS

Allergies

## WHAT IT HEALS

Weight gain

## NUTRIENTS

Trace amount of some minerals such as manganese, potassium, iron, and magnesium, depending on the variety

## BUYING

Choose:
- inexpensive white vinegar for making pickles
- sherry vinegar for vinaigrettes
- rice wine vinegar for sushi
- a shop that offers samples of different vinegars before buying

## STORING

**Where:** In a cool dark cabinet.
**How:** In a sealed bottle or jar.
**For how long:** Indefinitely if unopened; up to 6 months when opened.

## COOKING

- Add fresh herbs or fruit to distilled, cider, or wine vinegars to make flavored vinegars.
- Use white wine vinegar in recipes calling for lemon juice.
- Use sherry wine vinegar to dress a three-bean salad.
- Marinate beef chuck in cider vinegar for several hours before roasting.

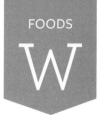

## RECIPES TO TRY

- Brussels Sprouts with Caraway Seeds
- Napa Cabbage Slaw with Peanut Dressing
- Buffalo Chicken Fingers

# WALNUTS

*See* Nuts and Seeds, page 76

# WATERCRESS

*See* Lettuce and Other Salad Greens, page 73

# WATERMELON

*See* Melons, page 73

# WHEAT AND WHEAT GERM

*See also* Grains, page 57

**Typical serving size:** 2 Tbsp wheat germ (14 g), 54 calories

## HOW THEY HARM

High blood sugar (refined wheat)

Allergies

## WHAT THEY HEAL

High cholesterol

Gastrointestinal distress

Weight gain

Cardiovascular disease

High blood pressure

Inflammation

Anemia

## NUTRIENTS

B vitamins

Copper

Fiber

Folate

Iron

Magnesium

Manganese

Phosphorous

Sterols (cholesterol-lowering compounds)

Protein

Thiamine

Vitamin E

Zinc

## BUYING

Choose:

- products labeled "100% whole wheat"

Avoid:

- refined products

## STORING

**Where:** In the refrigerator; defatted wheat germ can be kept in the cupboard.

**How:** In an airtight container.

**For how long:** 6 to 8 months.

## COOKING

- Cook wheat berries for a grain side dish.
- Sprinkle toasted wheat germ over creamy soups before serving.
- Toss some wheat germ into a salad.

## RECIPES TO TRY

- Whole Wheat Noodles with Peanut Sauce and Chicken
- Macaroni and Cheese with Spinach
- Wheat Berry Salad with Dried Apricots

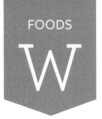
# WRAPS AND TORTILLAS

*See* Bread, page 28

# YAMS

*See* Sweet Potatoes and Yams, page 111

# YOGURT

*See also* Milk and Dairy Products, page 74

**Typical serving size:** 6 oz, 80 to 160 calories, depending on brand and type

### HOW IT HARMS
Phenylketonuria

### WHAT IT HEALS
Digestion
Bone health
High blood pressure

### NUTRIENTS
Calcium
Live or "active" bacteria
Phosphorus
Protein

## BUYING

Choose yogurt that is:
- plain
- low-fat or nonfat

Avoid yogurt with:
- fruit added
- sweeteners or flavoring

## STORING

**Where:** Refrigerator.
**How:** In its container.
**For how long:** Within a week of the "use-by" date.

## COOKING

- Use 2% Greek yogurt in recipes calling for sour cream.
- Blend a dip with plain yogurt, sundried tomatoes, garlic, and salt-free seasoning mix.
- Replace buttermilk in baked goods with yogurt thinned with milk or water.

### RECIPES TO TRY

- Mackerel Tandoori Style
- Lobster Salad with Lime Dressing
- Tomato Biscuits
- Carrot Soup with Dill
- Strawberry-Yogurt Smoothie

# YUCCA

(also known as cassava or manioc)

**Typical serving size:** ½ cup raw (103 g), 165 calories

### HOW IT HARMS
Bloating and flatulence

### WHAT IT HEALS
Immunity
Collagen production
Digestion
Celiac disease
Gluten intolerance

### NUTRIENTS
Fiber
Vitamin C

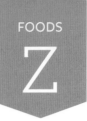

## BUYING

Choose yucca that is:

- firm

Avoid yucca that is:

- blemished
- soft

## STORING

**Where:** In a dry, cool, dark place.
**How:** Unwashed, uncut.
**For how long:** 1 week uncut. You can also peel yucca, place it in water, and refrigerate it for up to 3 days; or peel, wrap, and freeze it for up to about 3 months.

## COOKING

- Bake yucca sticks coated with olive oil and garlic until browned and crispy.
- Top a shepherd's pie with mashed cooked yucca.
- Toss a salad of cooked yucca cubes with corn kernels, red bell pepper, scallions. and cilantro in lime dressing.

## RECIPES TO TRY

- Shrimp and Yucca Salad
- Baked Yucca Chips

# ZUCCHINI

*See also* Squash, page 108

**Typical serving size:** 1 cup raw, chopped (124 g), 20 calories

## WHAT IT HEALS

High cholesterol
Weight gain

## NUTRIENTS

Fiber
Folate
Potassium
Vitamin C

## BUYING

Choose zucchini that are:

- firm
- heavy for their size
- small, about 6 to 9 in (15 to 22.5 cm) long

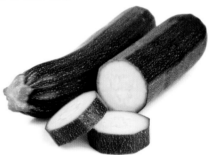

Avoid zucchini that are:

- blemished
- bruised
- moldy

**Best time to buy:** summer

## STORING

**Where:** Crisper drawer of refrigerator.
**How:** In a plastic bag.
**For how long:** Up to 1 week.

## COOKING

- Coarsely shred zucchini, place in a cold skillet, and cook until it's wilted; drain and sprinkle with parmesan cheese.
- Make a gratin of thinly sliced zucchini and fine dry bread crumbs drizzled with olive oil.
- Toss a salad of grilled zucchini strips, tomatoes, olives, and crumbled feta cheese.

## RECIPES TO TRY

- Zucchini Frittata
- Monkfish and Mussel Kebabs
- Beef and Blue Cheese Burgers
- Couscous-Stuffed Peppers
- Zucchini-Carrot Crustless Quiche Squares

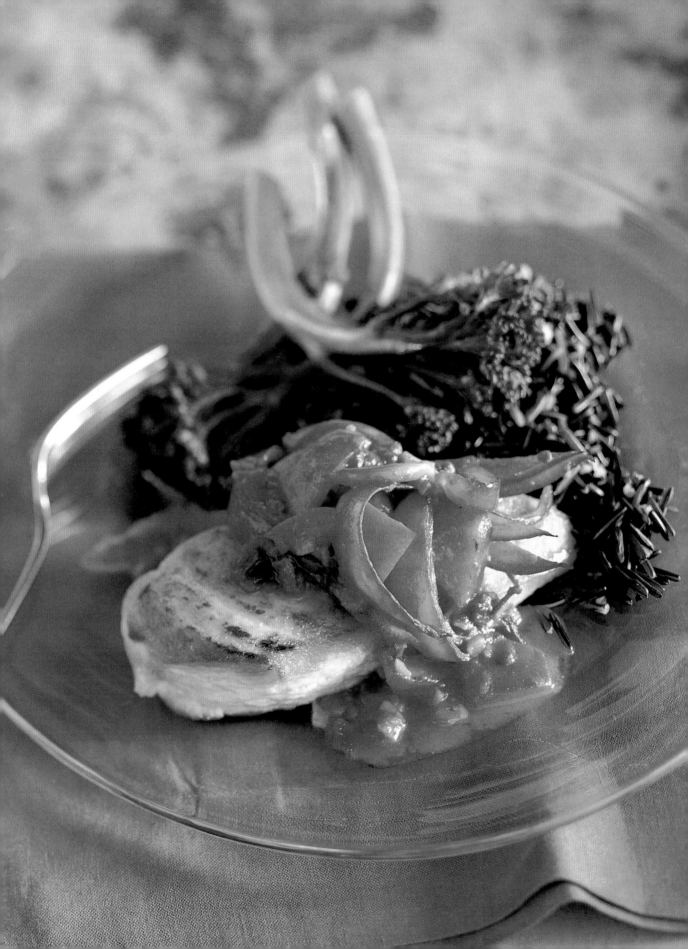

# (2)

# RECIPES

## 250 Delicious Recipes for Good Health

Healthy eating doesn't have to be time-consuming, expensive, bland, or boring. In this section, you're going to discover simple ways to get more foods that heal into your diet. It's easy when every recipe contains at least three healing foods—some have many more. (We've listed just the ones that are most abundant on these pages.) These recipes are packed with nutrients, but they don't have endless lists of ingredients. The foods you'll use, however, are specially selected to enhance the flavor of each dish without making preparation difficult. You'll be amazed at how tasty healthy cuisine can be.

More than 250 recipes cover Breakfasts, Soups and Stews, Sandwiches and Light Meals, Salads, Entrées, Sides, Snacks, Desserts, and Drinks—you can eat healthy all day long and keep your taste buds entertained with new dishes. While some of the recipes may seem exotic and use foods you're not familiar with, you'll also find some old favorites that have been made over to provide

more nutrients with less fat, calories, sugar, and sodium. There's something for everyone.

In addition to the healing foods, each recipe features a list of the ailments it may help. Again, this is not intended to be a complete listing but just a guide to help you identify recipes that address the health issues you face. For instance, fish and tomatoes are bursting with antioxidants that help prevent cancer, lower cholesterol, and combat mood disorders; you'll find them both in the Tuna and Tomato Pizzas. But these same ingredients may also benefit Alzheimer's disease, eye problems, and many other health issues that we didn't have room to put on these pages. Plus, we go beyond the ingredients to make sure that the sodium, saturated fat, fiber, and levels of other nutrients in each recipe are appropriate for the ailments listed.

Planning and preparing dishes that boost your health and improve your life just got easier and tastier. Bon appétit!

# NUTTY MUESLI

**Serves 6**
**Prep Time:** 15 minutes plus soaking
**Healing Foods:** bulgur, oats, nuts and seeds, persimmons, passion fruit
**Ailments It Heals:** atherosclerosis, chronic fatigue syndrome, lactose intolerance, neuralgia

½ cup bulgur
1 cup water
1½ cups rolled oats
1 cup apple juice
½ cup slivered unblanched almonds
¼ cup pine nuts
2 Tbsp shelled raw sunflower seeds
10 dried apricots, diced
10 dried figs, stalks removed, then diced
¼ cup brown sugar
2 green apples, cored and coarsely grated
1 large or 2 small persimmons, peeled and diced plus extra for serving
1 passion fruit
Few drops of pure almond essence (optional)
Pomegranate seeds or blueberries

**1.** In large bowl, combine bulgur with water and stir to combine. Cover and soak for 30 minutes to soften bulgur. Drain well in sieve and return to bowl.

**2.** Add oats, apple juice, almonds, pine nuts, sunflower seeds, apricots, figs, sugar, apples, and persimmon. Fold into bulgur.

**3.** Cut passion fruit in half. Place sieve over bowl of muesli, and spoon passion fruit pulp and seeds into it. Press until juice has gone through sieve and only seeds are left behind. Discard seeds.

**4.** Add almond essence, if using, and a little more apple juice if needed to make a moist but not sloppy consistency. Keep, tightly covered, in fridge until ready to eat. It can be kept for up to 2 days. To serve, stir muesli well, then top with pomegranate seeds or blueberries, whichever is in season, plus additional persimmon.

**Per serving:** 369 calories, 8 g protein, 62 g carbohydrates, 10 g fiber, 11 g total fat, 1 g saturated fat, 0 mg cholesterol, 25 mg sodium

# BLUEBERRY AND CRANBERRY GRANOLA

**Serves 8**
**Prep Time:** 10 minutes
**Cook Time:** 40 minutes plus cooling
**Healing Foods:** oats, wheat germ, nuts and seeds, blueberries, cranberries
**Ailments It Heals:** cardiovascular disease, colds and flu, peptic ulcers, urinary tract infections

2¾ cups oats
½ cup wheat germ
7 Tbsp millet flakes
2 Tbsp slivered almonds
2 Tbsp sunflower seeds
1 Tbsp sesame seeds
½ cup dried blueberries
½ cup dried cranberries
1 Tbsp soft light brown sugar
2 Tbsp maple syrup
2 Tbsp canola oil
2 Tbsp orange juice

**1.** Preheat oven to 325°F (160°C). In large bowl, combine oats, wheat germ, millet flakes, almonds, sunflower seeds, sesame seeds, dried berries, and sugar. Stir until well mixed.

**2.** In measuring cup, whisk together maple syrup, oil, and orange juice. Pour slowly into dry ingredients, stirring until liquid is evenly distributed and coats everything lightly.

**3.** In nonstick roasting pan, spread out mixture evenly. Bake, stirring every 10 minutes to encourage even browning, for 30 to 40 minutes, or until slightly crisp and lightly brown.

**4.** Remove roasting pan from oven and leave granola to cool. Store in airtight container up to 2 weeks. Serve with plain yogurt, milk, or fruit juice.

**Per serving:** 307 calories, 8 g protein, 48 g carbohydrates, 7 g fiber, 9 g total fat, 1 g saturated fat, 0 mg cholesterol, 22 mg sodium

# HOT CEREAL WITH APPLES AND DATES

Serves 4
**Prep Time:** 10 minutes
**Cook Time:** 10 minutes
**Healing Foods:** milk, apple, oats, bulgur, dates
**Ailments It Heals:** AIDS and HIV infections, constipation, hemmorrhoids, menstrual problems, PCOS, stroke

1½  cups low-fat milk
1½  cups water
 1  cup unpeeled chopped apple (¼ in or 0.5 cm pieces)
 ½  cup old-fashioned oats
 ½  cup coarse bulgur
 3  dates, pitted and snipped
 ½  tsp ground cinnamon

Stir together milk, water, apple, oats, bulgur, dates, and cinnamon in medium saucepan and heat, stir-

ring frequently, until boiling. Cover, reduce the heat to low, and cook, stirring occasionally, for 10 minutes, or until grains are tender.

**Per serving:** 185 calories, 7 g protein, 37 g carbohydrates, 6 g fiber, 2 g total fat, 1 g saturated fat, 5 mg cholesterol, 44 mg sodium

# ASPARAGUS, EGG, AND HAM SANDWICHES

Serves 4
**Prep Time:** 15 minutes
**Cook Time:** 8 minutes
**Healing Foods:** asparagus, eggs, tomatoes, cheese
**Ailments It Heals:** anemia, mood disorders, psoriasis

24  thin stalks asparagus or 12 thick stalks, trimmed
 4  slices seven-grain bread
 4  tsp Dijon mustard
 8  slices 97% fat-free ham
 2  hard-cooked eggs, peeled and sliced
 8  thin slices tomatoes
 2  slices provolone cheese, cut into thin strips

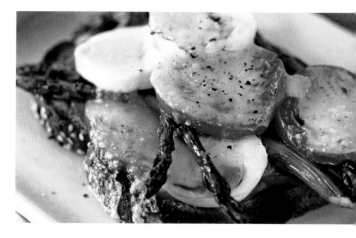

**1.** Preheat broiler.

**2.** In skillet of simmering water, cook asparagus for 3 to 4 minutes, or until crisp-tender. Drain well.

**3.** Place bread slices on baking sheet. Broil 3 to 4 in (7.5 to 10 cm) from heat for 1 minute each side, or until bread is toasted.

**4.** On each bread slice, spread 1 tsp mustard, then arrange 2 slices of ham, 6 thin or 3 thick asparagus spears, half of 1 sliced egg, 2 tomato slices, and a quarter of the provolone strips.

**5.** Broil sandwiches for 1 to 2 minutes, or until cheese is melted and golden brown and sandwich is heated through.

**Per serving:** 199 calories, 15 g protein, 17 g carbohydrates, 3 g fiber, 9 g total fat, 4 g saturated fat, 128 mg cholesterol, 738 mg sodium

# SPINACH AND GOAT CHEESE OMELET

Serves 1
**Prep Time:** 10 minutes
**Cook Time:** 2 minutes
**Healing Foods:** spinach, cheese, eggs
**Ailments It Heals:** ADHD, bleeding problems, celiac disease, hyperthyroidism, menopause

- 2   cups baby spinach, rinsed
- 2   Tbsp crumbled goat cheese or feta cheese
- 1   Tbsp chopped scallion
- 1   large egg
- 2   large egg whites
- ¼   tsp hot red-pepper sauce, such as Tabasco
- 1   tsp olive oil

Pinch of salt
Pinch of ground black pepper

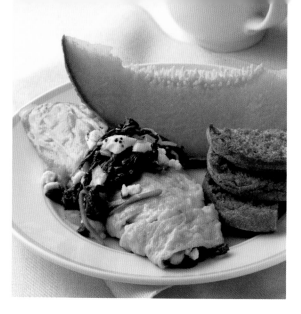

**1.** Bring about 1 in (2.5 cm) of water to a boil in large saucepan. Drop in spinach and cook for 30 seconds, or just until wilted. Drain, press out liquid, and chop coarsely. (Alternatively, place spinach in microwave-safe bowl, cover with vented plastic wrap, and microwave on high for 1 to 2 minutes.) Place spinach in small bowl. Stir in cheese and scallion.

**2.** Stir egg, egg whites, hot sauce, salt, and black pepper briskly with fork in medium bowl. Heat oil in 7- to 10-in (18 to 25 cm) nonstick skillet over medium-high heat until hot. Tilt skillet to spread oil over surface. Pour in egg mixture. Immediately stir with heat-resistant rubber spatula or fork for a few seconds. Then use spatula to push cooked portions at edges toward the center, tilting skillet to allow uncooked egg mixture to fill in areas around edges. Sprinkle spinach mixture over omelet. Continue to cook until almost set and bottom is golden. The entire cooking process should take about 1 minute.

**3.** Use spatula to fold one-third of omelet over filling. Tip skillet and, using spatula as a guide, slide omelet onto plate so that it lands, folded in thirds, seam side down.

**Per omelet:** 235 calories, 20 g protein, 4 g carbohydrates, 1 g fiber, 15 g total fat, 6 g saturated fat, 228 mg cholesterol, 471 mg sodium

# ONE-EGG OMELET WITH CHOPPED BROCCOLI, TOMATOES, AND CHEDDAR

**Per serving:** 129 calories, 9 g protein, 4 g carbohydrates, 1 g fiber, 7 g total fat, 3 g saturated fat, 188 mg cholesterol, 269 mg sodium

Serves 4
**Prep Time:** 10 minutes
**Cook Time:** 12 minutes
**Healing Foods:** broccoli, tomatoes, eggs, cheese
**Ailments It Heals:** anorexia, cancer, hepatitis, jet lag

1½   cups chopped broccoli florets
2   Tbsp water
¼   cup chopped tomato
1   Tbsp chopped fresh basil or cilantro
1   tsp extra-virgin olive oil
1   clove garlic, crushed or grated
¼   tsp coarse salt
⅛   tsp ground black pepper
4   large eggs
1   oz (30 g) shredded cheddar cheese

**1.** In small covered saucepan over medium-low heat, cook broccoli in water for 4 minutes, or until broccoli is fork-tender. Drain off excess moisture, then add tomato, basil or cilantro, oil, garlic, salt, and pepper. Stir to blend. Keep warm over low heat.

**2.** Heat small heavy nonstick skillet over medium heat until hot enough that a drop of water sizzles. Coat with cooking spray. Beat 1 egg until frothy and add to pan, tilting pan to let egg run to edges. Cook, undisturbed, for 2 minutes, or until egg is set along edges and center is moist but not runny.

**3.** Slide egg "pancake" onto plate. Place ¼ cup of the broccoli mixture on half of egg and top with one-quarter of the cheese. Fold egg over to make omelet. Repeat with remaining eggs.

# MUSHROOM AND BELL PEPPER FRITTATA

Serves 4
**Prep Time:** 10 minutes
**Cook Time:** 26 minutes
**Healing Foods:** peppers, mushrooms, eggs, cheese, basil
**Ailments It Heals:** alcoholism, diabetes, osteoporosis, stress

2   Tbsp olive oil
1   red or orange bell pepper, seeded and cut into ¼-in (0.5 cm) slices
1   yellow bell pepper, seeded and cut into ¼-in (0.5 cm) slices
2   cups sliced mushrooms
8   large eggs
¼   tsp salt
¼   tsp ground black pepper
⅓   cup grated parmesan cheese
10   fresh basil leaves, torn in small pieces

**1.** In large nonstick skillet over medium-high heat, heat oil. Add bell peppers. Sauté until softened, about 4 minutes. Add mushrooms. Sauté for 5 minutes, or until vegetables are lightly browned. Reduce heat to medium.

**2.** In medium bowl, stir together eggs, salt, and black pepper. Pour into skillet, spreading evenly. Cook, stirring frequently, for 3 to 4 minutes, or until soft-scrambled. Reduce heat to medium-low. Stir in cheese and basil. Smooth top. Cook for 5 minutes. Cover and cook for 8 minutes, or until eggs are firm and bottom is browned.

**3.** To serve, loosen frittata around edge with spatula. Invert onto large plate. Cut into 4 equal wedges. Serve warm or at room temperature.

**Per serving:** 269 calories, 17 g protein, 8 g carbohydrates, 2 g fiber, 19 g total fat, 5 g saturated fat, 430 mg cholesterol, 397 mg sodium

# ZUCCHINI FRITTATA

Serves 6
**Prep Time:** 5 minutes
**Cook Time:** 15 minutes
**Healing Foods:** eggs, garlic, zucchini, peppers
**Ailments It Heals:** Alzheimer's disease, hepatitis, jaundice, kidney disease

- 4  eggs
- 4  egg whites
- ¼  cup grated parmesan cheese
- ¼  tsp salt
- 2  Tbsp olive oil
- 1  clove garlic, minced
- 2  small zucchini, shredded
- 2  roasted red bell peppers, cut into thin strips

**1.** Preheat oven to 400°F (200°F). In medium bowl, whisk together eggs, egg whites, cheese, and salt.

**2.** Heat oil in large ovenproof nonstick skillet over medium heat. Add garlic and cook for 1 minute, or just until tender. Add zucchini and peppers and cook for 1 minute. Pour in egg mixture and cook for 3 minutes, or until bottom of frittata is set.

**3.** Bake for 10 minutes, until set.

**Per serving:** 138 calories, 9 g protein, 5 g carbohydrates, 1 g fiber, 9 g total fat, 2 g saturated fat, 144 mg cholesterol, 331 mg sodium

# HUEVOS RANCHEROS

Serves 4
**Prep Time:** 15 minutes plus 30 minutes for marinating
**Cook Time:** 13 minutes
**Healing Foods:** tomatoes, chiles, eggs, cheese
**Ailments It Heals:** colds and flu, cystic fibrosis, respiratory disorders

**Salsa**
- 5  medium tomatoes, finely chopped
- 1  mild fresh red chile, seeded and finely chopped
- 1  small red onion, finely chopped
- 1  small clove garlic, finely chopped
- 2  Tbsp finely chopped fresh cilantro
- 1  Tbsp olive oil
- 2  tsp lime juice

Salt and pepper

**Eggs**
- 4  (10 in or 25 cm) flour tortillas
- 1  tsp vinegar
- 4  eggs

**Garnish**
- 2  oz (60 g) coarsely grated reduced-fat cheddar cheese
- 6  Tbsp low-fat sour cream

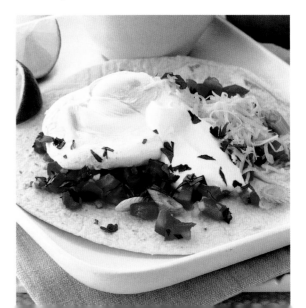

4 scallions, chopped
Chopped fresh cilantro
Lime wedges

**1.** To make salsa: Place tomatoes in bowl and stir in chile, red onion, garlic, and cilantro. Add oil and lime juice to taste. Set aside to marinate for about 30 minutes, then season lightly with salt and pepper to taste.

**2.** Preheat oven 350°F (180°C). Stack tortillas and wrap in foil. Place in oven to warm for 7 to 10 minutes.

**3.** To make eggs: Meanwhile, half-fill large skillet with water. Heat until just starting to simmer, then reduce heat so water does not boil. Add vinegar. Break eggs into water, one at a time, and poach for 3 minutes. Toward the end of cooking, spoon water over yolks. When cooked, remove eggs with slotted spoon and drain on paper towel–lined plate.

**4.** Place warmed tortillas on 4 plates. Spoon over a little salsa, then put eggs on top and season with salt and pepper to taste. Put cheese, sour cream, scallions, chopped cilantro, and lime wedges into small bowls, and serve, along with the remaining salsa.

**Per serving:** 459 calories, 20 g protein, 55 g carbohydrates, 5 g fiber, 19 g total fat, 7 g saturated fat, 231 mg cholesterol, 554 mg sodium

# INDIVIDUAL BREAKFAST TORTILLA

**Serves 1**
**Prep Time:** 12 minutes
**Cook Time:** 3 minutes
**Healing Foods:** eggs, beans, tomatoes, avocados
**Ailments It Heals:** diabetes, gallstones, sex drive (diminished)

1 large egg
⅛ tsp chili powder
1 corn or whole grain tortilla (6 in or 15 cm)
1 Tbsp shredded monterey jack, provolone, or cheddar cheese
2 Tbsp cooked or canned black beans, drained and mashed with a fork
1 thin slice tomato, halved
1 tsp chopped fresh cilantro
1 thin slice avocado
1½ tsp fat-free sour cream

**1.** Whisk together egg and chili powder in small bowl until well-blended.

**2.** Heat small heavy skillet over medium heat until hot enough that a drop of water sizzles. Coat with cooking spray and pour in egg. Cook, stirring with rubber spatula, for about 15 seconds, or until set. Transfer to plate and keep warm. Wipe out skillet and respray.

**3.** Increase heat to medium-high. Heat tortilla in skillet, turning, for 1 minute, or until heated. Turn, sprinkle with the cheese, and heat for 10 seconds, or until melted. Transfer to serving plate.

**4.** Spread beans on half of tortilla. Add egg, tomato, cilantro, avocado, and sour cream. Fold the tortilla to make a "sandwich."

**Per tortilla:** 238 calories, 12 g protein, 25 g carbohydrates, 5 g fiber, 10 g total fat, 3 g saturated fat, 188 mg cholesterol, 229 mg sodium

# SUMMER GREENS SCRAMBLE

Serves 4
**Prep Time:** 10 minutes
**Cook Time:** 11 minutes
**Healing Foods:** kale, eggs, cumin
**Ailments It Heals:** ADHD, celiac disease, mood disorders, osteoporosis

2  cups shredded, stemmed fresh kale
5  large eggs
5  large egg whites
¼  tsp ground cumin
¼  tsp salt
¼  cup chopped lean deli ham
2  scallions, trimmed and thinly sliced

**1.** In large saucepan of boiling salted water, cook kale, 3 to 5 minutes, or until tender. Drain. Rinse under cold water. Drain well.

**2.** In large bowl, whisk together eggs, egg whites, cumin, and salt.

**3.** Coat large nonstick skillet with cooking spray. Heat over medium heat. Add egg mixture. Cook, stirring constantly, for 2 to 3 minutes, or until eggs start to thicken slightly. Stir in kale, ham, and scallions. Cook, stirring occasionally, for 2 to 3 minutes, or until eggs are soft-scrambled.

**Per serving:** 145 calories, 15 g protein, 5 g carbohydrates, 1 g fiber, 7 g total fat, 2 g saturated fat, 270 mg cholesterol, 385 mg sodium

# BERRY SALAD WITH PASSION FRUIT

Serves 6
**Prep Time:** 10 minutes
**Healing Foods:** strawberries, raspberries, blackberries, blueberries, passion fruit
**Ailments It Heals:** cancer, colds & flu, irritable bowel syndrome, PCOS

4  cups ripe strawberries, hulled and cut in half
1  cup fresh red raspberries
1  cup fresh blackberries
½  cup fresh blueberries
½  cup mixed fresh red currants and black currants, removed from their stalks (optional)
2  passion fruits
3  Tbsp sugar, or to taste
1  Tbsp fresh lime or lemon juice

**1.** In large serving bowl, combine strawberries, raspberries, blackberries, blueberries, and red and black currants, if using.

**2.** Cut each passion fruit in half. Holding strainer over bowl of berries, spoon passion fruit and seeds into strainer. Press flesh and seeds with back of spoon to squeeze all of juice through strainer onto berries. Reserve a few seeds left in strainer and discard the rest.

**3.** Add sugar and lime juice to berries. Gently toss. Sprinkle with reserved passion fruit seeds. Serve salad immediately, or cover and chill briefly.

**Per serving:** 89 calories, 1 g protein, 22 g carbohydrates, 6 g fiber, 1 g total fat, 0 g saturated fat, 0 mg cholesterol, 4 mg sodium

# YOGURT PARFAIT

**Serves 1**

**Prep Time:** 5 minutes

**Healing Foods:** yogurt, berries, mangoes, coconuts

**Ailments It Heals:** osteoporosis, peptic ulcers, shingles, urinary tract infections

¾ cup nonfat plain or artificially sweetened yogurt

¼ cup mixed berries

¼ cup mango

¼ cup low-fat granola

1 Tbsp shredded coconut

In tall parfait glass, layer one-third of the yogurt, half of the fruit, all of the granola, another one-third of the yogurt, the remaining fruit, and the remaining yogurt. Top with coconut.

**Per serving:** 250 calories, 13 g protein, 44 g carbohydrates, 4 g fiber, 4 g total fat, 3 g saturated fat, 5 mg cholesterol, 210 mg sodium

# BLUEBERRY OATMEAL MUFFINS

**Makes 12**

**Prep Time:** 25 minutes

**Cook Time:** 22 minutes

**Healing Foods:** wheat, oats, blueberries

**Ailments It Heals:** constipation, diabetes, diverticulitis, hypoglycemia, irritable bowel syndrome, varicose veins

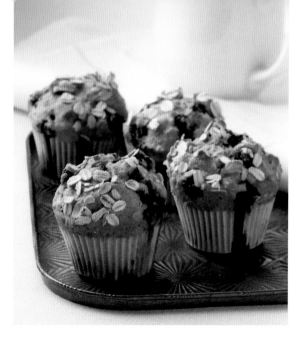

¾ cup plus 2 Tbsp whole wheat flour

¾ cup all-purpose flour

1½ tsp baking powder

½ tsp baking soda

¼ tsp salt

1 tsp ground cinnamon

1 cup plus 2 Tbsp old-fashioned rolled oats

1 large egg

2 large egg whites

½ cup maple syrup

¾ cup low-fat buttermilk

3 Tbsp canola oil

2 tsp grated orange zest

1 Tbsp orange juice

1 tsp vanilla extract

1½ cups fresh blueberries, rinsed and patted dry

**1.** Preheat oven to 400°F (200°C). Coat 12 standard-size muffin cups with cooking spray or insert paper liners.

**2.** In large bowl, whisk together flours, baking powder, baking soda, salt, and cinnamon. Stir in 1 cup rolled oats.

**3.** In medium bowl, whisk egg, egg whites, and syrup until smooth. Add buttermilk, oil, zest, orange juice, and vanilla and whisk until blended. Add to flour mixture and mix with rubber spatula just until dry ingredients are moistened. Fold in blueberries. Spoon batter into muffin cups, filling them almost to the top. Sprinkle tops with remaining 2 Tbsp rolled oats.

**4.** Bake for 18 to 22 minutes, or until muffins are lightly browned and tops spring back when touched lightly. Loosen edges of muffins, turn out onto wire rack, and let cool slightly before serving.

**Per muffin:** 180 calories, 5 g protein, 30 g carbohydrates, 3 g fiber, 5 g total fat, 0 g saturated fat, 18 mg cholesterol, 190 mg sodium

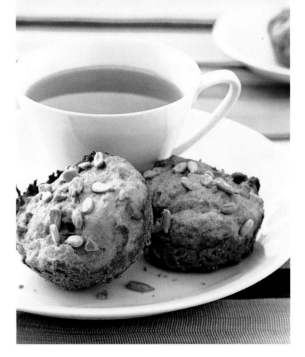

# PEAR RHUBARB MUFFINS

**Makes 12**
**Prep Time:** 10 minutes
**Cook Time:** 30 minutes
**Healing Foods:** pears, rhubarb, wheat, oats, ginger
**Ailments It Heals:** atherosclerosis, cardiovascular disease, cholesterol (high), hemorrhoids, PCOS

| | |
|---|---|
| 3.5 | oz (100 g) dried pears, cut into ¼ in (0.5 cm) cubes, tough parts removed |
| 3.5 | oz (100 g) rhubarb stalks, trimmed and chopped into ½ in (1 cm) lengths |
| 1 | cup low-fat milk |
| 1 | Tbsp soft brown sugar |
| 2 | Tbsp honey |
| 2 | Tbsp light olive oil |
| 1 | tsp baking soda |
| ⅔ | cup whole wheat flour |
| ⅔ | cup self-rising flour |
| ⅔ | cup oat bran |
| 1 | tsp baking powder |
| 1 | tsp ground cinnamon |
| 1 | tsp ground nutmeg |
| 2 | tsp ground ginger |

**1.** Preheat oven to 375°F (190°C). Coat 12 standard-size muffin cups with cooking spray or insert paper liners.

**2.** In large saucepan, add pears, rhubarb, milk, sugar, honey, and oil. Bring to a boil, then reduce heat to low and simmer for 2 minutes, or until rhubarb has softened. Mixture will look curdled, but this is normal. Add baking soda and stir until frothy.

**3.** In large bowl, combine flours, oat bran, baking powder, cinnamon, nutmeg, and ginger and stir to combine. Add fruit mixture and stir gently until just combined. Spoon into prepared muffin cups and bake for 30 minutes, or until muffins are brown and risen. Allow to cool slightly on a wire rack before serving.

**Per muffin:** 132 calories, 3 g protein, 26 g carbohydrates, 3 g fiber, 4 g total fat, 1 g saturated fat, 2 mg cholesterol, 250 mg sodium

# CARROT GINGER YOGURT MUFFINS

**Per muffin:** 118 calories, 4 g protein, 22 g carbohydrates, 3 g fiber, 2 g fat, 0 g saturated fat, 16 mg cholesterol, 186 mg sodium

**Makes 12**
**Prep Time:** 10 minutes
**Cook Time:** 25 minutes plus cooling
**Healing Foods:** flour, ginger, chia, oats, carrots, apples, yogurt
**Ailments It Heals:** arthritis, blood pressure, hives, interstitial cystitis

- 1 cup whole wheat flour
- 1 tsp ground ginger
- 1½ tsp baking soda
- ½ cup brown sugar
- ¼ cup chia seeds or flaxseed
- ½ cup rolled oats, plus extra to sprinkle
- 2 packed cups finely grated carrots (2 medium carrots)
- 1 packed cup grated apples (1 medium apple)
- 1 egg
- ½ cup low-fat plain yogurt
- ½ tsp vanilla extract

**1.** Preheat oven to 350°F (180°C). Coat 12 standard-size muffin cups with cooking spray or insert paper liners.

**2.** In large bowl, sift flour, ginger, and baking soda. Add sugar, chia seeds, and oats. Mix to combine, then mix in carrots and apples. Make a well in center of mixture.

**3.** In small bowl, whisk together egg and yogurt. Stir in vanilla. Add to well in large bowl and stir together until mixture is just combined (do not overstir).

**4.** Spoon evenly into muffin tin. Sprinkle each with extra oats.

**5.** Cook for 20 to 25 minutes, or until golden brown on top and a wooden pick inserted in center comes out clean. Cool in tin for 10 minutes, then transfer to wire rack.

# BUCKWHEAT PANCAKES WITH FRUIT SAUCE

**Serves 5**
**Prep Time:** 5 minutes
**Cook Time:** 20 minutes
**Healing Foods:** apples, buckwheat, eggs
**Ailments It Heals:** cardiovascular disease, cirrhosis, cholesterol (high), hypoglycemia, stroke

- 3 apples, pears, or plums, cored and sliced
- ⅓ cup pure maple syrup
- 1 cup buckwheat flour
- ⅓ cup brown rice flour
- 2 Tbsp brown sugar
- 1 tsp baking powder
- ½ tsp baking soda
- ½ tsp salt
- ½ tsp ground cinnamon
- ¾ cup milk
- 2 Tbsp canola oil
- 2 eggs

**1.** Coat nonstick skillet with cooking spray and heat over medium heat. Add apples and cook, turning, for 5 minutes, or until just tender. Add syrup and reduce heat to low to keep warm.

**2.** In large bowl, mix together flours, sugar, baking powder, baking soda, salt, and cinnamon. In measuring cup, whisk together milk, oil, and eggs. Stir into flour mixture just until blended.

**3.** Coat griddle or nonstick skillet with cooking spray and heat over medium heat. Drop 2 Tbsp batter onto griddle to form pancake. Cook for 3 minutes, or until browned on bottom and bubbles form on top. Turn and cook for 3 minutes, or until browned on bottom and firm to the touch. Place on plate and cover to keep warm. Repeat with remaining batter. Serve with fruit syrup.

**Per serving:** 328 calories, 7 g protein, 54 g carbohydrates, 7 g fiber, 10 g total fat, 2 g saturated fat, 88 mg cholesterol, 283 mg sodium

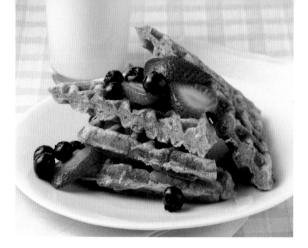

# MULTIGRAIN PANCAKES OR WAFFLES

**Serves 8**
**Prep Time:** 20 minutes
**Cook Time:** 15 to 20 minutes
**Healing Foods:** oats, wheat and wheat germ, eggs, strawberries
**Ailments It Heals:** depression, diabetes, muscle cramps, prostate problems

- 2 cups low-fat buttermilk
- ½ cup old-fashioned rolled oats
- ⅔ cup whole wheat flour
- ⅔ cup all-purpose flour
- ⅔ cup toasted wheat germ
- 1½ tsp baking powder
- ½ tsp baking soda
- ¼ tsp salt
- 1 tsp ground cinnamon
- 2 large eggs
- ¼ cup firmly packed brown sugar
- 1 Tbsp canola oil
- 2 tsp vanilla extract
- 1 cup maple syrup, warmed
- 1½ cups sliced strawberries or blueberries

**1.** Mix buttermilk and oats in small bowl. Let stand for 15 minutes.

**2.** In large bowl, whisk whole wheat flour, all-purpose flour, wheat germ, baking powder, baking soda, salt, and cinnamon.

**3.** In medium bowl, whisk eggs, sugar, oil, and vanilla. Add buttermilk mixture. Add this mixture to flour mixture and mix with rubber spatula just until flour mixture is moistened.

**4.** To make pancakes: Coat large nonstick skillet with cooking spray and heat over medium heat. Spoon about ¼ cup batter for each pancake into skillet. Cook for 3 minutes, or until bottoms are golden and small bubbles start to form on top. Flip the pancakes and cook for 1 to 2 minutes, or until browned and cooked through. (Adjust heat as necessary for even browning.) Keep the pancakes warm in 200°F (100°C) oven while you finish cooking remaining batter.

**5.** To make waffles: Coat waffle iron with cooking spray and heat iron. Spoon in enough batter to cover three-quarters of surface. Close iron and cook for 4 to 5 minutes, or until waffles are crisp and golden brown. Keep waffles warm in 200°F (100°C) oven while you finish cooking remaining batter.

**6.** Top with maple syrup and strawberries or blueberries. Wrap any leftover pancakes or waffles individually in plastic wrap, and refrigerate for up to 2 days or freeze for up to 1 month. Reheat in a toaster or toaster oven.

**Per serving:** 292 calories, 8 g protein, 60 g carbohydrates, 3 g fiber, 3 g total fat, 1 g saturated fat, 56 mg cholesterol, 331 mg sodium

# BERRY-FLAXSEED SMOOTHIE

Serves 2
**Prep Time:** 5 minutes
**Healing Foods:** flax, yogurt, berries, bananas
**Ailments It Heals:** cardiovascular disease, hay fever, irritable bowel syndrome, lupus, multiple sclerosis, osteoporosis

2 Tbsp whole flaxseeds
½ cup orange juice
½ cup nonfat vanilla yogurt
1 cup unsweetened frozen mixed berries or blueberries
1 small banana, sliced

In dry blender, place flaxseeds, cover, and blend until ground into fine powder. Add orange juice, yogurt, mixed berries (or blueberries), and banana. Cover and blend until smooth and creamy.

**Per serving:** 200 calories, 5 g protein, 36 g carbohydrates, 7 g fiber, 5 g total fat, 0 g saturated fat, 1 mg cholesterol, 33 mg sodium.

# RASPBERRY-BEET SMOOTHIE

Serves 4
**Prep Time:** 10 minutes
**Healing Foods:** beets, raspberries, yogurt
**Ailments It Heals:** asthma, menstrual problems, PCOS, urinary tract infections

2 cooked beets, cooled and coarsely chopped
2 oz (60 g) fresh or frozen raspberries
1 cup cranberry juice, chilled
1 cup low-fat plain yogurt
Chilled raspberries for garnish (optional)

**1.** In food processor or blender, puree beets, raspberries, and cranberry juice until smooth.

**2.** Pour through strainer into large pitcher. Whisk in most of the yogurt.

**3.** Pour into 4 glasses and top with remaining yogurt. Garnish with extra raspberries, if using. Serve immediately.

**Per serving:** 90 calories, 4 g protein, 18 g carbohydrates, 2 g fiber, 1 g total fat, 1 g saturated fat, 5 mg cholesterol, 75 mg sodium

# STRAWBERRY-YOGURT SMOOTHIE

Serves 4
**Prep Time:** 10 minutes
**Healing Foods:** strawberries, yogurt, oranges
**Ailments It Heals:** blood pressure, flatulence, infertility, sore throat, urinary tract infections, yeast infections

4 cups ripe strawberries
1 cup plain low-fat yogurt
½ cup fresh orange juice
1 Tbsp sugar, or to taste
4 small strawberries with leaves, optional
4 thin round slices unpeeled orange, optional

**1.** Rinse and drain strawberries and place in food processor or blender. Add yogurt, orange juice, and sugar. Process on highest speed until well-blended puree forms, about 15 seconds, stopping to scrape down sides of container once or twice. Taste and sweeten with more sugar, if you wish.

**2.** For a very smooth beverage, strain mixture, using wooden spoon to push the drink through a sieve. Discard strawberry seeds.

3. Pour into 4 tall glasses and serve immediately. If you wish to decorate the drinks, slit strawberries and orange slices halfway through centers. Attach one berry and one orange slice to rim of each glass.

**Per serving:** 108 calories, 4 g protein, 21 g carbohydrates, 4 g fiber, 2 g total fat, 1 g saturated fat, 5 mg cholesterol, 45 mg sodium

# WHEAT GERM SMOOTHIE

Serves 2
**Prep Time:** 5 minutes
**Healing Foods:** bananas, yogurt, peaches, wheat germ
**Ailments It Heals:** colds and flu, lupus, neuralgia, prostate problems, sex drive (diminished)

1 ripe medium banana, frozen and cut into chunks
1 cup low-fat or nonfat vanilla yogurt
1 cup fresh or frozen peaches
¼ cup fresh orange juice
¼ cup wheat germ
Skim milk
Peach or banana slices and wheat germ, for garnish

In blender, combine banana, yogurt, peaches, orange juice, and wheat germ. Blend until smooth, adding skim milk for desired consistency. Serve in 2 tall glasses. Garnish with sprinkle of wheat germ and a peach or banana slice.

**Per serving:** 220 calories, 10 g protein, 38 g carbohydrates, 7 g fiber, 3 g total fat, 1 g saturated fat, 8 mg cholesterol, 83 mg sodium

# SAVORY LAMB STEW WITH SWEET POTATOES

Serves 4
**Prep Time:** 15 minutes
**Cook Time:** 55 minutes
**Healing Foods:** lamb, sweet potatoes, peanut butter, okra
**Ailments It Heals:** ADHD, cystic fibrosis, dental problems, neuralgia

3 tsp olive oil
1 lb (500 g) well-trimmed lean leg of lamb, cut into 1-in (2.5 cm) chunks
1 medium onion, finely chopped
4 cloves garlic, minced
⅓ cup plus 1½ cups water
1 cup canned crushed tomatoes
1 lb (500 g) sweet potatoes, peeled and cut into ½-in (1 cm) chunks
2 Tbsp creamy peanut butter
½ tsp salt
½ tsp cayenne pepper
10 oz (300 g) frozen cut or whole okra, thawed

1. Preheat oven to 350°F (180°C). In large nonstick Dutch oven or flameproof casserole, heat 2 tsp oil over medium-high heat. Add lamb and sauté for 5 minutes, or until browned. With slotted spoon, transfer lamb to plate.

2. Reduce heat to medium and add remaining 1 tsp oil, onion, and garlic. Cook for 2 minutes. Stir in ⅓ cup water and cook until onion is golden brown and tender, about 5 to 8 minutes.

3. Stir in tomatoes, sweet potatoes, peanut butter, salt, cayenne, and 1½ cups water. Bring to a boil.

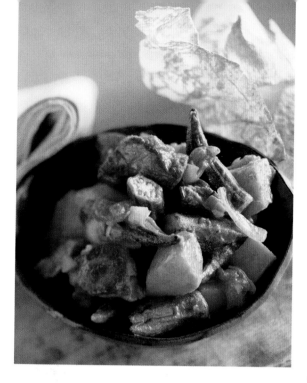

2 Tbsp olive oil

1 lb (500 g) pork tenderloin, cut into 1-in (2.5 cm) chunks

2 Tbsp flour

6 scallions, thinly sliced

3 cloves garlic, minced

1 large green bell pepper, cut into ½-in (1 cm) chunks

1 pickled jalapeño chile pepper, finely chopped

4.5 oz (140 g) chopped mild green chiles

¼ tsp salt

½ tsp ground coriander

1¼ cups water

1½ cups packed cilantro sprigs, chopped

1½ cups frozen peas, thawed

2 Tbsp fresh lime juice

1 red bell pepper, slivered

Return lamb to pan. Cover, transfer to oven, and bake for 25 minutes.

**4.** Stir in okra, return pan to oven, and bake for 15 minutes, or until lamb and okra are tender.

**Per serving:** 364 calories, 29 g protein, 32 g carbohydrate, 7 g fiber, 14 g total fat, 3 g saturated fat, 74 mg cholesterol, 618 mg sodium

# GREEN PORK CHILI

Serves 4

**Prep Time:** 15 minutes

**Cook Time:** 35 minutes plus stand time

**Healing Foods:** pork, peppers, chiles, cilantro, peas

**Ailments It Heals:** bleeding problems, depression, menstrual problems, shingles

**1.** Preheat oven to 350°F (180°C). In nonstick Dutch oven or flameproof casserole, heat oil over medium heat. Dredge pork in flour, shaking off excess. Sauté pork for 4 minutes, or until golden brown. With slotted spoon, transfer pork to plate.

**2.** Add scallions and garlic to pan and cook for 1 minute, or until scallions are tender. Add green bell pepper and jalapeño and cook for 4 minutes, or until bell pepper is crisp-tender. Stir in green chiles, salt, coriander, water, and half the cilantro. Bring to a boil.

**3.** Return pork to pan. Cover, place in oven, and bake for 25 minutes, or until pork is tender.

**4.** Stir in peas, lime juice, and remaining cilantro. Cover and let stand for 3 minutes. Serve topped with red bell pepper.

**Per serving:** 287 calories, 28 g protein, 20 g carbohydrate, 5 g fiber, 10 g total fat, 2 g saturated fat, 74 mg cholesterol, 338 mg sodium

# LENTIL SOUP WITH CANADIAN BACON

**Serves 8**
**Prep Time:** 10 minutes
**Cook Time:** 50 minutes
**Healing Foods:** olive oil, carrots, celery, tomatoes, lentils, yogurt
**Ailments It Heals:** atherosclerosis, constipation, irritable bowel syndrome, jaundice, memory loss

| | |
|---|---|
| 6 | tsp olive oil |
| 3 | oz (90 g) sliced Canadian bacon, cut into matchsticks |
| 3 | carrots, sliced |
| 2 | celery stalks, sliced |
| 1 | onion, chopped |
| 2 | cloves garlic, minced |
| 1 | tsp chili powder |
| ½ | tsp dried oregano |
| ½ | tsp ground cumin |
| ½ | tsp salt |
| 28 | oz (796 mL) crushed tomatoes, with juice |
| 1½ | cups lentils, sorted and rinsed |
| 6 | cups water |
| 2 | cups low-fat plain yogurt |

**1.** In stockpot, heat 1 tsp oil over medium heat. Add bacon and cook, stirring constantly, for 3 minutes, or until well browned. Transfer to a plate.

**2.** Add remaining 5 tsp oil to stockpot and heat. Add carrots, celery, and onion and cook, stirring, for 5 minutes, or until well browned. Add garlic, chili powder, oregano, cumin, and salt. Cook for 2 minutes, stirring constantly.

**3.** Add tomatoes with juice, lentils, and water and bring to a boil. Reduce heat to medium-low, partially cover, and simmer for 30 to 40 minutes, or until the lentils are tender.

**4.** To serve, ladle soup into 8 bowls and top each with ¼ cup yogurt and a few strips of bacon.

**Per serving:** 256 calories, 15 g protein, 38 g carbohydrates, 9 g fiber, 6 g total fat, 1 g saturated fat, 9 mg cholesterol, 506 mg sodium

# BASIC CHICKEN STOCK

**Makes 5 cups**
**Prep Time:** 10 minutes
**Cook Time:** 2 hours 10 minutes plus cooling
**Healing Foods:** chicken, onions, carrots, celery
**Ailments It Heals:** burns, diarrhea, fever, respiratory disorders

| | |
|---|---|
| 1 | chicken carcass, bones from 4 chicken pieces, or 1 leg with thigh |
| 1 | onion, quartered |
| 1 | large carrot, coarsely chopped |
| 1 | celery stalk, cut into chunks |
| 7 | cups water |
| 1 | bay leaf |
| 1 | parsley sprig |
| 1 | thyme sprig |
| 8 | whole black peppercorns |
| ½ | tsp salt |

**1.** Break up whole chicken bones; leave leg whole. In large saucepan over medium-high heat, combine bones or chicken, onion, carrot, and celery. Add water and bring to boil, skimming off foam.

**2.** Add bay leaf, parsley, thyme, peppercorns, and salt. Reduce heat, cover, and simmer for 2 hours.

**3.** Strain stock through sieve into heatproof bowl, discarding solids. Let cool, then refrigerate until cold and remove fat with spoon. Use refrigerated stock within 3 days or frozen stock within 3 months.

**Per serving:** 20 calories, 2 g protein, 1 g carbohydrate, 0 g fiber, .5 g total fat, 0 g saturated fat, 6 mg cholesterol, 247 mg sodium

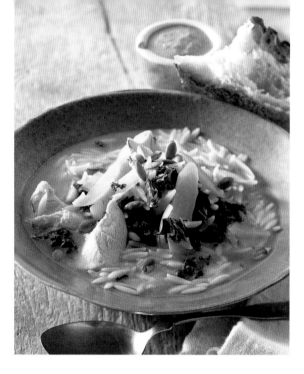

# CHICKEN-KALE SOUP WITH ROASTED PEPPER PUREE

**Serves 4**
**Prep Time:** 10 minutes
**Cook Time:** 20 minutes
**Healing Foods:** chicken, peppers, flax, kale
**Ailments It Heals:** colds and flu, eye problems, mood disorders, nail problems

- 4 cups water
- 1¼ lb (625 g) boneless skinless chicken thighs, cut into 1-in (2.5 cm) chunks
- 4 carrots, thinly sliced
- 3 large red onions, cut into ½-in (1 cm) chunks
- 5 cloves garlic, minced, plus 1 whole clove garlic
- 2 Tbsp finely chopped fresh ginger
- 1 tsp cayenne pepper
- ¾ tsp salt
- 2 red bell peppers, cut lengthwise into flat panels
- 1 Tbsp hulled roasted pumpkin seeds
- 1 Tbsp flaxseed oil
- ¾ cup orzo
- 8 cups shredded kale

**1.** In large saucepan or stockpot, combine water, chicken, carrots, onions, minced garlic, ginger, cayenne, and salt. Bring to a boil over high heat. Reduce to a simmer, partially cover, and cook for 25 minutes.

**2.** Meanwhile, preheat broiler. Place bell pepper pieces, skin side up, on broiler pan and broil 6 in (15 cm) from heat for 10 minutes, or until skin is well charred. When cool enough to handle, peel peppers and transfer them to food processor along with pumpkin seeds, flaxseed oil, and whole garlic clove. Process until pureed.

**3.** Add orzo to soup, and cook, uncovered, for 5 minutes. Stir in kale and cook for 5 minutes, or until kale and orzo are tender.

**4.** Serve soup with a dollop of roasted pepper puree on top.

**Per serving:** 439 calories, 35 g protein, 43 g carbohydrate, 8 g fiber, 15 g total fat, 3 g saturated fat, 94 mg cholesterol, 641 mg sodium

# QUICK CHICKEN NOODLE SOUP

**Serves 6**
**Prep Time:** 10 minutes
**Cook Time:** 25 minutes
**Healing Foods:** chicken, garlic, carrots, peppers, pasta
**Ailments It Heals:** colds and flu, inflammatory bowel disease, jaundice, Parkinson's disease, sore throat

2 Tbsp olive oil
¾ lb (375 g) boneless skinless chicken breasts, cut into 1-in (2.5 cm) pieces
1 large onion, chopped
2 cloves garlic, chopped
2 carrots, chopped
1 red bell pepper, chopped
1 tsp dried thyme
32 oz (1 L) chicken broth
1 cup water
8 oz (250 g) whole grain spaghetti, broken into 2-in (5 cm) pieces

1. In large saucepan, heat oil over high heat. Add chicken and cook, stirring, for 5 minutes, or until browned. With slotted spoon, transfer to bowl.

2. Add onion to saucepan and cook for 5 minutes, or until lightly browned. Add garlic, carrots, bell pepper, and thyme. Cook, stirring, for 3 minutes, or until lightly browned. Add broth, water, chicken, and any drippings in the bowl and bring to a boil. Add spaghetti and cook for 8 minutes, or until tender.

**Per serving:** 275 calories, 20 g protein, 37 g carbohydrates, 4 g fiber, 6 g total fat, 1 g saturated fat, 33 mg cholesterol, 345 mg sodium

# TURKEY, SPINACH, AND RICE IN ROASTED GARLIC BROTH

**Serves 4**
**Prep Time:** 15 minutes
**Cook Time:** 1 hour
**Healing Foods:** garlic, turkey, spinach
**Ailments It Heals:** arthritis, circulatory disorders, stroke

2 medium whole heads garlic, unpeeled
2 Tbsp tomato paste
29 oz (825 mL) reduced-sodium, fat-free chicken or turkey broth
1 cup cooked turkey cubes
1 cup cooked long-grain white rice
¾ lb (375 g) spinach, stemmed and coarsely chopped
¼ tsp ground black pepper
¼ tsp hot-pepper flakes, or to taste
1 Tbsp fresh-squeezed lemon juice

1. Preheat oven to 400°F (200°C).

2. Cut top third off garlic heads. Wrap each head in foil. Bake for 50 minutes, or until very soft. Let cool. Remove foil. Squeeze out pulp into small bowl.

3. In large saucepan, stir together garlic pulp and tomato paste. Stir in broth. Bring to a boil. Add turkey, rice, spinach, black pepper, and pepper flakes. Simmer, uncovered, for 8 minutes. Just before serving, stir in lemon juice.

**Per serving:** 197 calories, 19 g protein, 24 g carbohydrates, 3 g fiber, 4 g total fat, 1 g saturated fat, 30 mg cholesterol, 208 mg sodium

# COD AND VEGETABLE STEW

**Serves 4**
**Prep Time:** 15 minutes
**Cook Time:** 25 minutes
**Healing Foods:** onions, garlic, peppers, sweet potatoes, peas, fish
**Ailments It Heals:** AIDS and HIV infection, burns, cholesterol (high), obesity

2   Tbsp olive oil
2   medium onions, finely chopped
3   cloves garlic, thinly sliced
1   large red bell pepper, cut into matchsticks
1   lb (500 g) sweet potatoes, peeled and cut into ½-in (1 cm) chunks
1⅓  cups water
¾   tsp salt
½   tsp dried thyme
1½  cups frozen peas
1   cup frozen corn kernels
1½  lb (750 g) boneless skinless cod fillet, cut into bite-size pieces

**1.** In large skillet or Dutch oven, heat oil over medium heat. Add onions and garlic and cook, stirring frequently, for 5 minutes, or until onion is light golden.

**2.** Add bell pepper and sweet potatoes. Cover and cook for 5 minutes, or until sweet potatoes begin to soften. Stir in water, salt, and thyme and bring to a boil. Reduce to a simmer, cover, and cook for 5 minutes, or until sweet potatoes are tender. Stir in peas and corn.

**3.** Place cod on top of vegetables. Cover and cook for 7 minutes, or until fish is cooked through but still tender.

**Per serving:** 396 calories, 36 g protein, 42 g carbohydrate, 8 g fiber, 9 g total fat, 1 g saturated fat, 73 mg cholesterol, 584 mg sodium

# VEGETABLE STOCK

**Makes 12 cups**
**Prep Time:** 20 minutes
**Cook Time:** 1 hour 10 minutes plus cooling
**Healing Foods:** leeks, mushrooms, celeriac, parsnips, ginger
**Ailments It Heals:** diabetes, fever, gout, sore throat

2   Tbsp vegetable oil
3   large leeks with tops, rinsed and sliced
2   large carrots, scrubbed and coarsely chopped
1   medium onion, coarsely chopped
4   cloves garlic, crushed with the flat of a knife
14  cups water
8   oz (250 g) fresh mushrooms, halved
1   small celeriac, peeled and sliced
3   celery stalks with leaves, coarsely chopped
2   medium parsnips, peeled and thickly sliced
10  parsley sprigs
1½  Tbsp minced fresh ginger
2   bay leaves
¾   tsp dried marjoram
3   Tbsp tomato paste
½   tsp salt

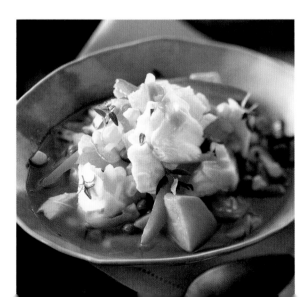

1. In 6-quart (6-L) stockpot, heat oil over medium-high heat. Add leeks, carrots, onion, and garlic and sauté, stirring occasionally, for 10 minutes, or just until tender.

2. Add water, mushrooms, celeriac, celery, parsnips, parsley, ginger, bay leaves, marjoram, tomato paste, and salt. Increase heat to high and bring to boil, then reduce heat and simmer, uncovered, for 1 hour.

3. Strain stock through a large sieve into heatproof bowl, discarding solids. When cool, cover and refrigerate up to 3 days or freeze up to 3 months.

**Per serving:** 5 calories, 0 g protein, 1 g carbohydrates, 0 g fiber, 0 g total fat, 0 g saturated fat, 0 mg cholesterol, 110 mg sodium

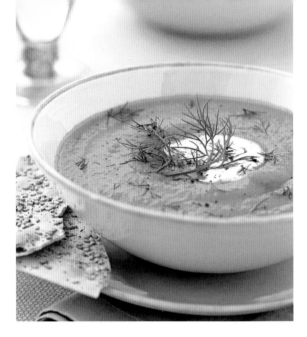

1. In medium saucepan, heat oil over medium heat. Add onion and garlic. Sauté for 5 minutes, or until softened. Add broth, carrots, and thyme. Simmer, uncovered, for 40 minutes, or until vegetables are very tender.

2. In batches, puree soup in blender. Add salt and pepper. To serve hot, ladle into 4 bowls and garnish each bowl with yogurt and dill. To serve cold, remove from heat and let cool to room temperature. Cover and refrigerate until cold. Garnish just before serving.

**Per serving:** 135 calories, 6 g protein, 20 g carbohydrates, 5 g fiber, 4 g total fat, 0 g saturated fat, 1 mg cholesterol, 628 mg sodium

# CARROT SOUP WITH DILL

Serves 4
**Prep Time:** 10 minutes
**Cook Time:** 45 minutes
**Healing Foods: carrots, yogurt, dill**
**Ailments It Heals: dental problems, hypothyroidism, interstitial cystitis, obesity**

1   Tbsp vegetable oil
1   onion, coarsely chopped
1   clove garlic, minced
29  oz (825 mL) reduced-sodium, fat-free chicken broth
4   cups carrots (about 1¼ lb or 625 g), peeled and coarsely chopped
½   tsp dried thyme, crumbled
Salt to taste
White pepper to taste
¼   cup low-fat plain yogurt
1   Tbsp finely chopped dill

# CELERIAC AND SPINACH SOUP

Serves 4
**Prep Time:** 15 minutes
**Cook Time:** 20 minutes
**Healing Foods: onions, garlic, celeriac, spinach**
**Ailments It Heals: fibroids, lactose intolerance, psoriasis**

1 large onion, thinly sliced

1 clove garlic, crushed

1 celeriac (about 1¼ lb or 625 g), peeled and grated

4 cups boiling water

1 reduced-sodium vegetable bouillon cube, crumbled, or 2 tsp vegetable bouillon powder

1 lb (500 g) fresh spinach, washed and trimmed

Pinch of nutmeg

Salt and ground black pepper

2 Tbsp fat-free half-and-half

Fresh chives

**1.** Coat large saucepan with cooking spray and heat over medium-high heat. Add onion and garlic, and cook until onion is softened but not browned, about 5 minutes. Add celeriac. Pour in water and add bouillon cube or powder. Bring to a boil, then reduce heat to low and cover pan. Cook until celeriac is tender, about 10 minutes.

**2.** Add spinach and stir well. Increase heat and bring soup to a boil, then remove pan from heat. Cool slightly, then puree it, in batches, in blender or food processor until smooth. (Alternatively, puree soup in pan using handheld blender.) Soup will be fairly thick.

**3.** Reheat soup, if necessary, then stir in nutmeg, salt, and pepper. Ladle into 4 bowls. Swirl a spoonful of half-and-half into each portion and garnish with fresh chives. Serve immediately.

**Per serving:** 95 calories, 5 g protein, 20 g carbohydrates, 5 g fiber, 1 g total fat, saturated fat, 0 mg cholesterol, 232 mg sodium

# GINGER BUTTERNUT SQUASH SOUP

Serves 4

**Prep Time:** 20 minutes

**Cook Time:** 45 minutes plus cooling

**Healing Foods:** turmeric, butternut squash, apples, ginger

**Ailments It Heals:** atherosclerosis, eczema, memory loss, motion sickness

2 Tbsp olive oil

1 large onion, chopped

2 cloves garlic, minced

1 tsp turmeric

1 butternut squash (about 2 lb or 1 kg), peeled, seeded, and cubed

4 cups vegetable or chicken broth

2 large apples, peeled, cored, and chopped

1 Tbsp grated fresh ginger or 1 tsp ground ginger

¼ tsp salt

**1.** In large saucepan, heat oil over medium heat. Add onion and cook, stirring, for 4 minutes, or until lightly browned. Stir in garlic and turmeric and cook for 1 minute. Add squash and broth and bring to a boil.

**2.** Reduce heat to low, cover, and simmer for 20 minutes, or until squash is just tender. Add apples, ginger, and salt and cook for 10 to 20 minutes, or until squash and apples are very tender. Remove from heat and let cool for about 10 minutes.

**3.** Working in batches, place the mixture in a food processor or blender and process until smooth.

**Per serving:** 267 calories, 4 g protein, 51 g carbohydrates, 6 g fiber, 8 g total fat, 1 g saturated fat, 0 mg cholesterol, 617 mg sodium

# BROCCOLI POTATO SOUP

Serves 4
**Prep Time:** 20 minutes
**Cook Time:** 1 hour 40 minutes
**Healing Foods:** broccoli, potatoes, yogurt
**Ailments It Heals:** hyperthyroidism, infertility, Parkinson's disease, urinary tract infections

  1   bulb garlic
  1   bunch broccoli
  2   Tbsp olive oil
  1   large onion, chopped
 32   oz (1L) vegetable or chicken broth
  1   russet potato, peeled and chopped
  1   cup water
  ½   cup low-fat plain yogurt

**1.** Preheat oven to 400°F (200°F). Cut top ¼ in (0.5 cm) off garlic to expose cloves. Wrap in a double thickness of foil and bake for 1 hour, or until very tender and browned.

**2.** Meanwhile, remove florets from broccoli and chop coarsely. Peel and chop stalks.

**3.** In large saucepan, heat oil over medium heat. Add onion and cook for 5 minutes, or until lightly browned. Add 3 cups broth, potato, and broccoli. Bring to a boil, then reduce heat to low, cover, and simmer for 30 minutes, or until broccoli stalks and potato are very tender.

**4.** Squeeze garlic into food processor. Add hot broccoli mixture and puree until smooth. Return to saucepan and add water and remaining broth. Simmer for 10 minutes, to blend flavors. Top each serving with a dollop of yogurt.

**Per serving:** 247 calories, 9 g protein, 37 g carbohydrates, 7 g fiber, 8 total fat, 1 g saturated fat, 2 mg cholesterol, 512 mg sodium

# MISO SOUP WITH TOFU

Serves 4
**Prep Time:** 5 minutes plus standing
**Cook Time:** 10 minutes
**Healing Foods:** seaweed, mushrooms, tofu
**Ailments It Heals:** fever, menopause, sore throat, yeast infections

  4   cups water
  1   piece (about 3½ in or 8.5 cm) kombu or kelp
  ¼   cup dried bonito flakes
  3   Tbsp light or dark miso
  6   shiitake mushrooms, stems removed, thinly sliced
  8   oz (250 g) soft tofu, cut into ½-in (1 cm) cubes
  1   scallion, trimmed and finely chopped

**1.** In medium soup pot, add water and kombu and bring almost to a boil.

**2.** Meanwhile, wrap bonito flakes in a clean coffee filter or tea ball. When water is just under a boil, remove pot from heat and add wrapped bonito flakes. Let stand for 5 minutes. Remove and discard kombu and bonito.

**3.** In small bowl, whisk together miso and a few Tbsp of soup broth until miso dissolves. Stir back into soup pot along with mushrooms, tofu, and scallion. Heat over low heat for 2 minutes. Let stand for 2 minutes before serving.

**Per serving:** 82 calories, 8 g protein, 4 g carbohydrates, 1 g fiber, 4 g total fat, 1 g saturated fat, 0 mg cholesterol, 563 mg sodium

# THREE-BEAN CHILI

Serves 8

**Prep Time:** 10 minutes

**Cook Time:** 7 hours 15 minutes

**Healing Foods:** carrots, celery, tomatoes, chiles, beans, peppers

**Ailments It Heals:** AIDS and HIV infections, burns, cancer, cardiovascular disease, constipation, diverticulitis

- 3 carrots, sliced
- 3 celery stalks, sliced
- 2 cloves garlic, minced
- 1 large onion, chopped
- 28 oz (796 mL), crushed tomatoes
- 16 oz (455 mL) salsa
- 2 tsp chili powder
- 1 tsp ground cumin
- 15.5 oz (440 mL) kidney beans, drained and rinsed
- 15 oz (425 mL) black beans, drained and rinsed
- 15 oz (425 mL) white beans, drained and rinsed
- 1 green bell pepper, chopped
- 1 red bell pepper, chopped

**1.** In a 3½- to 4-quart (3½- to 4-L) slow cooker, place carrots, celery, garlic, onion, tomatoes, salsa, chili powder, and cumin. Cover and cook on high for 5 to 7 hours, or until vegetables are tender.

**2.** Stir in beans and bell peppers and cook, uncovered, on high for 15 minutes, or until chili thickens slightly and peppers are tender.

**Per serving:** 299 calories, 19 g protein, 58 g carbohydrates, 16 g fiber, 2 g total fat, 0 g saturated fat, 0 mg cholesterol, 712 mg sodium

# TUSCAN BEAN SOUP

Serves 6

**Prep Time:** 15 minutes

**Cook Time:** 30 minutes

**Healing Foods:** onions, carrots, celery, tomatoes, beans

**Ailments It Heals:** atherosclerosis, celiac disease, colds and flu, hemorrhoids, obesity, PCOS

- 1 Tbsp olive oil
- 2 medium onions, coarsely chopped
- 2 medium carrots, coarsely chopped
- 2 celery ribs, chopped
- 29 oz (825 mL) reduced-sodium chicken broth
- 28 oz (796 mL), crushed tomatoes in puree
- ½ cup chopped fresh basil
- 2 Tbsp chopped fresh oregano, or 1 tsp dried
- 15.5 oz (440 mL) red kidney beans
- 15.5 oz (440 mL) cannellini beans
- 15.5 oz (440 mL) chickpeas
- 6 Tbsp freshly grated parmesan cheese

**1.** In large nonstick Dutch oven, heat oil over medium-high heat. Add onions, carrots, and celery and sauté for 5 minutes, or until soft. Add broth,

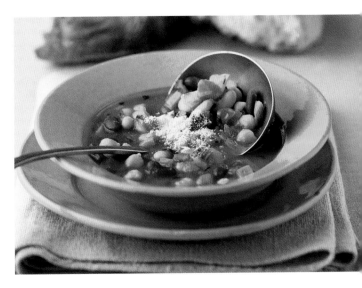

tomatoes in puree, basil, and oregano. Bring to a boil. Reduce heat to medium-low, partially cover, and cook for 10 minutes.

**2.** Put kidney and cannellini beans and chickpeas in colander. Rinse and drain. Stir into soup. Cook for 10 minutes, or until flavors develop. Remove from heat.

**3.** Very coarsely puree about one-fourth of soup using immersion blender. Or transfer about 2 cups soup to food processor, very coarsely puree, and return to pot. Serve 2 cups soup per person topped with 1 Tbsp parmesan.

**Per serving:** 290 calories, 15 g protein, 45 g carbohydrates, 10 g fiber, 6 g total fat, 1 g saturated fat, 4 mg cholesterol, 605 mg sodium

# CHUNKY GAZPACHO WITH GARLICKY CROUTONS

**Serves 4**
**Prep Time:** 20 minutes plus chilling
**Cook Time:** 15 minutes
**Healing Foods:** garlic, tomatoes, cucumbers, peppers
**Ailments It Heals:** chronic fatigue syndrome, respiratory disorders, rosacea

- 2  cloves garlic, peeled
- 4  slices French bread (1 in or 2.5 cm thick)
- 1  tsp ground black pepper
- ½  tsp salt
- ½  cup coarsely chopped red onion
- 28  oz (796 mL) no-salt-added diced tomatoes
- ¼  cup seasoned dry bread crumbs
- ¼  cup chopped parsley

- 3  Tbsp red wine vinegar
- 1  Tbsp olive oil
- 2  medium cucumbers, peeled and chopped
- 2  medium green bell peppers, chopped
- 2  medium red bell peppers, chopped

**1.** Preheat oven to 350°F (180°C). Cut 1 garlic clove in half and rub cut sides on inside of large bowl and on both sides of bread slices. Tear bread into 1-in (2.5 cm) pieces. Put in large bowl and lightly coat with cooking spray. Sprinkle with ½ tsp black pepper and ¼ tsp salt. Toss to coat and transfer to baking sheet. Bake for 15 minutes, or until golden. Cool croutons completely.

**2.** Pulse onion and remaining garlic clove in food processor or blender until finely chopped. Add half of tomatoes and all their juice. Puree. Add bread crumbs, parsley, vinegar, oil, and remaining ½ tsp black pepper and ¼ tsp salt. Process just until blended and pour into large nonreactive bowl.

**3.** Stir remaining tomatoes into tomato mixture with half of cucumbers and half of green and red peppers. Refrigerate for 1 hour, until chilled. Ladle into bowls and top with remaining cucumber, green and red peppers, and croutons.

**Per serving:** 250 calories, 8 g protein, 46 g carbohydrates, 6 g fiber, 5 g total fat, 1 g saturated fat, 0 mg cholesterol, 730 mg sodium

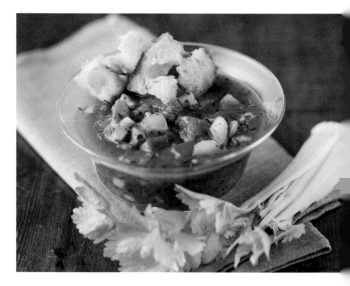

# CANTALOUPE AND ORANGE SOUP

**Serves 6**
**Prep Time:** 20 minutes plus chilling time
**Healing Foods:** oranges, cantaloupe, honey, yogurt, raspberries
**Ailments It Heals:** blood pressure, colds and flu, gout, memory loss, muscle cramps, osteoporosis

- 3 large orange
- 1 large cantaloupe, halved and seeded
- 2 cups orange juice
- Juice of 1 lime
- 1 Tbsp honey
- 1 cup fat-free plain yogurt
- 1 cup fresh raspberries

**1.** Finely grate zest from 1 or 2 oranges, according to taste, and reserve. With a sharp knife, peel cantaloupe. Cut flesh into chunks and place in food processor or blender. Peel and section oranges, then cut sections into pieces and add to melon. Puree until smooth.

**2.** Strain puree through medium-gauge sieve into large bowl, pressing fruit through sieve with back of wooden spoon.

**3.** Stir in orange juice, lime juice, honey, and yogurt until blended. Cover bowl and refrigerate for at least 2 hours.

**4.** Serve soup garnished with orange zest and fresh raspberries.

**Per serving:** 161 calories, 5 g protein, 37 g carbohydrate, 4 g fiber, 1 g total fat, 0 g saturated fat, 1 mg cholesterol, 54 mg sodium

# BEEF IN LETTUCE WRAPS

**Serves 4**
**Prep Time:** 5 minutes
**Cook Time:** 11 minutes
**Healing Foods:** beef, carrots, lettuce
**Ailments It Heals:** anemia, eczema, herpes, osteoporosis

- 3 Tbsp hoisin sauce
- 2 Tbsp wine vinegar
- 1 Tbsp soy sauce
- 1 tsp toasted sesame oil
- ½ tsp ground ginger
- 1 lb (500 g) lean ground beef
- 4 scallions, chopped
- 2 carrots, shredded
- 1 clove garlic, minced
- 12 Bibb or Boston lettuce leaves

**1.** In small bowl, whisk together hoisin sauce, vinegar, soy sauce, oil, and ginger.

**2.** In nonstick skillet over medium heat, cook beef for 5 minutes, or until browned. Add scallions, carrots, and garlic and cook for 3 minutes, or until tender. Stir in the hoisin mixture and cook for 3 minutes, or until thickened and flavors are blended.

**3.** Place 3 lettuce leaves on each of 4 plates and fill with beef mixture.

**Per serving:** 201 calories, 24 g protein, 13 g carbohydrates, 3 g fiber, 6 g total fat, 2 g saturated fat, 61 mg cholesterol, 619 mg sodium

# BEEF, ONION, AND PEPPER FAJITAS

**Serves 8**

**Prep Time:** 15 minutes plus marinating

**Cook Time:** 13 minutes

**Healing Foods:** beef, onions, peppers, garlic, chiles

**Ailments It Heals:** hepatitis, memory loss, nail problems

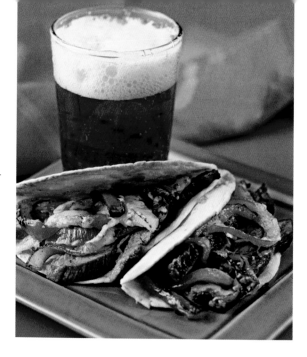

- 1 flank steak (about 1 lb or 500 g)
- 1 red onion, sliced
- 1 small red bell pepper, seeded and cut into thin strips
- 1 small green bell pepper, seeded and cut into thin strips
- 1 small yellow bell pepper, seeded and cut into thin strips
- 4 cloves garlic, minced
- ½ cup fresh lime juice
- 2 Tbsp olive oil
- 2 Tbsp balsamic vinegar
- 1 tsp ground cumin
- ½ tsp salt
- ¼ tsp ground black pepper
- 1 serrano or jalapeño chile pepper, seeded and finely chopped (wear gloves when handling; they burn)
- 8 flour tortillas (6 in or 15 cm), warmed following package directions
- ¼ lb (125 g) monterey jack cheese, shredded

**1.** In shallow baking dish, combine steak, onion, and bell peppers. In small bowl, whisk together garlic, lime juice, oil, vinegar, cumin, salt, black pepper, and chile pepper. Pour over steak mixture. Toss to coat. Refrigerate, covered, for 1 to 2 hours.

**2.** Preheat broiler.

**3.** Broil steak on broiler-pan rack 4 in (10 cm) from heat 2 minutes each side. Add onion and bell peppers to rack. Spoon remaining marinade over steak and vegetables. Broil, turning meat and vegetables occasionally, for 6 to 8 minutes, or until meat is cooked to desired doneness and vegetables are crisp-tender. Let meat stand for 5 minutes.

**4.** Cut meat diagonally across grain into thin slices. Place meat, onion, and peppers on warmed tortillas, dividing equally. Top with cheese. Place under broiler for 30 seconds, or just until cheese melts. Fold tortillas over filling and serve.

**Per serving:** 293 calories, 18 g protein, 24 g carbohydrates, 2 g fiber, 14 g total fat, 6 g saturated fat, 40 mg cholesterol, 411 mg sodium

# BEEF AND BLUE CHEESE BURGERS

**Serves 4**
**Prep Time:** 15 minutes plus soaking
**Cook Time:** 10 minutes
**Healing Foods:** beef, zucchini, cheese, spinach, wheat
**Ailments It Heals:** anemia, bleeding, burns, neuralgia

8 oz (250 g) 95% lean ground beef
1 large egg white, lightly beaten
1 cup shredded zucchini (½ small)
⅓ cup finely chopped onion (½ small)
⅔ cup whole wheat panko (Japanese-style bread crumbs) or fresh whole wheat bread crumbs
1 Tbsp Worcestershire sauce
2 tsp dijon mustard
¼ tsp salt
¼ tsp ground black pepper
¼ cup crumbled blue cheese
1 cup thinly sliced sweet onion or red onion
2 cups baby spinach or arugula, washed and dried
1 medium tomato, sliced
4 100% whole wheat English muffins, split

1. In large bowl, mix beef, egg white, zucchini, onion, panko, Worcestershire sauce, mustard, salt, and pepper. Form into 8 patties, ¼ in (0.5 cm) thick. Place about 1 Tbsp cheese on each of 4 patties and place a second patty on top to enclose cheese. Press to seal in cheese and form into ½-in-thick (1 cm) patties.

2. Place onion in medium bowl, cover with ice water, and soak for 10 to 20 minutes. Drain.

3. Preheat grill to medium-high. Lightly oil grill grate by rubbing it with a piece of oil-soaked paper towel (use tongs to hold paper towel when working over a hot grill). Grill patties for 5 minutes per side, or until browned and cooked through (an instant-read thermometer inserted in center should register 160°F or 71°C). About 1 minute before patties are done, place muffins, cut side down, on grill for 30 to 60 seconds, or until lightly toasted.

4. To assemble burgers, divide spinach and tomato slices among muffin bottoms. Add patties and top with onion slices. Replace muffin tops. One serving is 1 patty with 1 English muffin and garnishes.

**Per serving:** 322 calories, 23 g protein, 43 g carbohydrates, 7 g fiber, 7 g total fat, 3 g saturated fat, 41 mg cholesterol, 909 mg sodium

# SLOPPY JOES

**Serves 4**
**Prep Time:** 10 minutes
**Cook Time:** 15 minutes
**Healing Foods:** onions, beef, tomatoes, chiles, carrots, cabbage
**Ailments It Heals:** ADHD, jaundice, Parkinson's disease

1 Tbsp vegetable oil
1 medium onion, finely chopped
1 celery rib, finely chopped
1 small green bell pepper, finely chopped
1 lb (500 g) lean (95%) ground beef
4 sandwich buns, split
14.5 oz (410 mL) no-salt-added stewed tomatoes
½ cup chili sauce
2 tsp Worcestershire sauce
½ tsp ground black pepper
2 tsp cider vinegar
1 large carrot, cut into very thin matchsticks
¼ small head cabbage, slivered

1. Put rack in middle of oven and preheat to 350°F (180°C). In large nonstick skillet, heat oil over medium-high heat. Add onion, celery, and green pepper and sauté for 5 minutes, or until tender. Add ground beef and cook, breaking up meat with spoon, for 4 minutes, or until meat is no longer pink.

2. Meanwhile, put buns cut side up on baking sheet and heat in oven for 4 minutes, or until toasted.

3. Add tomatoes (with juice), chili sauce, Worcestershire, and black pepper to skillet. Cook, stirring often, for 4 minutes, or until flavors blend. Stir in vinegar.

4. Transfer buns to 4 plates. Spoon mixture on bottom of each bun. Top with several strips of carrot and cabbage. Cover with top of bun.

**Per serving:** 396 calories, 31 g protein, 42 g carbohydrates, 5 g fiber, 11 g total fat, 3 g saturated fat, 51 mg cholesterol, 767 mg sodium

# THAI-STYLE BEEF SANDWICH

Serves 4

**Prep Time:** 10 minutes plus marinating and standing
**Cook Time:** 8 minutes
**Healing Foods:** limes, beef, cabbage, carrots, herbs and spices
**Ailments It Heals:** acne, alcoholism, arthritis, hepatitis, prostate problems

- 2 Tbsp tomato paste
- ½ cup fresh lime juice (about 3 limes)
- 1½ tsp ground coriander
- 1 lb (500 g) well-trimmed flank steak
- 1 tsp sugar
- ½ tsp salt
- ¾ tsp red-pepper flakes
- 3 cups packed shredded green cabbage (about 12 oz or 375 g)
- 2 carrots, shredded
- 1 large red bell pepper, cut into matchsticks
- ¾ cup chopped cilantro
- ⅓ cup chopped fresh mint
- 4 whole grain rolls, halved crosswise

1. In shallow nonaluminum pan, stir together the tomato paste, ¼ cup lime juice, and coriander. Add flank steak, turning to coat. Refrigerate for 30 minutes.

2. In large bowl, whisk together sugar, salt, pepper flakes, and remaining ¼ cup lime juice. Add cabbage, carrots, bell pepper, cilantro, and mint and toss well to combine. Refrigerate until serving time.

3. Preheat broiler. Remove steak from marinade. Broil 6 in (15 cm) from heat for 4 minutes per side for medium-rare, brushing any remaining marinade over steak. Let stand for 10 minutes before thinly slicing across the grain on the diagonal.

4. To serve, place cabbage slaw on bottom half of each cut roll. Top with ribbons of sliced steak.

**Per serving:** 396 calories, 32 g protein, 48 g carbohydrates, 9 g fiber, 10 g total fat, 3 g saturated fat, 70 mg cholesterol, 723 mg sodium

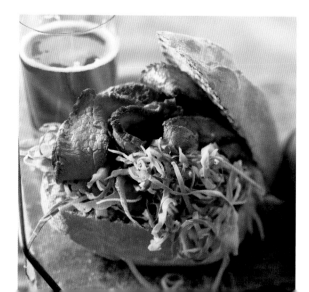

# LAMB BURGERS WITH FRUIT RELISH

Serves 4
**Prep Time:** 20 minutes
**Cook Time:** 10 minutes
**Healing Foods:** lamb, wheat, oranges
**Ailments It Heals:** anemia, multiple sclerosis, stress

1  lb (500 g) lean ground lamb
1  medium carrot, peeled and grated
1  small onion, finely chopped
½  cup fresh whole wheat bread crumbs
Pinch of freshly grated nutmeg
2  tsp fresh thyme leaves or 1 tsp dried
Salt and ground black pepper
1  large egg, beaten
2  tsp olive oil
1  orange
½  cup fresh or thawed frozen raspberries
2  tsp sugar
4  whole wheat English muffins
Shredded lettuce to garnish

1. Preheat grill or oven broiler. Put lamb into large bowl. Add carrot, onion, bread crumbs, nutmeg, and thyme. Season with salt and pepper to taste. Mix well. Add egg and use your hands to mix ingredients together thoroughly.

2. Divide mixture into 4 patties. Brush both sides of burgers with oil, then put in grill pan. Cook for 4 to 5 minutes on each side, depending on thickness.

3. Meanwhile, cut peel and pith from orange with sharp knife. Working over a bowl to catch juice, cut between membranes to release segments. Roughly chop segments and add to juice. Add raspberries and sugar, lightly crushing fruit with fork to mix relish together.

4. Split English muffins and toast lightly. Put a burger on each muffin and add some lettuce to garnish and a good spoonful of relish. Serve with remaining relish.

**Per serving:** 370 calories, 26 g protein, 40 g carbohydrates, 6 g fiber, 12 g total fat, 4 g saturated fat, 121 mg cholesterol, 328 mg sodium

# HAM AND CELERIAC PITAS

Serves 6
**Prep Time:** 15 minutes
**Cook Time:** 2 minutes
**Healing Foods:** celeriac, carrots, pork, onions, olives
**Ailments It Heals:** chronic fatigue syndrome, eye problems, hypothyroidism, memory loss, peptic ulcers

¼  cup Greek yogurt
½  tsp whole grain mustard
2  Tbsp mayonnaise
1  small celeriac
2  carrots
5  oz (150 g) thickly sliced lean low-sodium smoked ham, cut into ½-in (1 cm) pieces
1  small red onion, thinly sliced
8  pitted green olives, pimiento-stuffed if desired, halved
⅓  cup currants
2  Tbsp chopped fresh parsley
6  pita breads
1  Romaine lettuce heart, finely shredded
Fresh parsley sprigs to garnish

1. In medium-size bowl, mix together yogurt, mustard, and mayonnaise.

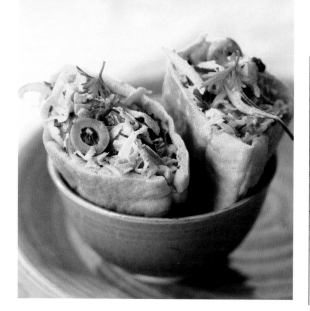

**2.** Preheat grill to high. Peel and coarsely grate the celeriac and carrots. Add to the bowl of dressing and mix well. Add the ham, onion, olives, currants, and chopped parsley and mix everything together.

**3.** Warm the pita breads on the grill for about 1 minute on each side. Cut each one across in half to make 2 pockets of bread. Divide the lettuce among the pita pockets, then add the ham and celeriac salad. Garnish with parsley sprigs and serve.

**Per serving:** 303 calories, 12 g protein, 46 g carbohydrates, 3 g fiber, 8 g total fat, 2 g saturated fat, 16 mg cholesterol, 797 mg sodium

# CURRIED CHICKEN SALAD SANDWICHES

**Serves 4**
**Prep Time:** 10 minutes
**Healing Foods:** yogurt, curry, chicken, apples, celery
**Ailments It Heals:** burns, colds and flu, jet lag

| | |
|---|---|
| ¼ | cup low-fat plain yogurt |
| 2 | Tbsp low-fat canola mayonnaise |
| 1½ | tsp curry powder |
| 1 | tsp honey |
| ¼ | tsp salt |
| 2 | cups chopped cooked chicken |
| 1 | apple, cored and chopped |
| 2 | celery stalks, chopped |
| 4 | lettuce leaves |
| 2 | whole grain pita breads (8 in or 20 cm), halved |

**1.** In large bowl, whisk together yogurt, mayonnaise, curry powder, honey, and salt. Add the chicken, apple, and celery.

**2.** Place a lettuce leaf in each pita half and fill with one-quarter of the chicken salad.

**Per serving:** 253 calories, 23 g protein, 27 g carbohydrates, 4 g fiber, 6 g total fat, 1 g saturated fat, 53 mg cholesterol, 440 mg sodium

# GRILLED CHICKEN SANDWICHES WITH BASIL MAYONNAISE

Serves 4

**Prep Time:** 10 minutes

**Cook Time:** 7 minutes

**Healing Foods:** lemons, basil, chicken, salad greens, tomatoes

**Ailments It Heals:** Alzheimer's disease, hyperthyroidism, obesity

1 large lemon
1/3 cup reduced-fat mayonnaise
2 Tbsp chopped fresh basil or 2 tsp dried
4 boneless, skinless chicken breast halves (4 oz or 125 g each)
1 Tbsp lemon-pepper seasoning
4 sandwich rolls (2 oz or 60 g each), split
1 small bunch watercress or arugula, trimmed
2 medium tomatoes, sliced

**1.** Grate zest from lemon into small bowl. Squeeze juice into measuring cup. Combine mayonnaise and basil with zest. Sprinkle chicken with lemon-pepper seasoning.

**2.** Generously coat nonstick ridged grill pan with cooking spray and set over medium-high heat until hot but not smoking. Cook chicken for 4 minutes, or until grill marks appear. Turn chicken and sprinkle with lemon juice. Cook for 3 minutes, or until juices run clear.

**3.** Cut chicken into thin slices. Spread rolls evenly with basil mayonnaise. Layer bottoms of rolls with half of watercress, all of tomato and chicken, then remaining watercress. Cover with tops of rolls.

**Per serving:** 378 calories, 33 g protein, 38 g carbohydrates, 4 g fiber, 11 g total fat, 2 g saturated fat, 66 mg cholesterol, 614 mg sodium

# HERBED CHICKEN AND APPLE BURGERS

Serves 4

**Prep Time:** 20 minutes plus chilling

**Cook Time:** 10 minutes

**Healing Foods:** chicken, apples, herbs, wheat, watercress

**Ailments It Heals:** diabetes, hypoglycemia, Parkinson's disease, PCOS

1 lb (500 g) ground chicken
1 large red onion, finely chopped
1/4 cup plain dry bread crumbs
2 large green apples, such as Granny Smith (for a tart taste) or Golden Delicious (for a sweet taste), peeled and coarsely grated
1 Tbsp chopped fresh sage leaves
1 Tbsp fresh thyme leaves
1/4 tsp salt
1/4 tsp ground black pepper
1/4 cup dijon mustard
1 Tbsp honey
4 whole wheat hamburger buns, split
3 oz (90 g) watercress sprigs, large stalks discarded

**1.** In large bowl, place chicken, onion, bread crumbs, apples, sage, thyme, salt, and pepper. Using your hands, mix ingredients together until evenly distributed. Wet your hands, then divide mixture into 4 equal portions and shape each into a burger about 4 in (10 cm) in diameter and 1½ in (4 cm) thick. Chill burgers for 1 hour to firm up meat and make it easier to hold together while it cooks.

**2.** Preheat grill or broiler to high. Place burgers on rack about 6 in (15 cm) from source of heat. Grill or broil about 5 minutes per side, turning once, until golden brown on both sides and still juicy but cooked through completely or until the burger reaches an internal temperature of 165°F or 74°C.

3. Meanwhile, mix mustard and honey in small cup. On flat surface, open 4 buns with soft cut sides up. Spread cut sides of tops and bottoms with honey mustard. Pile one-fourth of the watercress on bottom of each bun.

4. Place cooked burger on top of watercress. Cover with top of bun and serve immediately.

**Per serving:** 364 calories, 34 g protein, 49 g carbohydrates, 6 g fiber, 5 g total fat, 1 g saturated fat, 64 mg cholesterol, 872 mg sodium

# INDIAN-STYLE TURKEY BURGERS

Serves 4
**Prep Time:** 10 minutes
**Cook Time:** 18 minutes
**Healing Foods:** garlic, ginger, peppers, curry, mangoes, turkey, yogurt
**Ailments It Heals:** anemia, depression, mood disorders

| | |
|---|---|
| 1 | Tbsp olive oil |
| 1 | large red onion, finely chopped, |
| 3 | cloves garlic, minced |
| 2 | Tbsp minced fresh ginger |
| 1 | red bell pepper, diced |
| 1½ | tsp curry powder |
| ½ | cup tomato juice |
| 4 | Tbsp chopped mango chutney |
| 1 | lb (500 g) lean ground turkey breast |
| ⅓ | cup plain low-fat yogurt |
| ¼ | cup chopped cilantro |
| 1 | slice firm white sandwich bread, crumbled |
| ¼ | tsp salt |

1. In small skillet, heat oil over medium heat. Add onion, garlic, and ginger and cook, stirring frequently, for 5 minutes, or until onion is lightly browned. Measure out ½ cup onion-ginger mixture and transfer to large bowl.

2. To remaining mixture in skillet, add bell pepper and cook for 4 minutes, or until crisp-tender. Stir in 1 tsp curry powder and cook for 1 minute. Stir in tomato juice and 2 Tbsp chutney and bring to a boil. Boil for 1 minute.

3. To bowl with reserved onion-ginger mixture, add turkey, yogurt, cilantro, crumbled bread, salt, and remaining ½ tsp curry powder and 2 Tbsp chutney. Gently shape mixture into 4 patties.

4. Preheat broiler. Broil patties 6 in (15 cm) from heat for 3½ minutes per side, until cooked through or until the burger reaches an internal temperature of 165°F or 74°C. Serve burgers with the sautéed pepper mixture on top.

**Per serving:** 288 calories, 31 g protein, 28 g carbohydrates, 2 g fiber, 5 g total fat, 1 g saturated fat, 72 mg cholesterol, 540 mg sodium

# TURKEY COBB SALAD SANDWICHES

Serves 4
**Prep Time:** 15 minutes
**Cook Time:** 5 minutes
**Healing Foods:** chives, avocado, salad greens, turkey, tomatoes
**Ailments It Heals:** hives, insomnia, mood disorders

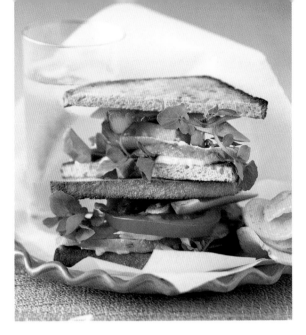

¼ cup nonfat mayonnaise
¼ cup blue cheese, crumbled
2 Tbsp snipped fresh chives
4 slices lean low-sodium bacon
8 slices whole wheat bread, toasted
4 oz (125 g) watercress, tough stems trimmed
12 oz (375 g) fresh-roasted turkey breast slices
2 medium tomatoes, sliced
4 scallions, thinly sliced
1 small avocado, peeled, pitted, and thinly
  sliced

**1.** In small bowl, combine mayonnaise, blue cheese, and chives.

**2.** In medium skillet over medium-high heat, cook bacon until crisp. Transfer to paper towels to drain, then tear into small pieces.

**3.** Spread blue cheese mixture evenly on bread. Layer 4 slices with watercress, turkey, tomatoes, scallions, avocado, and bacon. Top with remaining bread and cut sandwiches diagonally in half.

**Per serving:** 450 calories, 37 g protein, 39 g carbohydrates, 7 g fiber, 14 g total fat, 4 g saturated fat, 85 mg cholesterol, 660 mg sodium

# JAPANESE SUSHI ROLLS

Makes 32
**Prep Time:** 20 minutes plus cooling
**Cook Time:** 20 minutes
**Healing Foods:** rice, vinegar, cucumbers, fish, seaweed
**Ailments It Heals:** anorexia, jet lag, rosacea

10 oz (300 g) sushi rice
1 Tbsp fine granulated sugar
3 Tbsp rice wine vinegar
2 scallions, very finely chopped
1 cucumber, seeded and finely chopped
4 oz (125 g) smoked salmon
4 sheets sushi nori
2 tsp wasabi paste
Gari (pickled ginger)
Reduced-sodium soy sauce

**1.** In saucepan of boiling water, cook sushi rice according to packet instructions.

**2.** Meanwhile, place sugar and vinegar in small pan and heat gently until sugar dissolves. When rice is cooked, drizzle mixture over it, then add spring onions and cucumber and mix. Cover with tea towel and leave to cool.

**3.** Divide sushi rice into 4 equal portions. Cut salmon into strips about ½ in (1 cm) wide. Place a sheet of nori, shiny side down, on a bamboo mat or on a sheet of parchment paper on a board. Spread a portion of rice over nori, pressing it down evenly and leaving a ½ in (1 cm) space at top and bottom. Place one-quarter of salmon along middle of layer of rice, then spread salmon with ½ tsp wasabi paste.

**4.** Using the bamboo mat or the paper, roll up nori, rice, and salmon into a neat tube. Roll tightly to ensure rice sticks together and holds filling in place. Make 3 more rolls in the same way.

**5.** Using a wet knife, cut each roll across into 8 slices and stand them upright on a serving plate. Rinse knife between cuts. Garnish with pieces of gari and offer a small dish of soy sauce for dipping.

**Per serving:** 109 calories, 3 g protein, 23 g carbohydrates, 0 g fiber, 0 g total fat, 0 g saturated fat, 2 mg cholesterol, 187 mg sodium

# SALMON AND FENNEL LETTUCE WRAPS

Serves 4
**Prep Time:** 15 minutes
**Healing Foods:** lemons, fish, fennel, lettuce
**Ailments It Heals:** cardiovascular disease, hay fever, stroke

3   Tbsp reduced-fat mayonnaise
1   Tbsp reduced-fat sour cream
2   Tbsp fresh lemon juice
1   Tbsp chopped fresh dill
12  oz (375 g) canned Alaskan pink or sockeye salmon, drained
½   fennel bulb, trimmed and finely chopped
4   large Boston lettuce leaves

**1.** In medium bowl, whisk together mayonnaise, sour cream, lemon juice, and dill. Stir in salmon and fennel.

**2.** For each wrap, start about 1 in (2.5 cm) up from bottom of lettuce leaf and mound one-fourth of salmon mixture in horizontal row along bottom third of lettuce.

**3.** Fold bottom of lettuce over filling, then fold in about 1 in (2.5 cm) of sides. Roll firmly away from you.

**4.** Cut each wrap in half on a diagonal.

**Per serving:** 179 calories, 21 g protein, 5 g carbohydrates, 1 g fiber, 8 g total fat, 2 g saturated fat, 39 mg cholesterol, 422 mg sodium

# SALMON CAKE SANDWICHES

Serves 4
**Prep Time:** 15 minutes plus chilling
**Cook Time:** 6 minutes
**Healing Foods:** fish, wheat, lettuce, tomatoes
**Ailments It Heals:** cancer, lactose intolerance, menstrual problems, multiple sclerosis

¼   cup mild salsa
2   egg whites
¼   cup low-fat canola mayonnaise
½   tsp ground cumin
¼   to 1 tsp hot red-pepper sauce
2   pouches (7 oz or 200 g each) salmon, patted dry
1   cup fresh whole wheat bread crumbs
4   lettuce leaves
4   whole wheat sandwich rolls
1   large tomato, cut into 4 slices

**1.** Drain salsa by placing it in a sieve over a bowl for about 10 minutes. Shake sieve to release any remaining liquid.

**2.** Line baking sheet with parchment paper. In medium bowl, whisk egg whites. Stir in salsa, mayonnaise, cumin, and red-pepper sauce. Add salmon and bread crumbs and gently fold in just until combined. Shape mixture into 4 cakes, place on baking sheet, and refrigerate for at least 30 minutes.

**3.** Coat nonstick skillet with cooking spray. Add cakes and cook over medium heat, turning once, for 6 minutes, or until browned and crisp.

4. Place lettuce leaf on each roll. Top with salmon cake and tomato slice.

**Per serving:** 367 calories, 30 g protein, 39 g carbohydrates, 6 g fiber, 11 g total fat, 1 g saturated fat, 81 mg cholesterol, 779 mg sodium

# ASIAN GRILLED TUNA BURGERS

Serves 4
**Prep Time:** 25 minutes
**Cook Time:** 5 minutes
**Healing Foods:** fish, peppers, cucumbers, limes
**Ailments It Heals:** AIDS and HIV infections, cholesterol (high), halitosis, sex drive (diminished),

12  oz (375 g) water-packed albacore tuna, drained
 1  large egg
 4  scallions, thinly sliced
 ½  cup chopped cilantro
 3  Tbsp plain dried bread crumbs
 2  Tbsp low-fat mayonnaise
 1  Tbsp minced fresh ginger
 2  tsp dark sesame oil
 ¼  tsp salt
 1  red bell pepper, cut into matchsticks
 1  cucumber, peeled, halved lengthwise, seeded, and cut into matchsticks
 2  Tbsp reduced-sodium soy sauce
 2  Tbsp fresh lime juice
 2  tsp sugar

1. In large bowl, combine tuna, egg, scallions, cilantro, bread crumbs, mayonnaise, ginger, sesame oil, and salt. Stir until well combined.

2. Form mixture into four 4-in (10 cm) patties, a scant ½ in (1 cm) thick. (Patties can be made ahead and refrigerated for several hours.)

3. In medium bowl, combine bell pepper, cucumber, soy sauce, lime juice, and sugar.

4. Preheat broiler. Broil patties 4 in (10 cm) from heat, carefully turning once, for 2½ minutes per side, or until firm and lightly golden. Top the finished burgers with pepper-cucumber relish.

**Per serving:** 216 calories, 24 g protein, 13 g carbohydrates, 2 g fiber, 8 g total fat, 2 g saturated fat, 38 mg cholesterol, 862 mg sodium

# TUNA AND CARROT SANDWICH ON RYE

Serves 2
**Prep Time:** 15 minutes
**Healing Foods:** carrots, lemons, olive oil, fish, rye
**Ailments It Heals:** eye problems, hyperthyroidism, mood disorders, rosacea

 ⅔  cup shredded carrot (1 medium)
 2  tsp lemon juice
 2  tsp extra-virgin olive oil
 1  Tbsp chopped scallions
 1  Tbsp chopped fresh dill or parsley
 ⅛  tsp salt, or to taste
 3  oz (90 g) water-packed chunk light tuna, drained and flaked
 ¼  cup finely chopped celery
 2  Tbsp reduced-fat mayonnaise
 4  slices rye or pumpernickel bread
 4  lettuce leaves, rinsed and dried

1. In small bowl, combine carrot, lemon juice, oil, scallions, dill or parsley, and salt. Mix with fork.

2. In another small bowl, mix tuna, celery, and 1 Tbsp of mayonnaise.

3. Spread remaining 1 Tbsp mayonnaise over bread slices. Spread half of tuna mixture over 2 bread slices. Top with carrot salad and lettuce. Set remaining bread slices over filling. Cut each sandwich in half. One serving equals 2 sandwich halves. Sandwiches will keep, well wrapped, in refrigerator or cooler packed with ice packs for up to 1 day.

**Per serving:** 303 calories, 17 g protein, 38 g carbohydrates, 5 g fiber, 9 g total fat, 2 g saturated fat, 13 mg cholesterol, 758 mg sodium

# OPEN-FACED SARDINE SANDWICHES

Serves 2
**Prep Time:** 5 minutes
**Cook Time:** 5 minutes
**Healing Foods:** lemons, fish, cheese
**Ailments It Heals:** Alzheimer's disease, atherosclerosis, asthma, circulatory disorders

1   Tbsp low-fat canola mayonnaise
½   tsp fresh lemon juice
¼   tsp grated lemon zest
2   slices (each ¾ in or 1.5 cm thick) whole grain bread, such as 12-grain
1   small tomato, cut into 4 slices
3.75  oz (106 g) sardines in olive oil
2   slices (2 oz or 60 g) low-fat Jarlsberg cheese

1. Preheat the broiler. In a small bowl, combine the mayonnaise, lemon juice, and lemon zest. Spread half of the mixture onto each slice of bread.

2. Top each slice with 1/2 of the tomatoes, sardines, and cheese. Place on a broiler pan or baking sheet and broil until the cheese melts, about 3 minutes.

**Per serving:** 228 calories, 20 g protein, 17 g carbohydrates, 5 g fiber, 9 g total fat, 1 g saturated fat, 72 mg cholesterol, 637 mg sodium

# FISH TACOS

Serves 4
**Prep Time:** 10 minutes plus standing
**Cook Time:** 7 minutes
**Healing Foods:** limes, fish, mangoes, lettuce
**Ailments It Heals:** cholesterol (high), chronic fatigue syndrome, jaundice, obesity, multiple sclerosis

1   Tbsp olive oil
2   cloves garlic, minced
1   tsp ground cumin
½   tsp salt
3   Tbsp lime juice
1½  lb (750 g) halibut fillets
1   ripe mango, peeled, seeded, and chopped
½   small red bell pepper, seeded and finely chopped
½   jalapeño chile pepper, seeded and finely chopped (wear gloves when handling; they burn)
¼   cup chopped cilantro (optional)
8   soft corn tortillas (6 in or 15 cm)
1   cup shredded lettuce

1. Preheat broiler. Coat broiler pan with cooking spray. In medium bowl, combine oil, garlic, cumin, salt, 1 Tbsp lime juice, and fish and toss to coat. Let stand 15 minutes.

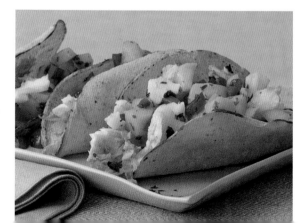

2. In small bowl, combine mango, bell pepper, chile pepper, cilantro (if using), and remaining 2 Tbsp lime juice. Set salsa aside.

3. Wrap tortillas in foil. Remove fish from marinade and place on broiler pan. Broil for 3 to 6 minutes, or until opaque. Transfer to plate and place tortillas in oven for 1 minute, to warm slightly. Flake the fish.

4. Top tortillas with equal amounts of lettuce, fish, and salsa.

**Per serving:** 380 calories, 39 g protein, 36 g carbohydrates, 5 g fiber, 9 g total fat, 1 g saturated fat, 54 mg cholesterol, 430 mg sodium

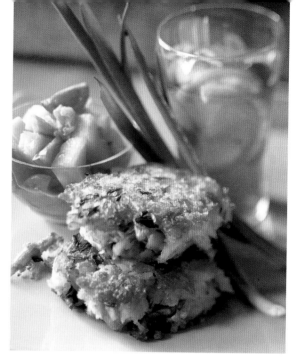

# CRAB CAKES WITH MELON RELISH

Serves 4
**Prep Time:** 10 minutes
**Cook Time:** 12 minutes
**Healing Foods:** limes, cantaloupe, tomatoes, shellfish, olive oil
**Ailments It Heals:** burns, cancer, psoriasis, respiratory disorders

¼  cup fresh lime juice
2  Tbsp honey
1  Tbsp plus 2 tsp dijon mustard
2  cups cantaloupe chunks (½ in or 1 cm)
1  green bell pepper, diced
1  cup cherry tomatoes, quartered
1  lb (500 g) lump crabmeat, picked over to remove any cartilage
4  scallions, thinly sliced
¼  tsp salt
2  egg whites
½  cup plain dry bread crumbs
2  Tbsp olive oil

1. In medium bowl, whisk together lime juice, honey, and 1 Tbsp mustard. Add cantaloupe, bell pepper, and tomatoes and toss to combine. Refrigerate until ready to serve.

2. In separate bowl, combine crabmeat, scallions, salt, and remaining 2 tsp mustard. Beat egg whites until stiff peaks form and gently fold into crabmeat mixture. Gently shape into 8 patties.

3. Dip patties in bread crumbs. In large nonstick skillet, heat 1 Tbsp oil over medium heat. Add 4 crab cakes and cook for 2 to 3 minutes per side, or until hot and cooked through. Transfer crab cakes to a plate. Repeat with remaining 1 Tbsp oil and 4 crab cakes. Serve crab cakes with melon relish alongside.

**Per serving:** 315 calories, 26 g protein, 32 g carbohydrates, 3 g fiber, 9 g total fat, 2 g saturated fat, 88 mg cholesterol, 768 mg sodium

# GRILLED EGGPLANT SANDWICHES WITH RED PEPPER–WALNUT SAUCE

**Serves 4**
**Prep Time:** 20 minutes
**Cook Time:** 12 minutes
**Healing Foods:** nuts, peppers, eggplant, cheese
**Ailments It Heals:** Alzheimer's disease, eye problems, prostate problems

## Red Pepper–Walnut Sauce

¼ cup walnuts
1 Tbsp fine dry unseasoned bread crumbs
1 clove garlic, minced (½ tsp)
1 tsp ground cumin
⅛ tsp red-pepper flakes
Salt to taste
7 oz (200 g) roasted red peppers, drained and rinsed
1 tablespoon lemon juice

## Sandwich

2 medium-large baby eggplants, cut crosswise into ⅜-in-thick (1 cm) slices
Salt to taste
Ground black pepper to taste
8 small slices sourdough bread, toasted if desired
4 oz (125 g) creamy goat cheese, cut into ⅜-in-thick (1 cm) slices
¾ cup arugula leaves, washed and dried

**1.** To make sauce: In food processor, combine walnuts, bread crumbs, garlic, cumin, red pepper, and salt. Process until walnuts are ground. Add roasted red peppers and lemon juice and process until smooth.

**2.** Preheat grill or broiler.

**3.** To make sandwich: Spritz both sides of eggplant slices with cooking spray and season with salt and pepper. Lightly oil grill or broiler rack by rubbing it with a piece of oil-soaked paper towel (use tongs to hold paper towel when working over a hot grill). Grill or broil eggplant for 4 to 6 minutes per side, or until very tender and browned.

**4.** Spread about 1½ Tbsp Red Pepper–Walnut Sauce over one side of each bread slice. Layer eggplant slices and goat cheese slices on 4 bread slices. Top with arugula. Set remaining bread slices on top and cut sandwiches in half. One serving is 2 sandwich halves. Sandwiches will keep, wrapped in plastic wrap or foil, in refrigerator or cooler packed with ice packs for up to 2 days.

**Per serving:** 425 calories, 16 g protein, 60 g carbohydrates, 7 g fiber, 18 g total fat, 6 g saturated fat, 13 mg cholesterol, 960 mg sodium

# OPEN-FACED GRILLED VEGETABLE SANDWICH

**Serves 4**
**Prep Time:** 15 minutes
**Cook Time:** 14 minutes
**Healing Foods:** olive oil, mushrooms, asparagus, peppers, cheese
**Ailments It Heals:** cardiovascular disease, diabetes, kidney disease

2 Tbsp olive oil
1 Tbsp balsamic vinegar
¼ tsp salt
⅛ tsp ground black pepper

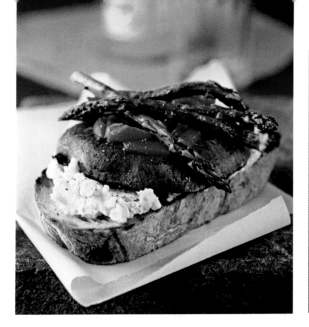

4 portobello mushrooms, stems removed

1 small bunch asparagus, trimmed and spears cut in half

1 large red bell pepper, halved and seeded

4 slices Italian bread

3 oz (90 g) goat cheese

**1.** Preheat grill or broiler.

**2.** In small bowl, whisk together oil, balsamic vinegar, salt, and black pepper. Brush mushrooms, asparagus, and bell pepper with oil mixture.

**3.** Grill or broil vegetables 4 in (10 cm) from heat, turning once, until tender, about 10 minutes for asparagus and bell pepper, and about 12 minutes for mushrooms. When cool enough to handle, peel and slice pepper.

**4.** Turn off grill or broiler. Place bread on grill or broiler rack for 2 minutes, or until warm. Spread goat cheese on bread. Place mushrooms on each slice. Top with bell pepper and asparagus. Serve warm.

**Per serving:** 274 calories, 11 g protein, 26 g carbohydrates, 4 g fiber, 15 g total fat, 6 g saturated fat, 17 mg cholesterol, 443 mg sodium

# ZUCCHINI-CARROT CRUSTLESS QUICHE SQUARES

Serves 16

**Prep Time:** 15 minutes

**Cook Time:** 1 hour plus cooling

**Healing Foods:** zucchini, eggs, carrots, cheese

**Ailments It Heals:** ADHD, anemia, cystic fibrosis

1 tsp olive oil

1 large onion, finely chopped

1 large zucchini, cut into ½-in (1 cm) cubes

½ tsp salt

2 large eggs

¼ cup milk

3 medium carrots, peeled, grated, blotted dry

1 cup shredded cheddar cheese

1 Tbsp chopped dill

**1.** Heat oven to 375°F (190°C). Lightly coat 8-in (2 L) square or round baking pan with cooking spray. In large nonstick skillet, heat oil over medium heat. Add onion and sauté for 3 minutes, or until slightly softened. Add zucchini. Increase heat to medium-high and sauté for 7 to 10 minutes, or until zucchini is soft and all liquid has evaporated. Stir in ¼ tsp salt. Remove from heat.

**2.** In large bowl, beat eggs, milk, and remaining ¼ tsp salt. Add zucchini, carrots, cheese, and dill. Spread in prepared pan.

**3.** Bake for 45 minutes, or until quiche is just set in center. Transfer to wire rack. Let cool for at least 10 minutes before cutting. Serve warm.

**Per serving:** 54 calories, 3 g protein, 3 g carbohydrates, 1 g fiber, 3 g total fat, 2 g saturated fat, 35 mg cholesterol, 128 mg sodium

# COUSCOUS-STUFFED PEPPERS

Serves 6
**Prep Time:** 20 minutes
**Cook Time:** 28 minutes
**Healing Foods:** peppers, zucchini, chickpeas, cheese
**Ailments It Heals:** cancer, cirrhosis, stress

 6  large bell peppers (red, yellow, orange, or green)
 1  Tbsp vegetable oil
 1  small zucchini, finely chopped
 2  cloves garlic, minced
 1  Tbsp fresh-squeezed lemon juice
 2  cups cooked couscous
15  oz (450 mL) chickpeas, drained and rinsed
 1  ripe tomato, seeded and finely chopped
 1  tsp dried oregano, crumbled
½  tsp salt
¼  tsp ground black pepper
½  cup crumbled feta cheese

**1.** Slice tops off peppers to make lids. Scoop out membranes and seeds and discard. In large saucepan of lightly salted boiling water, simmer peppers and lids, covered, for 5 minutes. Drain.

**2.** Preheat oven to 350°F (180°C).

**3.** In medium saucepan, heat oil over medium heat. Add zucchini and garlic and sauté for 2 minutes. Stir in lemon juice. Cook for 1 minute and remove from heat. Stir in couscous, chickpeas, tomato, oregano, salt, and black pepper. Stir in cheese. Fill each pepper with couscous mixture. Place upright in shallow baking dish. Cover with pepper tops.

**4.** Bake for 20 minutes, or just until filling is heated through.

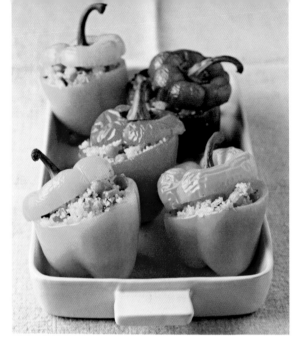

**Per serving:** 207 calories, 8 g protein, 36 g carbohydrates, 7 g fiber, 4 g total fat, 1 g saturated fat, 3 mg cholesterol, 307 mg sodium

**SALADS**

# BEEF-FILLET SALAD WITH MUSTARD VINAIGRETTE

Serves 4
**Prep Time:** 20 minutes
**Cook Time:** 45 minutes plus chilling, standing
**Healing Foods:** beef, vinegar, mustard, potatoes, green beans, peas, leeks
**Ailments It Heals:** ADHD, anemia, infertility

1    lb (500 g) beef fillet
1    tsp plus 1½ Tbsp olive oil
1    Tbsp red wine vinegar
1½  tsp dijon mustard
Pinch of sugar
Salt and ground black pepper
¾    lb (375 g) new potatoes, scrubbed
¼    lb (125 g) haricots verts (French green beans)
       or regular green beans, halved
½    cup shelled fresh or frozen peas
1    large leek, finely chopped
2    Tbsp snipped fresh chives

**1.** Preheat oven to 450°F (230°C). Rub fillet with 1 tsp oil and set on a rack in a roasting pan. Roast for 15 minutes for rare beef or up to 25 minutes for well done.

**2.** Meanwhile, in large mixing bowl, whisk together vinegar, mustard, sugar, salt, pepper, and 1½ Tbsp oil.

**3.** When beef is done, remove from oven and let stand for 5 minutes, then cut into thin slices against the grain. Add to bowl with dressing and let cool.

**4.** In saucepan of boiling water, cook potatoes for 15 minutes, or until tender. Drain well. When cool enough to handle, cut in half or into thick slices and add to bowl.

**5.** Drop green beans into another pan of boiling water and cook for 1 minute. Add peas and cook for 3 minutes, or until vegetables are tender. Drain vegetables and refresh briefly under cold running water, then add to bowl. Toss well. Cover and refrigerate for 30 minutes.

**6.** About 15 minutes before serving, remove salad from refrigerator and stir in leek and chives.

**Per serving:** 318 calories, 24 g protein, 25 g carbohydrates, 4 g fiber, 14 g total fat, 4 g saturated fat, 60 mg cholesterol, 117 mg sodium

# PORK, PEAR AND POTATO SALAD

Serves 6
**Prep Time:** 35 minutes
**Cook Time:** 22 minutes
**Healing Foods:** pecans, potatoes, radishes, pears, salad greens, pork
**Ailments It Heals:** infertility, memory loss, menstrual problems, neuralgia

### Salad

⅓    cup halved pecans
1½  lb (750 g) new potatoes (even sized), washed
2    Tbsp finely minced fresh ginger
2    tsp coarse mustard
2    tsp white wine vinegar
2    Tbsp canola oil
2    tsp hazelnut oil
Salt and ground black pepper
1    small daikon radish (Japanese white radish), peeled and thinly sliced
8    red radishes, cut into quarters
2    firm ripe pears
1    oak leaf lettuce or other greens, separated into leaves
1    bunch watercress, tough stalks discarded
12  oz (375 g) cooked roast pork loin, trimmed of fat and thinly sliced

**1.** Heat small skillet over medium-high heat and toast pecans for 6 to 7 minutes. Cool, then chop roughly. Set aside.

**2.** In saucepan of boiling water, cook potatoes for 15 minutes, or until tender. Drain. When cool enough to handle, cut into quarters and place in mixing bowl.

**3.** Put ginger in garlic crusher and press to squeeze out juice (this will have to be done in three or four batches). You need 2 tsp of this ginger juice. In small jar or container with a tight-fitting lid, add ginger, mustard, vinegar, oils, and salt and pepper to taste. Shake well to mix. Pour about one-third of dressing over warm potatoes and toss gently to coat. Leave to cool.

**4.** In another bowl, toss the daikon and red radishes with half of remaining dressing, to prevent them from browning. Halve pears lengthways and scoop out cores, then cut into long wedges. Toss with radishes.

**5.** Arrange lettuce leaves and watercress in shallow salad bowl. Add radish mixture to potatoes and gently mix together. Pile mixture onto the middle of the salad leaves and arrange pork slices on top.

**6.** Stir toasted pecans into remaining dressing and drizzle over top of salad. Serve immediately.

**Per serving:** 355 calories, 21 g protein, 34 g carbohydrates, 5 g fiber, 16 g total fat, 3 g saturated fat, 48 mg cholesterol, 93 mg sodium

# ROAST PORK AND QUINOA SALAD

Serves 4
**Prep Time:** 25 minutes
**Cook Time:** 25 minutes
**Healing Foods:** mustard, lemons, pork, grains, grapefruits, salad greens
**Ailments It Heals:** AIDS and HIV infection, celiac disease, jaundice

¼ cup apricot jam
2 Tbsp dijon mustard
1 tsp grated lemon zest
2 Tbsp fresh lemon juice
1 tsp chili powder
1 lb (500 g) well-trimmed pork tenderloin
¾ tsp salt
2 cups water
1 cup quinoa, well rinsed
1 Tbsp olive oil
3 pink grapefruits
8 cups arugula (about 2 bunches)

**1.** Preheat oven to 400°F (200°C). In large bowl, whisk together jam, mustard, lemon zest, lemon juice, and ½ tsp chili powder. Measure out 3 Tbsp of jam mixture and reserve.

**2.** Place pork in small roasting pan. Rub with ¼ tsp salt and remaining ½ tsp chili powder. Roast for 15 minutes. Brush 3 Tbsp jam mixture over pork and roast for 10 minutes, or until cooked through but still juicy.

**3.** Meanwhile, in large saucepan, bring water to a boil. Add quinoa and remaining ½ tsp salt and return to a boil. Reduce to a simmer, cover, and cook for 12 minutes, or until tender. Drain.

**4.** Whisk oil with remaining jam mixture in bowl. Add quinoa, tossing to combine.

**5.** With paring knife, cut off skin from grapefruits. Working over a bowl to catch juice, cut between membranes to release sections. Add sections and ¼ cup grapefruit juice to bowl with quinoa.

**6.** Place quinoa salad on bed of arugula. Thinly slice pork and arrange on top.

**Per serving:** 450 calories, 31 g protein, 59 g carbohydrates, 5 g fiber, 10 g total fat, 2 g saturated fat, 65 mg cholesterol, 697 mg sodium

# ASIAN CHICKEN SALAD

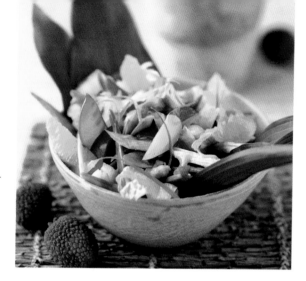

Serves 4

**Prep Time:** 20 minutes

**Cook Time:** 10 minutes

**Healing Foods:** lettuce, peas, oranges, plums, chicken, peanut butter

**Ailments It Heals:** acne, hepatitis, obesity

| | |
|---|---|
| 1 | lb (500 g) romaine lettuce |
| 4 | oz (125 g) snow peas |
| 20 | oz (568 mL) canned lychees, drained and cut in half |
| 1 | large navel orange, peeled and cut into sections |
| 1 | red plum, pitted and sliced |
| 4 | scallions, thinly sliced |
| 12 | oz (375 g) boneless, skinless chicken breast halves |
| ⅓ | cup nonfat mayonnaise |
| 3 | Tbsp creamy peanut butter |
| 1 | clove garlic, minced |

**Per serving:** 378 calories, 27 g protein, 53 g carbohydrates, 7 g fiber, 9 g total fat, 2 g saturated fat, 49 mg cholesterol, 378 mg sodium

**1.** Finely shred lettuce and put into large salad bowl. Trim snow peas and remove strings with fingers. Cut peas in half on the diagonal and add to salad bowl. Add lychees, orange, plum, and scallions and toss to mix.

**2.** Coat nonstick ridged grill pan with cooking spray and set over medium-high heat for 2 minutes, or until hot. Grill chicken breasts for 4 minutes on each side, or until cooked through.

**3.** Meanwhile, in small measuring cup, whisk mayonnaise, peanut butter, and garlic until blended. Diagonally cut chicken into thin slices and add to salad bowl. Right before serving, drizzle salad with dressing and toss to coat.

# CHICKEN SALAD WITH CITRUS

Serves 4

**Prep Time:** 30 minutes

**Healing Foods:** oranges, grapefruits, chicken, olives, salad greens

**Ailments It Heals:** anemia, fibroids, prostate problems, varicose veins

| | |
|---|---|
| 3 | navel oranges |
| 2 | ruby red grapefruits |
| 3 | Tbsp olive oil |
| 1 | Tbsp balsamic vinegar |
| 2 | tsp dijon mustard |
| ½ | tsp salt |
| 2 | generous cups shredded cooked chicken breasts or thighs, leftover or poached |
| ½ | cup kalamata olives, pitted and sliced |
| ½ | cup slivered red onion |
| 2 | bunches arugula, tough stems trimmed (about 6 cups) |

1. With paring knife, cut off and discard skin, white pith, and outer membrane of oranges and grapefruits. Working over a bowl to catch juices, section oranges and grapefruits: Use paring knife to cut along both sides of each dividing membrane to release segments, transferring them to smaller bowl. Squeeze any juice left in membranes into bowl. Measure out 3 Tbsp of citrus juice and transfer to large salad bowl (reserve any extra juice for another use).

2. Whisk oil, vinegar, mustard, and salt into citrus juice in bowl. Add chicken, olives, onion, arugula, and orange and grapefruit sections and toss well.

**Per serving:** 385 calories, 27 g protein, 29 g carbohydrates, 5 g fiber, 19 g total fat, 3 g saturated fat, 70 mg cholesterol, 619 mg sodium

# CHICKEN-MELON SALAD

Serves 4
**Prep Time:** 15 minutes
**Cook Time:** 13 minutes
**Healing Foods:** chicken, limes, salad greens, cantaloupe, tomato
**Ailments It Heals:** colds and flu, diabetes, hives, respiratory disorders

1 Tbsp chili powder
1 tsp dried oregano
1 lb (500 g) boneless, skinless chicken breasts
1 Tbsp olive oil
5 Tbsp fresh lime juice
½ tsp salt
2 corn tortillas (6-in or 15 cm diameter), cut into 8 wedges each
2 Tbsp light mayonnaise
2 tsp dijon mustard
2 bunches watercress, tough stems trimmed (about 6 cups)
3 cups cantaloupe chunks (½ in or 1 cm)
2 cups cherry tomatoes, halved
2 scallions, thinly sliced

1. Preheat oven to 450°F (230°C). In small bowl, stir together chili powder and oregano. Measure out 1 tsp of mixture and set aside. Rub remaining mixture into chicken.

2. In small bowl, whisk together oil, reserved 1 tsp spice mixture, 1 Tbsp lime juice, and ¼ tsp salt. Dip tortilla wedges into mixture. Transfer wedges to baking sheet and bake for 5 minutes, or until crisp. Remove from oven and preheat broiler.

3. Broil chicken 6 in (15 cm) from heat for 4 minutes per side, or until cooked through. When cool enough to handle, slice into bite-size pieces.

4. Meanwhile, in large bowl, whisk together mayonnaise, mustard, and remaining 4 Tbsp lime juice and ¼ tsp salt. Add chicken, watercress, cantaloupe, tomatoes, and scallions. Serve topped with tortilla wedges.

**Per serving:** 286 calories, 28 g protein, 23 g carbohydrates, 4 g fiber, 10 g total fat, 2 g saturated fat, 75 mg cholesterol, 616 mg sodium

# JAMAICAN JERKED CHICKEN SALAD

Serves 4
**Prep Time:** 15 minutes
**Cook Time:** 8 minutes
**Healing Foods:** vinegar, chicken, pineapples, kiwi, peppers, jicama
**Ailments It Heals:** arthritis, chronic fatigue syndrome, colds and flu

3 cloves garlic, minced
1¼ tsp dried thyme
1 tsp ground black pepper
¾ tsp ground allspice
4 scallions, thinly sliced
¾ tsp salt
2 tsp dark brown sugar
4 Tbsp red wine vinegar
2 Tbsp dijon mustard
1 lb (500 g) boneless, skinless chicken breasts
1 Tbsp olive oil
2 cups pineapple chunks
4 kiwi, peeled and cut into wedges
1 large red bell pepper, cut into matchsticks
1 cup jicama matchsticks

**1.** In large bowl, stir together garlic, thyme, black pepper, allspice, half the scallions, and ½ tsp salt. Stir in brown sugar, 2 Tbsp vinegar, and 1 Tbsp mustard and mix well. Add chicken, rubbing mixture into chicken. Cover and set aside.

**2.** In separate bowl, whisk together oil and remaining 2 Tbsp vinegar, 1 Tbsp mustard, ¼ tsp salt. Add pineapple, kiwi, bell pepper, jicama, and remaining scallions. Toss to combine.

**3.** Preheat broiler. Broil chicken 6 in (15 cm) from heat for 4 minutes per side, or until cooked through. When cool enough to handle, slice chicken on diagonal. Add to bowl with salad and toss.

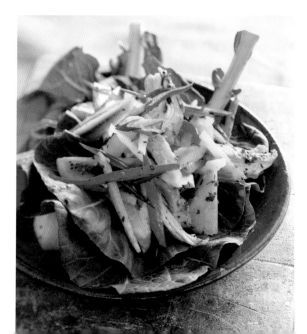

**Per serving:** 287 calories, 28 g protein, 31 g carbohydrates, 5.9 g fiber, 6 g total fat, 1 g saturated fat, 66 mg cholesterol, 701 mg sodium

# WARM KASHA AND SEAFOOD SALAD

Serves 4
**Prep Time:** 15 minutes
**Cook Time:** 1 hour 15 minutes
**Healing Foods:** buckwheat, fish, cucumbers, peas, fennel, seaweed
**Ailments It Heals:** cancer, flatulence, sore throat

8 oz (250 g) kasha (toasted buckwheat)
2½ cups vegetable stock
3 Tbsp sunflower oil
2 Tbsp extra-virgin olive oil
1 Tbsp white wine vinegar
1 tsp dijon mustard
2 Tbsp chopped fresh mixed herbs, such as basil, marjoram, oregano, rosemary, sage, and thyme
14 oz (420 g) frozen mixed seafood, thawed
1 English cucumber, diced
7 oz (210 g) sugar snap peas, sliced
1 fennel bulb, about (8 oz or 250 g), halved and thinly sliced
4 oz (125 g) radishes, thinly sliced
1 sheet toasted nori
Salt and ground black pepper

**1.** Put kasha in nonstick saucepan, pour in stock, and bring to a boil. Cover and simmer for 5 minutes, or until kasha has absorbed the stock.

**2.** Stir in 2 Tbsp sunflower oil, cover, and cook for 10 minutes. Remove lid and fluff kasha with a fork, tossing and turning to separate grains. Cook over very low heat, uncovered, for 1 hour, tossing the kasha with a fork every 10 minutes to separate grains. When done, place in large salad bowl.

**3.** Meanwhile, in medium bowl, whisk together olive oil, vinegar, mustard, and mixed herbs until thoroughly mixed.

**4.** Heat remaining 1 Tbsp sunflower oil in wok or large frying pan. Add seafood and stir-fry over medium heat for 2 to 3 minutes, or until hot. Add hot seafood to kasha together with cucumber, sugar snap peas, fennel, and radishes. Drizzle dressing over top and toss gently to mix.

**5.** Snip nori into fine strips with scissors, sprinkle over salad, and serve immediately.

**Per serving:** 500 calories, 27 g protein, 56 g carbohydrates, 10 g fiber, 20 g total fat, 3 g saturated fat, 135 mg cholesterol, 682 mg sodium

# GRILLED SALMON SALAD

Serves 4

**Prep Time:** 30 minutes plus marinating

**Cook Time:** 5 minutes

**Healing Foods:** cardamom, fish, salad greens, mangoes, papayas, oranges

**Ailments It Heals:** acne, cholesterol (high), psoriasis

 8 cardamom pods, crushed
 1 tsp cumin seeds
Finely grated zest and juice of 1 lime
Juice of 1 large orange
 1 Tbsp light soy sauce
 1 Tbsp honey
Salt and ground black pepper

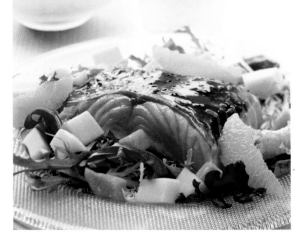

 4 pieces (4 oz or 125 g each) skinless salmon fillet
 4 cups mixed salad leaves, such as oak leaf, red leaf lettuce, and baby chard, or use romaine
 1 mango, peeled and cut into 1-in (2.5 cm) cubes
 1 papaya, peeled, seeded, and cut into 1-in (2.5 cm) cubes
 1 orange, peeled and segmented

**1.** Heat small nonstick skillet over medium heat. Scrape seeds from cardamom pods and add to hot pan with cumin seeds. Toast for a few seconds to release aromas and remove seeds to shallow nonmetallic dish.

**2.** Add lime zest and juice, orange juice, soy sauce, and honey to seeds. Season lightly with salt and pepper. Lay salmon pieces in dish and turn to coat both sides. Cover and let marinate for 30 minutes.

**3.** Preheat grill or oven broiler. Lift salmon out of marinade, place on grill rack or broiler pan, and grill or broil for 4 to 5 minutes on one side only. The fillets should still be slightly translucent in the center. Meanwhile, pour marinade into small saucepan and bring just to a boil.

**4.** Arrange salad leaves in middle of 4 plates. Scatter mango and papaya cubes and orange segments over salad. Place cooked salmon on top of salad and drizzle with warm marinade. Serve immediately.

**Per serving:** 313 calories, 26 g protein, 30 g carbohydrates, 4 g fiber, 10 g total fat, 2 g saturated fat, 77 mg cholesterol, 223 mg sodium

# TOSSED TUNA SALAD NIÇOISE

Serves 4
**Prep Time:** 15 minutes
**Cook Time:** 20 minutes
**Healing Foods:** potatoes, lemons, green beans, fish, tomatoes, salad greens
**Ailments It Heals:** Alzheimer's disease, hives, hyperthyroidism, mood disorders

1 lb (500 g) small red-skinned potatoes, cut into eighths
⅓ cup fresh lemon juice
2 Tbsp olive oil
2 Tbsp dijon mustard
½ tsp salt
12 oz (375 g) green beans, cut into 2-in (5 cm) lengths
2 tuna steaks (1 in or 2.5 cm thick, 1½ lb or 750 g total)
½ tsp ground black pepper
1 pint cherry tomatoes, halved
1 bunch watercress, tough stems trimmed
1 belgian endive, cut crosswise into ½-in (1 cm) slices

**1.** In large pot of boiling water, cook potatoes for 10 minutes, or until tender. Drain.

**2.** Meanwhile, in large bowl, whisk together lemon juice, oil, mustard, and ¼ tsp salt. Add potatoes while still warm, tossing to coat.

**3.** In vegetable steamer, steam green beans for 4 minutes, or until crisp-tender. Add to bowl with potatoes and toss to combine.

**4.** Meanwhile, preheat broiler. Place tuna on broiler pan and sprinkle with pepper and remaining ¼ tsp salt. Broil 6 in (15 cm) from heat for 3 minutes per side for medium-rare.

**5.** Add tomatoes, watercress, and endive to bowl, tossing well. To serve, slice tuna and place on top.

**Per serving:** 427 calories, 41 g protein, 32 g carbohydrates, 6 g fiber, 15 g total fat, 3 g saturated fat, 58 mg cholesterol, 566 mg sodium

# TUNA AND CANNELLINI SALAD WITH LEMON

Serves 4
**Prep Time:** 25 minutes
**Healing Foods:** beans, fish, lemons, salad greens, tomatoes
**Ailments It Heals:** depression, cholesterol (high), PCOS

**DRESSING**
3 Tbsp lemon juice
1 clove garlic, minced
¼ tsp salt, or to taste
⅛ tsp crushed red-pepper flakes
¼ cup extra-virgin olive oil
Ground black pepper

**SALAD**
19 oz (540 mL) cannellini beans, drained and rinsed
6 oz (175 g) water-packed chunk light tuna, drained and flaked
⅓ cup finely diced red onion
2 tsp chopped fresh rosemary
1½ tsp freshly grated lemon zest
6 cups arugula, washed, dried, and torn into bite-size pieces
1 cup cherry tomatoes, quartered

**1.** In small bowl, combine lemon juice, garlic, salt, and red pepper. Gradually whisk in the oil. Season to taste with pepper.

**2.** To make the salad: In medium bowl, combine beans, tuna, onion, rosemary, and lemon zest. Add ¼ cup dressing (save remaining dressing for the arugula). Toss to coat well. (The tuna-bean salad will keep, covered, in the refrigerator for up to 1 day.)

**3.** Just before serving, place arugula in large bowl. Add reserved dressing and toss to coat well. Divide arugula mixture among 4 plates. Top with tuna-bean salad and garnish with cherry tomatoes. One serving is 2/3 cup tuna-bean salad and 1½ cups arugula.

**Per serving:** 305 calories, 18 g protein, 25 g carbohydrates, 7 g fiber, 15 g total fat, 2 g saturated fat, 26 mg cholesterol, 500 mg sodium

# SHRIMP AND YUCCA SALAD

Serves 4
**Prep Time:** 15 minutes
**Cook Time:** 15 minutes
**Healing Foods:** yucca, shrimp, garlic, green beans
**Ailments It Heals:** Alzheimer's disease, burns, cancer

1  bag (24 oz or 750 g) frozen yucca
1  Tbsp olive oil
1  lb (500 g) shrimp, peeled and deveined
2  cloves garlic, sliced thin
3  bunches scallions, cut into 1½-in (3.5 cm) pieces
½  lb (250 g) fresh string beans, steamed
Salt and ground black pepper

**1.** In large pot of boiling water, boil yucca for 10 minutes, or until soft. Do not overcook, or it will be mushy.

**2.** Remove and drain in colander. Cut into slices.

**3.** Heat large skillet or wok over high heat. When hot, add oil and coat pan. Add shrimp and cook, stirring, for 2 to 3 minutes, or until almost entirely pink. Add garlic and scallions and cook, stirring, for 2 minutes, or until scallions are bright green. Pour over yucca. Serve with string beans. Season to taste with salt and pepper.

**Per serving:** 429 calories, 19 g protein, 74 g carbohydrates, 5 g fiber, 6 g total fat, 1 g saturated fat, 143 mg cholesterol, 661 mg sodium

# SHELLFISH SALAD WITH HERBED LEMON DRESSING

Serves 4
**Prep Time:** 15 minutes
**Cook Time:** 11 minutes
**Healing Foods:** shellfish, lemons, mustard, celery, peppers
**Ailments It Heals:** burns, halitosis, shingles

1  cup dry white wine
1  tsp dried tarragon
½  tsp dried oregano
1  dozen littleneck clams, well scrubbed
12  oz (375 g) large shrimp, shelled and deveined
8  oz (250 g) sea scallops, halved horizontally
½  cup fresh lemon juice
1  Tbsp olive oil
1½  tsp dijon mustard
2  celery stalks, halved lengthwise and cut crosswise into ¼-in (0.5 cm) slices
2  red bell peppers, diced
⅓  cup chopped parsley

**1.** In large saucepan, combine white wine, tarragon, and oregano and bring to a boil over high heat. Add clams, cover, and cook for 4 to 5 minutes, or until clams open (check after 3 minutes as some will open before others). Remove clams as they open (discard any that do not open). Reserve liquid in pan. When clams are cool enough to handle, remove clam meat and place in large bowl. Discard shells.

**2.** Heat liquid in pan over medium-low heat. Add shrimp and cook for 3 to 4 minutes, or until cooked through. With slotted spoon, remove shrimp, reserving liquid in pan. When shrimp are cool enough to handle, halve them horizontally and add to bowl with clams.

**3.** Heat liquid in pan over medium-low heat. Add scallops and cook for 2 minutes, or until cooked through. With slotted spoon, transfer scallops to bowl, reserving liquid in pan. Cool liquid to room temperature and measure out ½ cup.

**4.** In medium bowl, whisk together lemon juice, oil, mustard, and ½ cup reserved cooking liquid. Pour over shellfish. Add celery, bell peppers, and parsley and toss to combine. Chill salad until serving time.

**Per serving:** 208 calories, 30 g protein, 9 g carbohydrates, 1 g fiber, 6 g total fat, 1 g saturated fat, 138 mg cholesterol, 285 mg sodium

# CRAB AND AVOCADO SALAD

**Serves 6**
**Prep Time:** 20 minutes
**Cook Time:** 15 minutes plus cooling
**Healing Foods:** bulgur, tomatoes, shellfish, avocados, apples, bean sprouts, lettuce
**Ailments It Heals:** atherosclerosis, chronic fatigue syndrome, menstrual problems

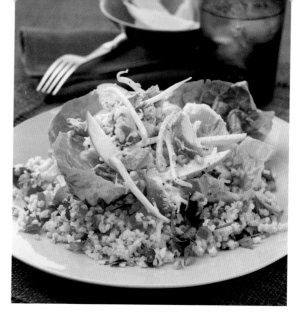

|   |   |
|---|---|
| 1 | cup bulgur wheat |
| 2½ | cups boiling water |
| 1 | Tbsp olive oil |
| 3 | Tbsp chopped fresh flat-leaf parsley |
| 1 | Tbsp snipped fresh chives |
| 2 | medium tomatoes, diced |
| 4 | Tbsp lemon juice |

Salt and ground black pepper

|   |   |
|---|---|
| 12 | oz (375 g) fresh white crabmeat |
| 2 | avocados |
| 2 | crisp green apples |
| ½ | cup bean sprouts |
| 3 | Tbsp low-fat mayonnaise |
| 3 | Tbsp low-fat plain yogurt |

Pinch of cayenne pepper

|   |   |
|---|---|
| 1 | head butter (Bibb or Boston) lettuce, separated into leaves |
| ¼ | cup walnut halves, toasted and roughly chopped |

**1.** Put bulgur wheat and boiling water in large saucepan. Bring to a boil over high heat, then reduce heat and simmer for 10 to 15 minutes, or until grains are just tender. Drain in a large sieve, pressing down well to squeeze out excess water. Let cool.

**2.** Combine oil, parsley, chives, diced tomatoes, and 3 Tbsp lemon juice in large mixing bowl. Add bulgur wheat and mix thoroughly, then season with salt and pepper to taste. Let stand at room temperature while preparing crab salad.

3. Pick over and flake crabmeat, discarding any fragments of shells. Place crabmeat in large bowl. Halve, pit, and peel avocados, then chop flesh and add to crab. Quarter and core apples, then thinly slice. Add apple slices and bean sprouts to crabmeat.

4. In small bowl, mix mayonnaise and yogurt until smooth. Add cayenne and remaining 1 Tbsp lemon juice and stir. Spoon into crab mixture and toss very gently until just combined.

5. Pile bulgur onto serving platter and arrange lettuce leaves on top. Spoon crab salad onto leaves and scatter walnuts over top. Serve immediately.

**Per serving:** 341 calories, 18 g protein, 39 g carbohydrates, 10 g fiber, 15 g total fat, 2 g saturated fat, 57 mg cholesterol, 254 mg sodium

# LOBSTER SALAD WITH LIME DRESSING

**Serves 4**
**Prep Time:** 20 minutes
**Cook Time:** 15 minutes
**Healing Foods:** potatoes, peas, grapes, salad greens, lobster
**Ailments It Heals:** cardiovascular disease, depression, varicose veins, yeast infections

½ lb (250 g) baby red-skinned new potatoes, scrubbed
2 Tbsp low-fat mayonnaise
2 Tbsp low-fat plain yogurt
Finely grated zest of 1 lime
Salt and ground black pepper
2 small shallots, thinly sliced
½ cup snow peas, sliced
½ cup halved seedless red grapes
½ cup halved seedless green grapes

2 cups arugula, washed
1 cup watercress, washed
1 lb (500 g) cooked lobster meat

1. Put potatoes in a saucepan and cover with boiling water. Cook over medium-high heat for 15 minutes, or until just tender. Drain and leave to cool, then cut potatoes in half. Place in large bowl.

2. While potatoes are cooling, mix together mayonnaise, yogurt, and lime zest, and season with salt and pepper to taste.

3. Toss potatoes with shallots, snow peas, grapes, and lime dressing.

4. Arrange arugula on 4 large plates, and add watercress and potato salad. Scatter lobster on top.

**Per serving:** 219 calories, 26 g protein, 25 g carbohydrates, 2 g fiber, 2 g total fat, 0 g saturated fat, 81 mg cholesterol, 518 mg sodium

# BARLEY AND BEET SALAD

**Serves 5**
**Prep Time:** 15 minutes
**Cook Time:** 45 minutes
**Healing Foods:** barley, olive oil, beets, dill
**Ailments It Heals:** AIDS and HIV infection, diabetes, gallstones

2½ cups water
½ cup pearl barley
½ tsp salt
⅓ cup extra-virgin olive oil
3 Tbsp red wine vinegar
Ground black pepper to taste
1½ cups (8 oz or 250 g) diced cooked beets
½ cup chopped scallions
½ cup crumbled feta cheese
3 Tbsp chopped fresh dill

1. In small saucepan, combine water, barley, and ¼ tsp salt. Cover and simmer over medium-low heat for 40 to 45 minutes, or until tender. Transfer to large bowl and let cool.

2. In small bowl, whisk oil, vinegar, remaining ¼ tsp salt, and pepper. Add to barley along with beets, scallions, cheese, and dill. Toss to coat.

**Per serving:** 273 calories, 5 g protein, 23 g carbohydrates, 4 g fiber, 18 g total fat, 4 g saturated fat, 13 mg cholesterol, 444 mg sodium

# BROCCOLI AND PEARL BARLEY SALAD

**Serves 4**

**Prep Time:** 15 minutes plus cooling

**Cook Time:** 30 minutes

**Healing Foods:** barley, broccoli, zucchini, peas, apricots, seeds

**Ailments It Heals:** hemorrhoids, hypoglycemia, lactose intolerance, obesity

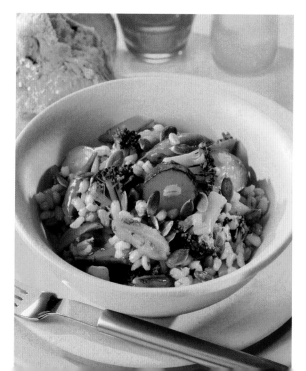

**Spicy tomato dressing**
- 3 Tbsp extra-virgin olive oil
- 1 Tbsp tomato paste
- Juice of 1 lime
- 2 tsp ground cumin
- Dash of Tabasco sauce
- 1 clove garlic, crushed
- 2 Tbsp chopped fresh coriander or flat-leaf parsley (optional)

**Salad**
- ⅔ cup pearl barley
- 3 cups cold water
- 7 oz (200 g) broccoli, cut into small florets
- 3 zucchini, thickly sliced
- 3.5 oz (100 g) sugar snap peas, halved
- ¼ cup dried apricots, thinly sliced
- Salt and ground black pepper
- ¼ cup pepitas (pumpkin seeds)

1. In large bowl, whisk together oil, tomato paste, lime juice, cumin, Tabasco, garlic, and coriander or parsley, if using. Set dressing aside.

2. Rinse barley in one or two changes of water—do this in a bowl, swirling grains with your fingers and pouring off cloudy water. Drain barley in a sieve, then place in saucepan and pour in 3 cups water. Bring to a boil, then reduce heat and cover. Simmer very gently for 30 minutes, or until most of the water has been absorbed and grains are tender but still firm. Drain well.

3. While barley is cooking, bring a second pan of water to a boil. Add broccoli, zucchini, and peas and bring to a boil. Reduce heat and simmer for 3 to 4 minutes, or until just tender but still crisp. Drain well and rinse briefly with cold water to refresh and stop the cooking.

4. Stir apricots into dressing. Add barley and vegetables to dressing as soon as they are cooked, and mix well to coat. Check the seasoning, then cover and allow to cool until just warm.

5. Add pepitas to salad just before serving, warm or cold.

**Per serving:** 315 calories, 9 g protein, 46 g carbohydrates, 11 g fiber, 13 g total fat, 2 g saturated fat, 0 mg cholesterol, 65 mg sodium

# WHEAT BERRY SALAD WITH DRIED APRICOTS

Serves 6
**Prep Time:** 25 minutes
**Cook Time:** 1 hour 45 minutes
**Healing Foods:** wheat, apricots, olive oil, mint, almonds
**Ailments It Heals:** atherosclerosis, diabetes, nail problems

- ¾ cup hard wheat berries or spelt berries, rinsed
- ½ cup dried apricots, diced
- ¼ cup extra-virgin olive oil
- 3 Tbsp orange juice
- 2 Tbsp lemon juice
- ½ tsp honey
- ½ tsp ground cinnamon
- 1 clove garlic, minced
- ½ tsp salt, or to taste
- Ground black pepper to taste
- ½ cup chopped scallions
- ⅓ cup chopped fresh mint
- ⅓ cup slivered almonds or chopped peeled pistachios, toasted

**1.** In large saucepan, place wheat berries and cover generously with water. Bring to a simmer over medium-high heat. Reduce heat to medium-low, partially cover, and cook until wheat berries are tender, 1½ to 1¾ hours. (Add more water, if necessary.) Drain and rinse with cold running water.

**2.** Meanwhile, place apricots in small bowl. Cover with boiling water and let soak for 5 to 10 minutes. Drain.

**3.** In medium bowl or jar with tight-fitting lid, combine oil, orange juice, lemon juice, honey, cinnamon, garlic, salt, and pepper. Whisk or shake to blend.

**4.** In large bowl, combine wheat berries, apricots, scallions, and mint. Add orange juice dressing and toss to coat well. Just before serving, sprinkle with nuts. The salad will keep, covered, in the refrigerator for up to 2 days.

**Per serving:** 262 calories, 6 g protein, 32 g carbohydrates, 5 g fiber, 13 g total fat, 2 g saturated fat, 0 mg cholesterol, 200 mg sodium

# ASIAN NOODLE SALAD

Serves 6
**Prep Time:** 15 minutes
**Cook Time:** 10 minutes
**Healing Foods:** wheat, peas, carrots, basil, peppers, peanuts
**Ailments It Heals:** anorexia, blood pressure, cirrhosis, eye problems

- 12 oz (375 g) whole wheat linguine
- ½ lb (250 g) snow peas, halved lengthwise
- 3 medium carrots, peeled, cut into 2-in (5 cm) lengths, and cut lengthwise into thin slices
- 2 cups packed fresh basil leaves
- ½ cup packed fresh mint leaves
- ¼ cup packed fresh cilantro leaves
- 2 cloves garlic
- 2 Tbsp dark sesame oil
- 1 Tbsp vegetable oil
- ¼ tsp red-pepper flakes
- ½ tsp salt

1 red bell pepper, seeded and cut into slivers
3 scallions, finely chopped
2 Tbsp chopped unsalted dry-roasted peanuts

**1.** Cook linguine in large pot of lightly salted boiling water until tender, following package directions. For last 2 minutes of cooking, add snow peas and carrots. Drain in colander. Rinse under cold running water. Drain well.

**2.** Meanwhile, in small food processor, combine basil, mint, cilantro, garlic, oils, pepper flakes, and ¼ tsp salt. Pulse until a paste forms.

**3.** In large bowl, combine linguine, snow peas, carrots, bell pepper, scallions, basil mixture, and remaining ¼ tsp salt. Serve at room temperature or chilled. Garnish with peanuts.

**Per serving:** 321 calories, 12 g protein, 52 g carbohydrates, 11 g fiber, 10 g total fat, 1 g saturated fat, 0 mg cholesterol, 355 mg sodium

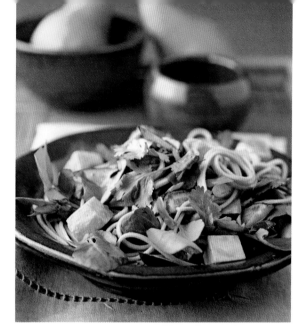

# BUCKWHEAT NOODLES WITH TOFU AND GREEN VEGETABLES

Serves 4
**Prep Time:** 15 minutes
**Cook Time:** 15 minutes
**Healing Foods:** garlic, zucchini, tofu, buckwheat, salad greens
**Ailments It Heals:** atherosclerosis, diabetes, memory loss, menopause, menstrual problems, osteoporosis

1 Tbsp vegetable oil
4 scallions, chopped
4 cloves garlic, minced
1 medium zucchini, halved lengthwise and cut crosswise into ¼-in-thick (0.5 cm) slices
½ cup vegetable broth or reduced-sodium, fat-free chicken broth
2 Tbsp reduced-sodium soy sauce
2 tsp cornstarch
1 tsp dark sesame oil
6 oz (175 g) extra-firm tofu, cut in cubes
6 oz (175 g) buckwheat (soba) noodles
1 cup packed watercress, tough stems removed
2 Tbsp chopped cilantro
½ cup roasted unsalted soy nuts

**1.** In large nonstick skillet, heat oil over medium-high heat. Reserve some dark green parts of scallions for garnish. Add remaining scallions, garlic, and zucchini to skillet. Sauté for 5 minutes, or until softened.

**2.** In small bowl, whisk together broth, soy sauce, cornstarch, and sesame oil until smooth. Add to skillet along with tofu. Heat to a boil and cook, stirring constantly, for 1 to 2 minutes, or until sauce thickens. Remove from heat.

**3.** In large pot of lightly salted boiling water over medium-high heat, cook noodles until tender, following package directions. Reserve ¼ cup cooking liquid. Drain noodles and rinse under cold running water.

**4.** Combine noodles, zucchini-tofu mixture, reserved cooking liquid, watercress, and cilantro in large bowl. Toss gently. Divide into 4 portions. Garnish with reserved scallions, and soy nuts.

**Per serving:** 322 calories, 20 g protein, 45 g carbohydrates, 10 g fiber, 9 g total fat, 2 g saturated fat, 0 mg cholesterol, 647 mg sodium

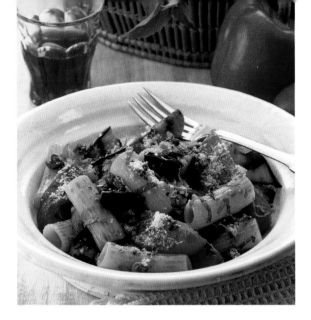

# RUSTIC GRILLED VEGETABLE AND RIGATONI SALAD

**Serves 4**

**Prep Time:** 15 minutes plus cooling and marinating

**Cook Time:** 27 minutes

**Healing Foods:** peppers, tomatoes, eggplant, vinegar, olive oil

**Ailments It Heals:** Alzheimer's disease, blood pressure, memory loss

<br>

- 8 oz (250 g) rigatoni
- 1 large red bell pepper, seeded and halved
- 2 medium tomatoes, cut into wedges
- 1 medium eggplant, trimmed and sliced lengthways
- 2 Tbsp balsamic vinegar or lemon juice
- 2 Tbsp olive oil
- 2 Tbsp chopped fresh basil
- 1 Tbsp chopped capers
- 1 large clove garlic, crushed (optional)
- ¼ cup grated parmesan cheese

Salt and ground black pepper

**1.** Cook rigatoni in boiling water for 10 to 12 minutes, or according to package directions, until al dente. Drain and rinse under cold running water, then drain thoroughly and set aside to cool.

**2.** Preheat broiler or grill to high. Broil or grill pepper halves, skin side up, for 5 to 10 minutes, or until blistered and blackened. Place in resealable plastic bag, then leave until cool enough to handle.

**3.** Broil or grill tomatoes and eggplant for 5 minutes, turning so that they cook evenly and removing pieces as they are ready. Place tomato wedges in large salad bowl. Set eggplant slices aside on plate to cool slightly.

**4.** Cut eggplant slices into 1-in (2.5 cm) strips and add to salad bowl. Peel peppers and cut into 1-in (2.5 cm) strips, then add to bowl. Mix in pasta.

**5.** In small bowl, mix vinegar or lemon juice, oil, basil, capers, garlic (if using), and cheese. Lightly toss with salad. Season lightly with salt and pepper. Set salad aside to marinate for about 30 minutes so that the flavors can infuse before serving.

**Per serving:** 242 calories, 8 g protein, 38 g carbohydrates, 4 g fiber, 7 g total fat, 2 g saturated fat, 5 mg cholesterol, 137 mg sodium

# SICILIAN PASTA SALAD

Serves 4
**Prep Time:** 15 minutes
**Cook Time:** 10 minutes
**Healing Foods:** lemons, fennel, raisins, fish
**Ailments It Heals:** halitosis, lactose intolerance, menstrual problems

  8  oz (250 g) medium pasta shells
 ½  cup fresh lemon juice
  3  Tbsp tomato paste
  1  tsp fennel seeds
 ½  tsp salt
  1  fennel bulb, stalks removed (fronds reserved), bulb cut into ½-in (1 cm) chunks
 ⅓  cup raisins
13.5 oz (400 g) sardines packed in oil, drained

**1.** In large pot of boiling water, cook pasta according to package directions. Drain, reserving ½ cup of pasta cooking liquid.

**2.** Meanwhile, in large bowl, whisk together lemon juice, tomato paste, fennel seeds, and salt. Whisk in the reserved pasta liquid.

**3.** Add drained pasta, fennel chunks, and raisins to bowl and toss well.

**4.** Mince enough reserved fennel fronds to get ½ cup. Add minced fronds and sardines to bowl, and toss gently to combine. Serve at room temperature or chilled.

**Per serving:** 452 calories, 29 g protein, 61 g carbohydrates, 15 g fiber, 10 g total fat, 1 g saturated fat, 114 mg cholesterol, 830 mg sodium

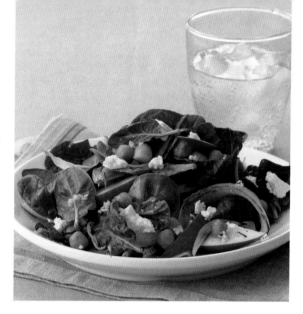

# SPINACH SALAD WITH CHICKPEAS

Serves 4
**Prep Time:** 10 minutes
**Cook Time:** 20 minutes
**Healing Foods:** onions, chickpeas, flax, spinach, apples
**Ailments It Heals:** eye problems, menopause, obesity, psoriasis, stroke

  2  medium onions, cut into ½-in (1 cm) slices
 15  oz (425 mL) chickpeas, drained, rinsed, and patted dry
 ¼  cup lemon juice
  2  Tbsp flaxseed oil
  1  Tbsp olive oil
  1  clove garlic, minced
 ½  tsp salt
 ½  cup crumbled feta cheese
  5  oz (150 g) baby spinach
  2  apples, cored and sliced
  2  Tbsp ground flaxseed

1. Preheat oven to 400°F (200°C). Coat baking sheet with sides with olive oil cooking spray. Add onion slices and coat each with spray. Roast for 10 minutes. Add chickpeas and roast for 10 minutes, or until onions are tender and browned.

2. Meanwhile, in measuring cup, whisk together lemon juice, oils, garlic, and salt. Stir in cheese.

3. Place spinach in large bowl and toss with onions, chickpeas, apples, and flaxseed. Drizzle with the vinaigrette.

**Per serving:** 292 calories, 9 g protein, 37 g carbohydrates, 10 g fiber, 14 g total fat, 3 g saturated fat, 8 mg cholesterol, 476 mg sodium

# THREE-BEAN SALAD WITH MANCHEGO CHEESE

Serves 4
**Prep Time:** 15 minutes
**Cook Time:** 5 minutes
**Healing Foods:** peppers, green beans, corn, beans, cheese
**Ailments It Heals:** depression, diverticulitis, hemorrhoids

¼ cup red wine vinegar
2 Tbsp olive oil
1 Tbsp honey
1 chipotle pepper in adobo, finely chopped (2 tsp)
Salt to taste
12 oz (375 g) green beans, halved
1 cup frozen corn kernels
15 oz (425 mL) black beans, drained and rinsed

15 oz (425 mL) red kidney beans, drained and rinsed
1 celery stalk, diced
⅓ cup finely chopped red onion
4 oz (125 g) manchego or monterey jack cheese, cut into ¼-in-wide (0.5 cm) matchsticks

1. In large bowl, whisk together vinegar, oil, honey, chipotle, and salt.

2. Meanwhile, in large vegetable steamer, steam green beans for 5 minutes, or until crisp-tender. Add corn during the final minute of steaming. Transfer hot vegetables to bowl with dressing and toss to coat.

3. Add black beans, kidney beans, celery, onion, and cheese and toss to combine. Serve at room temperature or chilled.

**Per serving:** 404 calories, 20 g protein, 43 g carbohydrates, 10 g fiber, 18 g total fat, 8 g saturated fat, 30 mg cholesterol, 510 mg sodium

# AVOCADO, JICAMA, AND ORANGE SALAD

Serves 6
**Prep Time:** 15 minutes plus chilling
**Healing Foods:** jicama, oranges, avocados, lettuce
**Ailments It Heals:** acne, diabetes, muscle cramps, psoriasis

3 Tbsp olive oil
1 Tbsp fresh-squeezed lime juice
1 clove garlic, minced
1½ tsp white wine vinegar

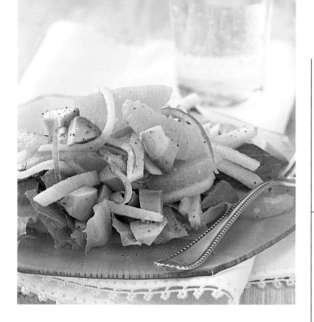

# BROCCOLI SALAD WITH ALMONDS AND DRIED CRANBERRIES

**Serves 6**
**Prep Time:** 20 minutes
**Healing Foods:** vinegar, flax, broccoli, almonds, cranberries, cheese
**Ailments It Heals:** herpes, obesity, prostate problems

¼ tsp ground cumin
⅛ tsp salt
Pinch of chili powder
8 oz (250 g) jicama, peeled and cut into 3 x ¼-in (7.5 x 0.5 cm) strips
2 oranges, peeled and cut into sections
1 avocado, peeled, pitted, and cut into chunks
½ small red onion, thinly sliced crosswise
8 cups torn romaine lettuce

**1.** In small bowl, whisk together oil, lime juice, garlic, vinegar, cumin, salt, and chili powder to make vinaigrette.

**2.** In large bowl, toss together jicama, oranges, avocado, onion, and vinaigrette. Refrigerate for 15 minutes.

**3.** Serve salad on bed of romaine leaves.

**Per serving:** 156 calories, 3 g protein, 14 g carbohydrates, 7 g fiber, 12 g total fat, 2 g saturated fat, 0 mg cholesterol, 57 mg sodium

¼ cup balsamic vinegar
2 Tbsp dijon mustard
2 Tbsp honey
¼ tsp salt
¼ tsp ground black pepper
2 Tbsp flaxseed oil
2 Tbsp extra-virgin olive oil
2 heads broccoli
1 small red onion, cut into thin wedges
½ cup whole almonds, toasted and coarsely chopped
½ cup dried cranberries
4 oz (125 g) chèvre goat cheese, crumbled

**1.** In large bowl, whisk together vinegar, mustard, honey, salt, and pepper. Whisk in oils until well blended. Set aside.

**2.** Remove florets from broccoli and add to bowl with vinaigrette. Trim ends of broccoli stalks and, with a vegetable peeler, peel off the thick outer layer. Shred stalks with a food processor or by hand.

**3.** Add shredded stalks, onion, almonds, and cranberries to bowl and toss to coat well. Top with cheese.

**Per serving:** 333 calories, 12 g protein, 33 g carbohydrates, 7 g fiber, 20 g total fat, 4 g saturated fat, 9 mg cholesterol, 303 mg sodium

# CAULIFLOWER SALAD WITH CASHEWS

**Serves 4**

**Prep Time:** 15 minutes plus marinating

**Cook Time:** 5 minutes

**Healing Foods:** cauliflower, nuts and seeds, bananas, persimmons

**Ailments It Heals:** blood pressure, bulimia, irritable bowel syndrome, muscle cramps, prostate problems

10 oz (300 g) tiny cauliflower florets

⅓ cup cashew nuts, roughly chopped

1 tsp cumin seeds

2 Tbsp fresh thyme leaves

2 bananas

Juice of ½ lemon

1 Tbsp olive oil

3 persimmons, peeled and cut into small chunks

⅓ cup snipped fresh chives

Fresh thyme sprigs

**1.** Bring saucepan of water to a boil, add cauliflower, and bring back to a full rolling boil. Drain immediately in a colander and refresh under cold running water. Leave to drain thoroughly.

**2.** In heavy-bottom frying pan, roast cashews with cumin seeds and thyme for 30 to 60 seconds, or until cashews are lightly browned. Place in bowl and set aside to cool.

**3.** Slice bananas. Put in large bowl, add lemon juice, and toss to coat. Add cauliflower, nut mixture, and oil. Toss gently to mix.

**4.** Add persimmons and chives to bowl and fold in. Cover bowl with plastic wrap and let marinate for 15 to 30 minutes.

**5.** Spoon salad into shallow serving dish and garnish with thyme sprigs.

**Per serving:** 200 calories, 4 g protein, 30 g carbohydrates, 4 g fiber, 9 g total fat, 2 g saturated fat, 0 mg cholesterol, 24 mg sodium

# FRUIT SALAD WITH SPICED COCONUT

**Serves 6**

**Prep Time:** 20 minutes plus chilling

**Healing Foods:** mangoes, cherries, grapes, strawberries, apricots, coconuts

**Ailments It Heals:** anorexia, constipation, eczema, PCOS

1 large mango, peeled and sliced

8 oz (250 g) cherries, pitted

3.5 oz (100 g) seedless green grapes

8 oz (250 g) strawberries, hulled and cut in half

3 large apricots, halved, stoned, and sliced

¾ cup unsweetened desiccated coconut

1 Tbsp sugar

Pinch of cayenne pepper

Pinch of mustard powder

**1.** In large serving bowl, place mango, cherries, grapes, strawberries, and apricots.

**2.** Finely grind the coconut in spice mill or with mortar and pestle. Add sugar, cayenne pepper, and mustard powder and mix well.

**3.** Add spiced coconut mixture to fruit and stir well to combine. Cover and refrigerate at least 2 hours, or overnight if time permits, to allow flavors to blend and develop.

**Per serving:** 181 calories, 2 g protein, 28 g carbohydrates, 4 g fiber, 8 g total fat, 6 g saturated fat, 0 mg cholesterol, 4 mg sodium

# ENDIVE, APPLE, AND WATERCRESS SALAD

Serves 6
**Prep Time:** 10 minutes
**Healing Foods:** yogurt, salad greens, apples, almonds
**Ailments It Heals:** blood pressure, cancer, depression, fibroids, sex drive (diminished)

⅓ cup low-fat plain yogurt
1 Tbsp reduced-fat mayonnaise
2 tsp honey
1 tsp Dijon mustard
¼ tsp curry powder
⅛ tsp ground ginger
1 bunch watercress, tough stems removed
1 large endive, halved lengthwise and cut crosswise into ½-in-thick (1 cm) slices
1 McIntosh apple, halved, cored, and thinly sliced
2 Tbsp sliced or slivered almonds, toasted

**1.** In small bowl, whisk together yogurt, mayonnaise, honey, mustard, curry powder, and ginger to make dressing.

**2.** In large bowl, toss together watercress, endive, apple, and dressing. Top with almonds.

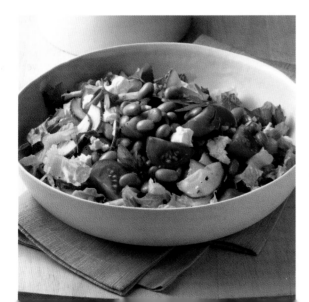

**Per serving:** 54 calories, 2 g protein, 8 g carbohydrates, 1 g fiber, 2 g total fat, 0 g saturated fat, 2 mg cholesterol, 62 mg sodium

# MEDITERRANEAN SALAD WITH EDAMAME

Serves 8
**Prep Time:** 25 minutes
**Cook Time:** 4 minutes
**Healing Foods:** edamame, garlic, lettuce, tomatoes, olives, cheese
**Ailments It Heals:** atherosclerosis, Alzheimer's disease, hyperthyroidism, menopause, stroke

1 cup frozen shelled edamame beans
⅓ cup extra-virgin olive oil
3 Tbsp lemon juice
2 cloves garlic, minced
Salt to taste
¼ tsp sugar
Ground black pepper to taste
2 cups shredded romaine lettuce
2 cups cherry tomatoes, halved
1 cup sliced English cucumber
⅔ cup chopped scallions
½ cup pitted kalamata olives, halved
½ cup fresh mint leaves, washed, dried, and torn into ½-in (1 cm) pieces
½ cup fresh flat-leaf parsley leaves, washed, dried, and torn into ½-in (1 cm) pieces
1 cup crumbled feta cheese

**1.** Bring large saucepan of lightly salted water to a boil. Add edamame beans and cook, covered, over medium heat for 3 to 4 minutes, or until tender. Drain and rinse with cold running water.

**2.** In screw-top jar with tight-fitting lid, combine oil, lemon juice, garlic, salt, sugar, and pepper. Shake to blend.

**3.** In large bowl, combine lettuce, tomatoes, cucumber, scallions, olives, mint, parsley, and edamame beans. Just before serving, drizzle lemon dressing over salad and toss to coat well. Sprinkle each serving with cheese.

**Per serving:** 220 calories, 7 g protein, 10 g carbohydrates, 3 g fiber, 17 g total fat, 5 g saturated fat, 15 mg cholesterol, 427 mg sodium

# PAPAYA AND AVOCADO SALAD

Serves 4
**Prep Time:** 15 minutes
**Cook Time:** 1 minute
**Healing Foods:** peppers, avocados, papayas, olive oil, seeds
**Ailments It Heals:** cirrhosis, diabetes, gallstones, hypothyroidism, multiple sclerosis

**Salad**

1   romaine lettuce head
2   scallions, thinly sliced
1   large orange or yellow bell pepper, seeded and cut into thin strips
1   medium avocado, peeled, pitted, and cut into 1-in (2.5 cm) slices
1   medium papaya, peeled, seeded, and cut into 1-in (2.5 cm) slices
Juice of 1 lime
1½  Tbsp olive oil
¼   tsp paprika
⅛   tsp ground cumin
1   tsp light brown sugar
4   Tbsp pumpkin seeds

**1.** Shred lettuce leaves and place in large shallow dish or on 4 individual dishes. Sprinkle scallions over lettuce.

**2.** Arrange peppers over lettuce. Scatter avocado and papaya over pepper.

**3.** In small bowl, whisk together lime juice, oil, paprika, cumin, and sugar. Pour over salad.

**4.** Heat small heavy saucepan over medium heat and add pumpkin seeds. Stir for 1 minute, or until lightly toasted. Sprinkle seeds over salad and serve.

**Per serving:** 242 calories, 8 g protein, 19 g carbohydrates, 5 g fiber, 17 g total fat, 3 g saturated fat, 0 mg cholesterol, 18 mg sodium

# POTATO SALAD WITH SUN-DRIED TOMATOES, SCALLIONS, AND BASIL

Serves 6
**Prep Time:** 10 minutes
**Cook Time:** 15 minutes
**Healing Foods:** potatoes, onions, tomatoes
**Ailments It Heals:** jet lag, menstrual problems, prostate problems

1½  lb (750 g) small red potatoes, unpeeled and halved
2   Tbsp reduced-fat mayonnaise
2   tsp dijon mustard
¼   cup low-fat buttermilk
2   scallions, thinly sliced
¼   cup chopped sun-dried tomatoes (not oil-packed)

8 basil leaves, shredded or finely chopped

½ tsp salt

¼ tsp ground black pepper

**1.** In large pot of lightly salted boiling water, cook potatoes over medium-high heat for 10 to 15 minutes, or until tender. Drain well.

**2.** In small bowl, stir together mayonnaise and mustard. Stir in buttermilk.

**3.** In large bowl, combine potatoes, scallions, sun-dried tomatoes, basil, salt, and pepper. Add buttermilk dressing. Toss to coat.

**Per serving:** 103 calories, 4 g protein, 17 g carbohydrates, 3 g fiber, 2 g total fat, 0 g saturated fat, 2 mg cholesterol, 340 mg sodium

# ROMAINE LETTUCE WITH CHUNKY TOMATO VINAIGRETTE

Serves 6

**Prep Time:** 12 minutes

**Healing Foods:** tomatoes, basil, olive oil, lettuce, cheese

**Ailments It Heals:** gout, osteoporosis, prostate problems, urinary tract infections

2 large ripe tomatoes, halved, seeded, and coarsely chopped

⅓ cup loosely packed fresh basil leaves

2 Tbsp ketchup

2 Tbsp olive oil

1 Tbsp balsamic vinegar

1 small clove garlic, minced

½ tsp salt

1 large head romaine lettuce, torn into bite-size pieces

¼ cup crumbled feta cheese

**1.** In food processor, combine tomatoes, basil, ketchup, oil, vinegar, garlic, and salt to make vinaigrette. Pulse until blended but still chunky.

**2.** In large bowl, toss romaine with vinaigrette. Sprinkle with cheese. Serve at once.

**Per serving:** 82 calories, 3 g protein, 5 g carbohydrates, 2 g fiber, 6 g total fat, 2 g saturated fat, 6 mg cholesterol, 237 mg sodium

# SPINACH, SWEET POTATO, AND SHIITAKE SALAD

Serves 4

**Prep Time:** 10 minutes

**Cook Time:** 30 minutes

**Healing Foods:** sweet potatoes, nuts, olive oil, mushrooms, spinach

**Ailments It Heals:** alcoholism, depression, hypothyroidism, memory loss

1 lb (500 g) sweet potatoes, peeled, halved lengthwise, and cut crosswise into ½-in (1 cm) slices

⅓ cup walnuts

1 Tbsp plus 4 tsp olive oil

2 cloves garlic, slivered

12 oz (375 g) fresh shiitake mushrooms, stems discarded and caps thickly sliced

½ tsp salt

12 cups spinach leaves

½ cup red wine vinegar

1 Tbsp dijon mustard

**1.** Preheat oven to 400°F (200°C). Place sweet potatoes on lightly oiled baking sheet and bake for 15 to 20 minutes, or until tender. Toast walnuts in separate pan in oven for 5 to 7 minutes, or until crisp. When cool enough to handle, coarsely chop nuts.

**2.** In large skillet, heat 1 Tbsp oil over medium heat. Add garlic and cook for 30 seconds, or until fragrant.

**3.** Add half the mushrooms, sprinkle with ¼ tsp salt, and cook for 4 minutes, or until they begin to soften. Add remaining mushrooms and ¼ tsp salt, and cook for 5 minutes, or until mushrooms are tender.

**4.** Place spinach in large bowl. Add sweet potatoes and walnuts. Remove mushrooms from skillet with slotted spoon and add to bowl.

**5.** In same s til warm. Pour dressing over salad and toss to combine.

**Per serving:** 283 calories, 9 g protein, 32 g carbohydrates, 8 g fiber, 15 g total fat, 2 g saturated fat, 0 mg cholesterol, 524 mg sodium

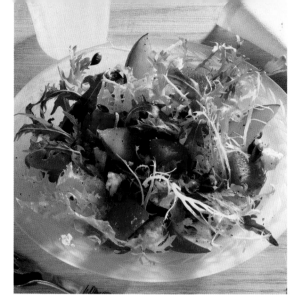

3  Tbsp olive oil
2  Tbsp fresh-squeezed lemon juice
¼  tsp salt
¼  tsp ground black pepper
1  small watermelon (about 1 lb or 500 g)
2  large nectarines or peaches
6  cups mixed salad greens, including arugula, endive, and leaf lettuce
1  cup crumbled feta cheese
2  Tbsp toasted pumpkin seeds or sunflower seeds

**1.** In 2-cup jar or container with tight-fitting lid, place oil, lemon juice, salt, and pepper. Cover and shake until well blended.

**2.** Using serrated knife, cut watermelon into bite-size chunks, discarding rind and seeds. Toss into large salad bowl.

**3.** Cut nectarines in half (do not peel) and pit them. Place nectarines on cutting board, cut side down, and cut lengthwise into thin slices. Toss with watermelon. Tear salad greens into bite-size pieces, add to fruit, and toss to mix.

**4.** Crumble cheese over salad. Sprinkle seeds over top, drizzle with lemon dressing, and serve.

**Per serving:** 198 calories, 6 g protein, 13 g carbohydrates, 2 g fiber, 15 g total fat, 5 g saturated fat, 22 mg cholesterol, 386 mg sodium

# WATERMELON AND FETA SALAD

**Serves 4**
**Prep Time: 20 minutes**
**Healing Foods: watermelon, nectarines, salad greens, cheese, seeds**
**Ailments It Heals: bulimia, chronic fatigue syndrome, jet lag, prostate problems**

# CARAWAY-COATED PEPPER STEAK WITH CHERRY SAUCE

**Serves 4**
**Prep Time:** 20 minutes
**Cook Time:** 20 minutes
**Healing Foods:** seeds, beef, cherries
**Ailments It Heals:** anemia, shingles, yeast infections

1 Tbsp coarsely cracked black peppercorns
2 tsp caraway seeds
4 lean sirloin steaks (about 4 oz or 125 g each)
1 Tbsp olive oil
1 medium red onion, finely chopped
1 cup dry red wine
20 oz (600 g) frozen pitted sweet cherries, thawed, drained, and coarsely chopped
2 tsp dijon mustard
1 Tbsp red wine vinegar
½ tsp salt
¼ tsp ground ginger
¼ cup chopped parsley

**1.** In shallow bowl, combine peppercorns and caraway seeds. Dip steaks in spice mixture, pressing it into both sides.

**2.** In large nonstick skillet, heat oil over medium heat. Add steaks and cook for 3 minutes per side for medium-rare. Transfer steaks to platter and keep warm.

**3.** Add onion to skillet and sauté for 4 minutes, or until tender. Add wine, increase heat to high, and cook for 2 minutes. Stir in cherries, mustard, vinegar, salt, and ginger. Cook for 5 minutes, or until cherries are very tender.

**4.** Return steaks to skillet and cook for 1 minute per side to heat through. Transfer steaks to 4 plates. Stir parsley into sauce and spoon sauce over steaks.

**Per serving:** 351 calories, 27 g protein, 30 g carbohydrate, 4 g fiber, 10 g total fat, 3 g saturated fat, 69 mg cholesterol, 425 mg sodium

# FLANK STEAK ROLL WITH CARROTS AND RED PEPPERS

**Serves 6**
**Prep Time:** 15 minutes plus marinating and standing
**Cook Time:** 40 minutes
**Healing Foods:** beef, spinach, onions, carrots, peppers
**Ailments It Heals:** hepatitis, memory loss, obesity

½ cup red wine
⅓ cup reduced-sodium soy sauce
2 Tbsp sugar
1 tsp garlic powder
1½ lb flank steak, butterflied
6 oz (175 g) fresh baby spinach leaves
4 scallions, coarsely chopped
⅛ tsp salt
2½ cups grated peeled carrots (1 lb or 500 g)
12 oz (375 g) roasted red peppers, drained

**1.** In large resealable plastic bag or container, combine red wine, soy sauce, sugar, and garlic powder. Add steak. Turn to coat. Refrigerate for at least 2 hours or up to 4 hours.

**2.** Meanwhile, rinse spinach and leave some water clinging to leaves. Place in large pot over medium

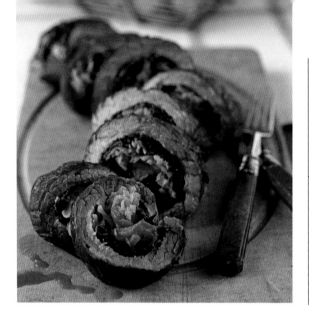

# POT ROAST WITH ROOT VEGETABLES

**Serves 6**
**Prep Time:** 30 minutes
**Cook Time:** 3 hours 5 minutes plus resting
**Healing Foods:** beef, onions, potatoes, celeriac, turnips, carrots
**Ailments It Heals:** anemia, herpes, menstrual problems

heat. Cook, stirring often, for 1 minute, or just until wilted. Transfer to plate. Let cool.

**3.** Preheat oven to 375°F (190°C).

**4.** Remove meat from marinade. Pat dry and lay on work surface. Set marinade aside. Spread spinach in even layer over steak. Top with scallions. Sprinkle with salt. Layer carrots on top, then red peppers. Starting at one long side of steak, roll up meat tightly to enclose filling. Secure seam in several spots with wooden picks. Place roll, seam side down, in shallow baking pan. Brush top with marinade.

**5.** Roast for 15 minutes. Spoon any juices in pan over top of meat. Roast for 20 minutes longer for medium-rare, or until desired doneness. Let meat stand for 10 minutes.

**6.** Meanwhile, in small saucepan, boil remaining marinade just until it's thick enough to coat a spoon. Strain and set aside.

**7.** Cut meat diagonally into ¼-in-thick (0.5 cm) slices. Drizzle a little marinade on each plate. Top with steak slices.

**Per serving:** 229 calories, 21 g protein, 15 g carbohydrates, 2 g fiber, 9 g total fat, 4 g saturated fat, 48 mg cholesterol, 738 mg sodium

1   tsp extra-virgin olive oil
2   lb (1 kg) boneless beef chuck, about 3 in or 7.5 cm thick, trimmed of fat and tied
2   large onions, finely chopped
1   celery stalk, finely chopped
3   cloves garlic, crushed
1   cup dry red or white wine
1   cup canned chopped tomatoes
1   large carrot, grated, and 4 medium carrots, sliced
1   tsp chopped fresh thyme
2   cups beef stock, preferably homemade
21  oz (625 g) new potatoes, scrubbed and quartered
12  oz (375 g) celeriac, cut into 1-in (2.5 cm) cubes
12  oz (375 g) rutabaga, cut into 1-in (2.5 cm) cubes
Salt and ground black pepper
¼   cup chopped fresh parsley

**1.** Preheat oven to 325°F (160°C). Heat oil in large flameproof casserole dish. Add beef and brown over a medium-high heat for 6 to 8 minutes, or until well colored. Remove to plate.

**2.** Reduce heat to medium. Add onions, celery, and garlic and cook, stirring frequently, for 3 minutes, or until onions begin to soften. Add wine and let it bubble for about 1 minute, then add tomatoes and grated carrot. Cook for 2 minutes.

3. Return beef to casserole dish, together with any juices, and add thyme. Tuck a piece of foil around top of meat, turning back corners so it doesn't touch liquid, then cover with a tight-fitting lid. Transfer to oven and cook for 2½ hours.

4. About 20 minutes before end of cooking time, bring stock to a boil in deep saucepan with a lid. Add potatoes, celeriac, rutabaga, and sliced carrots. Cover and simmer gently for 12 to 15 minutes, or until just starting to become tender.

5. Remove beef from casserole dish and set aside. Remove any fat from cooking liquid. In blender, combine cooking liquid and vegetables from casserole dish. Puree until smooth. Season with salt and pepper to taste.

6. Drain potatoes and other root vegetables, reserving liquid. In casserole dish, layer half the root vegetables on bottom, put beef on top, and add remaining root vegetables and their cooking liquid. Pour pureed sauce over top. Cover casserole, return to oven, and cook for 20 minutes, or until root vegetables are tender.

7. Remove beef to carving board, cover, and let rest for 10 minutes. Keep vegetables and sauce warm. Carve beef and arrange on warmed plates with vegetables and sauce. Sprinkle with parsley and serve immediately.

**Per serving:** 393 calories, 39 g protein, 35 g carbohydrates, 7 g fiber, 8 g total fat, 3 g saturated fat, 98 mg cholesterol, 688 mg sodium

# SPINACH-STUFFED MEAT LOAF

Serves 8
**Prep Time:** 45 minutes plus standing
**Cook Time:** 58 minutes
**Healing Foods:** onions, tomatoes, spinach, beef, pork, carrots
**Ailments It Heals:** bleeding problems, diabetes, Parkinson's disease, stress

- 1 tsp olive oil
- 2 large onions, finely chopped
- 6 cloves garlic, crushed, or to taste
- 24 oz (680 mL) chopped tomatoes
- ⅔ cup low-fat, reduced-sodium chicken broth
- 1 tsp dried mixed herbs (try basil, oregano, and thyme)

Salt and ground black pepper

- 1 lb (500 g) fresh spinach leaves
- 2 Tbsp low-fat plain yogurt
- ½ tsp freshly grated nutmeg
- 1 lb (500 g) lean (93%) ground beef
- 1 lb (500 g) lean ground pork
- 1 celery stalk, finely chopped
- 1 large carrot, grated
- ½ cup rolled oats
- 2 tsp chopped fresh thyme
- 5 Tbsp low-fat milk
- 1 egg, beaten
- 2 tsp dijon mustard

1. Heat oil in saucepan over medium heat. Add onions and garlic and cook for 5 minutes, or until onions are soft.

2. Transfer half of onion mixture to large bowl and set aside. Stir tomatoes (with their juice), broth, and mixed herbs into onions in saucepan. Season lightly with salt and pepper. Bring to a boil, then cover, reduce heat, and simmer sauce very gently.

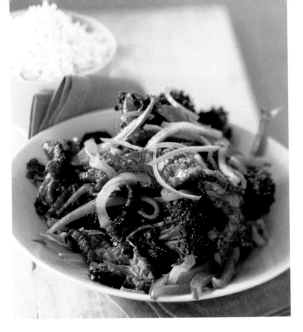

**3.** Preheat oven to 350°F (180°C). Put spinach in large saucepan, cover with tight-fitting lid, and cook over high heat for 2 to 3 minutes, or until the leaves are wilted. Drain spinach, squeeze it dry with your hands, then chop it roughly and put into a bowl. Stir in yogurt and season with ¼ tsp nutmeg and salt and pepper to taste.

**4.** Put beef and pork into bowl with reserved onion mixture. Add celery, carrot, oats, thyme, milk, egg, mustard, and remaining ¼ tsp nutmeg. Season with salt and pepper. Mix ingredients together with your hands.

**5.** Lay large sheet of plastic wrap on work surface and place meat mixture in center. With a spatula, spread meat into a 9 x 7-in (23 x 18 cm) rectangle. Spread spinach mixture evenly over meat, leaving a ½-in (1 cm) border. Starting at a short end, roll up meat and spinach. Pat sides and place on nonstick baking sheet, discarding plastic wrap.

**6.** Place meat loaf, uncovered, in the center of oven and cook for 45 minutes, then remove and brush lightly with a little tomato sauce. Return to oven and cook for 5 minutes to set glaze and brown slightly. To check if meat loaf is cooked through, insert a skewer into the center and remove after a few seconds. It should feel very hot when lightly placed on the back of your hand. When meat loaf is ready, remove from oven, cover loosely with foil, and leave to stand for 10 minutes.

**Per serving:** 250 calories, 30 g protein, 17 g carbohydrates, 5 g fiber, 7 g total fat, 2 g saturated fat, 99 mg cholesterol, 380 mg sodium

# ORANGE BEEF WITH BROCCOLI AND JICAMA

Serves 4
**Prep Time:** 20 minutes plus marinating
**Cook Time:** 11 minutes
**Healing Foods:** beef, broccoli, peppers, jicama
**Ailments It Heals:** anemia, hepatitis, herpes

| | |
|---|---|
| 12 | oz (375 g) flank steak |
| 2 | tsp cornstarch |
| ¼ | cup dry sherry |
| 2 | Tbsp reduced-sodium soy sauce |
| ¼ | tsp baking soda |
| 4 | tsp olive oil |
| 4 | Tbsp finely slivered orange zest |
| ¼ | tsp crushed red-pepper flakes |
| 5 | cups broccoli florets and stems |
| 1 | red bell pepper, cut into matchsticks |
| 4 | scallions, thinly sliced |
| 3 | cloves garlic, minced |
| ½ | cup plus 1/3 cup water |
| 1 | cup jicama matchsticks |

1. Halve flank steak lengthwise (with grain), then cut each piece crosswise (against grain) into thin slices.

2. In medium bowl, whisk together cornstarch, sherry, soy sauce, and baking soda until well combined. Add flank steak, tossing to coat. Refrigerate for 30 minutes.

3. In large nonstick skillet, heat 3 tsp oil over medium heat. Remove beef from marinade, reserving marinade. Add beef, 2 Tbsp orange zest, and pepper flakes and cook for 3 minutes, or until beef is just cooked through. Transfer beef to a plate.

4. Add remaining 1 tsp oil to skillet along with broccoli, bell pepper, scallions, and garlic. Cook for 3 minutes, or until broccoli begins to soften. Add ½ cup water and cook for 2 to 3 minutes, or until broccoli is crisp-tender.

5. Stir ⅓ cup water into reserved marinade and add to skillet. Bring to a boil and cook, stirring constantly, for 1 minute, or until sauce is slightly thickened. Return beef to skillet. Add jicama and cook for 1 minute, just until beef is heated through. Serve garnished with remaining 2 Tbsp orange zest.

**Per serving:** 255 calories, 23 g protein, 18 g carbohydrate, 6 g fiber, 10 g total fat, 2 g saturated fat, 53 mg cholesterol, 601 mg sodium

# CALF'S LIVER WITH RIGATONI

Serves 6
**Prep Time:** 40 minutes
**Cook Time:** 20 minutes
**Healing Foods:** broccoli, liver, oranges, pasta,
**Ailments It Heals:** anemia, bleeding problems, dental problems, infertility, sex drive (diminished)

10 oz (300 g) calf's liver, trimmed
2 large oranges
14.5 oz (435 g) rigatoni, penne, or other pasta shapes
8 oz (250 g) broccoli, cut into 1-in (2.5 cm) pieces
2 Tbsp extra-virgin olive oil
1 clove garlic, crushed
1 small fresh red chile, seeded and finely chopped
4 Tbsp marsala or medium sherry
Salt and ground black pepper
1 tsp balsamic vinegar
2 tsp butter
1 tsp crushed roasted coriander seeds (optional)

1. Cut liver into strips about ½ in (1 cm) wide and 2 in (5 cm) long. Use citrus zester to take zest off one orange in short strips. Set strips aside. Peel and segment both oranges, working over a bowl to catch juice. Squeeze juice from peel, too. Set aside the 12 best segments, then squeeze remaining segments into juice bowl to get about 4 Tbsp juice in total.

2. Drop pasta into large saucepan of boiling water. When water returns to a boil, cook for 10 minutes. Add broccoli and cook for 2 to 3 minutes, or until pasta and broccoli are just tender.

3. Meanwhile, heat 1 Tbsp oil in frying pan large enough to cook liver in one layer. Sprinkle in garlic and chile and cook, stirring, over medium-high heat for 1 minute. Add liver and toss for 1 minute, or until browned. Add marsala (or sherry) and orange zest strips and juice and cook for 1 minute.

4. Drain pasta and broccoli and return them to saucepan off heat. Remove liver from sauce and add to pasta and broccoli. Add remaining 1 Tbsp oil and salt and pepper to taste. Toss well.

5. Bring sauce to a boil and boil to reduce by half, about 5 minutes. Stir in vinegar and butter to make sauce glossy. Add reserved orange segments

and warm through for 30 seconds, then spoon over liver, pasta, and broccoli and toss gently to combine. Sprinkle with coriander seeds, if using, and serve immediately.

**Per serving:** 418 calories, 21 g protein, 62 g carbohydrates, 4 g fiber, 9 g total fat, 2 g saturated fat, 133 mg cholesterol, 59 mg sodium

# GREEK LAMB KEBABS

Serves 4
**Prep Time:** 20 minutes plus soaking
**Cook Time:** 8 minutes
**Healing Foods:** garlic, lamb, tomatoes, cabbage, mint, wheat
**Ailments It Heals:** ADHD, alcoholism, hepatitis, prostate problems

### Kebabs
1  Tbsp olive oil
2  large cloves garlic, crushed
Juice of 1 lemon
1  Tbsp chopped fresh oregano
1  lb (500 g) boneless leg of lamb, trimmed of all fat and cut into 1-in (2.5 cm) cubes
4  white or whole wheat pita breads, cut into triangles

### Salad
3  tomatoes, thickly sliced
1  small red onion, finely chopped
½  cup shredded green cabbage
4  Tbsp chopped fresh mint
1  cucumber, halved and thinly sliced
Juice of 1 lemon
2  tsp olive oil
Salt and ground black pepper

1. To make kebabs: Soak 4 wooden skewers in cold water for 30 minutes. Drain. Preheat grill or heat ridged cast-iron grill pan. Put oil, garlic, lemon juice, and oregano in bowl and stir to mix together. Add lamb and turn until very well coated. Thread cubes onto skewers.

2. Cook lamb on grill or grill pan, turning frequently, for 7 to 8 minutes, or until tender. Toward end of cooking, warm pita bread on grill or grill pan.

3. To make salad: In salad bowl, combine tomatoes, onion, cabbage, mint, cucumber, lemon juice, and oil and season to taste with salt and pepper. Toss together gently.

4. Serve kebabs with salad, and pita bread.

**Per serving:** 408 calories, 27 g protein, 46 g carbohydrates, 4 g fiber, 13 g total fat, 3 g saturated fat, 62 mg cholesterol, 389 mg sodium

# HONEY-ROASTED RACK OF LAMB

Serves 4
**Prep Time:** 20 minutes plus standing
**Cook Time:** 40 minutes to 1 hour
**Healing Foods:** zucchini, parsnips, carrots, peppers, lamb
**Ailments It Heals:** anemia, burns, shingles

3  Tbsp honey
3  Tbsp lemon juice
3  Tbsp reduced-sodium soy sauce
2  cloves garlic, crushed
4  zucchini, cut into strips
4  parsnips, peeled and cut into strips
4  carrots, peeled and cut into strips
1  celery stalk, halved lengthways then cut into 4-in (10 cm) lengths

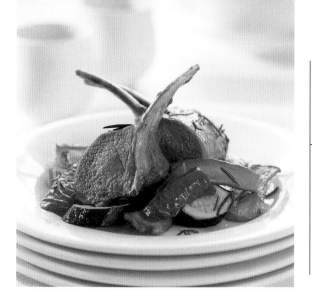

# SKILLET OKRA AND LAMB

**Serves 4**
**Prep Time:** 10 minutes
**Cook Time:** 31 minutes
**Healing Foods:** onions, garlic, lamb, tomatoes, okra
**Ailments It Heals:** constipation, obesity, prostate problems

| | |
|---|---|
| 1 | red bell pepper, cut into strips |
| 6 | sprigs fresh rosemary |
| 2 | cups lamb or beef stock |
| 2 | well-trimmed (frenched) lamb racks (8 cutlets each) |

**1.** Preheat oven to 400°F (200°C). In medium bowl, combine honey, lemon juice, soy sauce, and garlic. Set aside.

**2.** Lightly coat large baking dish with cooking spray. Add zucchini, parsnips, carrots, celery, and peppers and roast for 20 minutes, or until vegetables are lightly browned.

**3.** Top vegetables with rosemary and pour on stock. Arrange lamb racks on top of vegetables, baste with reserved honey sauce, and roast for 20 minutes for rare (lamb will be pink), 30 minutes for medium, or 40 minutes for well done. Continue basting with sauce occasionally while cooking.

**4.** Remove baking dish from oven and put lamb racks and vegetables on a platter. Cover and let rest for 10 minutes before carving meat.

**5.** Boil pan sauce and juices until they thicken slightly. Serve with lamb and vegetables.

**Per serving:** 435 calories, 42 g protein, 42 g carbohydrates, 7 g fiber, 11 g total fat, 5 g saturated fat, 109 mg cholesterol, 856 mg sodium

| | |
|---|---|
| 1 | Tbsp olive oil |
| 2 | onions, finely chopped |
| 2 | cloves garlic, minced |
| ½ | lb (250 g) ground lamb |
| 1 | tomato, seeded and finely chopped |
| 1 | cup water |
| ¼ | cup tomato paste |
| ¾ | tsp salt |
| ⅛ | tsp ground black pepper |
| 1 | lb (500 g) okra, trimmed |
| 2 | Tbsp fresh-squeezed lemon juice |
| 1 | Tbsp finely chopped cilantro (optional) |

**1.** In large nonstick skillet, heat oil over medium heat. Add onions and sauté for 5 minutes, or until softened. Add garlic and sauté for 1 minute. Add lamb and cook, breaking up meat with wooden spoon, for 5 minutes, or until browned. Drain off any fat.

**2.** Stir in tomato, water, tomato paste, salt, and pepper. Top with okra and sprinkle with lemon juice. Cover and cook for 15 minutes, or until okra is tender. Uncover and simmer for 5 minutes to reduce liquid. Sprinkle with cilantro before serving, if desired.

**Per serving:** 245 calories, 15 g protein, 21 g carbohydrates, 6 g fiber, 12 g total fat, 4 g saturated fat, 41 mg cholesterol, 492 mg sodium

# TUSCAN VEAL CHOPS

**Per serving:** 219 calories, 24 g protein, 16 g carbohydrates, 5 g fiber, 6 g total fat, 2 g saturated fat, 110 mg cholesterol, 501 mg sodium

**Serves 2**
**Prep Time:** 15 minutes
**Cook Time:** 15 minutes
**Healing Foods:** veal, carrots, tomatoes, green beans, onions
**Ailments It Heals:** anemia, lactose intolerance, obesity

2   bone-in rib or loin veal chops (¾ in or 1.5 cm thick, about 5 oz or 150 g each)
¼   tsp ground black pepper
1   large carrot, cut into matchsticks
1   medium tomato, cut into 8 wedges
4   oz (125 g) green beans
1   small red onion, thinly sliced
¼   cup fat-free Italian dressing
2   Tbsp dry white wine
1   tsp chopped rosemary

**1.** Season chops on both sides with pepper. Put in shallow dish with carrot, tomato, green beans, and onion. In jar with tight-fitting lid, shake dressing and wine until mixed. Drizzle over chops and vegetables and toss to coat. Let stand at room temperature for 5 minutes.

**2.** Coat nonstick ridged grill pan or grill rack with cooking spray. Set grill pan over medium heat or preheat grill to medium. Cook or grill chops until golden brown but still slightly pink in center, about 7 minutes on each side for medium.

**3.** Meanwhile, coat large nonstick skillet with cooking spray. Transfer vegetables and any liquid remaining in dish to skillet and sprinkle with rosemary. Sauté over medium-high heat for 6 minutes, or just until vegetables are tender. To serve, divide vegetables evenly between 2 plates and top with veal chop.

# PORK CHOPS AND CABBAGE

**Serves 4**
**Prep Time:** 20 minutes
**Cook Time:** 25 minutes
**Healing Foods:** pork, onions, cabbage, carrots
**Ailments It Heals:** alcoholism, celiac disease, herpes, osteoporosis, shingles

1   tsp dried thyme
¼   tsp salt
¼   tsp ground black pepper plus more to taste
1   lb (500 g) thin-cut boneless pork chops, trimmed
1   Tbsp canola oil
1   cup sliced onion (1 medium)
5   cups shredded green cabbage (½ medium head)
½   cup sliced carrots (2 medium)
1¾  cups reduced-sodium chicken broth
¾   cup water
2   tsp coarse-grain mustard
1   tsp apple cider vinegar

**1.** In small bowl, combine thyme, salt, and pepper. Rub mixture over pork chops. Heat 2 tsp oil in large nonstick skillet over medium heat. Add chops and cook for 2 to 3 minutes per side, or until browned and just cooked through. Transfer to plate, cover loosely with foil, and keep warm.

**2.** Add remaining 1 tsp oil to skillet. Add onion and cook over medium heat, stirring frequently, for 1 to 2 minutes, or until softened. Add cabbage and carrots and cook, stirring, for 2 minutes, or until cabbage is wilted. Add broth and water and bring to a simmer. Cover and cook for 10 to 15 minutes,

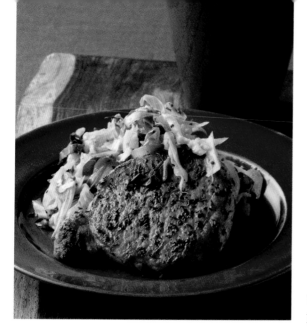

or until cabbage is tender. Stir in mustard and vinegar and season with pepper.

**3.** Serve pork chops over cabbage mixture.

**Per serving:** 224 calories, 24 g protein, 9 g carbohydrates, 3 g fiber, 10 g total fat, 2 g saturated fat, 57 mg cholesterol, 564 mg sodium

# ROASTED PORK WITH POMEGRANATE SAUCE

**Serves 4**
**Prep Time:** 10 minutes
**Cook Time:** 51 minutes
**Healing Foods:** butternut squash, onions, pork, pomegranates
**Ailments It Heals:** alcoholism, burns, herpes

- 4 cups cubed (1 in or 2.5 cm pieces) peeled butternut squash (1 lb 2 oz or 560g)
- 2 cups whole shallots or cipollini onions, peeled

- 1 Tbsp plus 2 tsp olive oil
- ½ tsp salt
- ½ tsp ground black pepper
- 1 tsp ground cumin
- 1 tsp brown sugar
- ½ tsp ground coriander
- ¼ tsp cayenne pepper
- 1 lb (500 g) pork tenderloin, trimmed
- ¾ cup unsweetened pomegranate juice
- ¾ cup reduced-sodium chicken broth
- 3 Tbsp water
- 1 tsp cornstarch

**1.** Preheat oven to 425°F (220°C). Coat large roasting pan or baking sheet with sides with cooking spray.

**2.** In medium bowl, combine squash, shallots, 1 Tbsp oil, ¼ tsp salt, and ¼ tsp pepper and toss to coat. Spread vegetables in pan and bake for 15 minutes.

**3.** Meanwhile, in small bowl, mix cumin, brown sugar, coriander, cayenne, and remaining ¼ tsp salt and ¼ tsp pepper. Pat pork dry and rub with spice mixture.

**4.** Heat remaining 2 tsp oil in large nonstick skillet over medium-high heat. Add pork and cook, for 4 minutes, turning occasionally, until browned on all sides.

**5.** Stir vegetables and push them to sides of pan. Place pork in center. Bake, stirring vegetables occasionally, for 20 to 25 minutes, or until pork is just cooked through (an instant-read thermometer inserted in center should register 155°F or 68°C; temperature will rise to 160°F or 71°C during resting) and vegetables are tender.

**6.** Meanwhile, add pomegranate juice and chicken broth to skillet and bring to a boil. Boil for 10 minutes, or until reduced to ⅔ cup. In small bowl, mix 3 Tbsp water and cornstarch, then add to sauce and cook, stirring, for 1 minute, or until slightly thickened.

**7.** Transfer vegetables to a bowl and pork to a cutting board. Let pork rest for 5 minutes before carving. Cut into ½-in-thick (1 cm) slices and serve with vegetables and sauce.

**Per serving:** 316 calories, 27 g protein, 31 g carbohydrates, 4 g fiber, 11 g total fat, 3 g saturated fat, 65 mg cholesterol, 452 mg sodium

# WHOLE WHEAT PASTA WITH SAUSAGE AND GREENS

**Serves 6**
**Prep Time:** 25 minutes
**Cook Time:** 23 minutes
**Healing Foods:** turkey, garlic, tomatoes, beans, pasta, cooking greens
**Ailments It Heals:** menstrual problems, obesity, sex drive (diminished)

- 1 link (4 oz or 125 g) hot Italian turkey sausage, casing removed
- 1 tsp olive oil
- ¾ cup chopped onion (1 small)
- 3 cloves garlic, minced
- 15 oz (425 mL) no-salt-added diced tomatoes
- 8 oz (225 mL) no-salt-added tomato sauce
- 15.5 oz (440 mL) cannellini beans, drained and rinsed
- ¼ cup water
- Ground black pepper to taste
- 4 cups whole wheat pasta, fusilli, penne, or rigatoni
- 1 bunch (1 lb or 500 g) Swiss chard, stems trimmed, leaves washed, and torn into bite-size pieces
- 6 Tbsp grated parmesan cheese

**1.** Bring large pot of lightly salted water to a boil. In large nonstick skillet, cook sausage over medium heat, crumbling it with wooden spoon, for 3 to 5 minutes, or until browned. Transfer sausage to paper towel–lined plate to drain.

**2.** Add oil to skillet. Add onion and cook over medium heat, stirring often, for 1 to 2 minutes, or until softened. Add garlic and cook, stirring, for 10 to 20 seconds. Add diced tomatoes and mash with wooden spoon. Add tomato sauce, beans, water, and sausage. Bring to a simmer. Cook, uncovered, at a lively simmer over medium-low heat, stirring occasionally, for 10 to 15 minutes, or until flavors have blended. Season with pepper.

**3.** Meanwhile, add pasta to boiling water and cook for 5 minutes. Add Swiss chard and stir to immerse. Cook for 3 to 5 minutes, or until pasta is just tender and chard has wilted. Drain well and transfer to large bowl. Toss with the tomato mixture. Sprinkle each serving with cheese.

**Per serving:** 390 calories, 19 g protein, 65 g carbohydrates, 11 g fiber, 6 g total fat, 1 g saturated fat, 22 mg cholesterol, 409 mg sodium

# ASPARAGUS AND CHICKEN STIR-FRY

**Serves 4**
**Prep Time:** 15 minutes
**Cook Time:** 10 minutes
**Healing Foods:** onions, chicken, asparagus, peas
**Ailments It Heals:** indigestion and heartburn, nail problems, peptic ulcers

- 1 Tbsp vegetable oil
- 3 scallions, thinly sliced
- ¾ lb (375 g) boneless, skinless chicken breasts, cut for stir-fry

12 oz (375 g) asparagus, trimmed and cut into
   long lengths on the diagonal
8 oz (250 g) sugar snap peas or snow peas
½ cup chicken stock
½ tsp grated lemon zest, plus extra to garnish
1 Tbsp light soy sauce
½ cup plus 1 Tbsp water
1 tsp cornstarch

**1.** In wok or large frying pan, heat half of oil over medium heat. Add spring onions and stir-fry for 1 minute, or until just wilted. Add chicken and stir-fry for 3 minutes, or until chicken is no longer pink.

**2.** Add remaining oil and asparagus and toss for 2 minutes to coat.

**3.** Add peas, stock, lemon zest, soy sauce, and ½ cup water and bring to a boil. Reduce to a simmer and stir-fry for 2 minutes, or until chicken and asparagus are just cooked through.

**4.** Mix cornstarch with 1 Tbsp water to make smooth paste. Add to wok and stir until blended. Bring to a boil and cook, stirring constantly, for 1 minute, or until sauce is slightly thickened. Divide among bowls, garnish with extra lemon zest, and serve.

**Per serving:** 191 calories, 23 g protein, 12 g carbohydrates, 3 g fiber, 6 g total fat, 1 g saturated fat, 55 mg cholesterol, 270 mg sodium

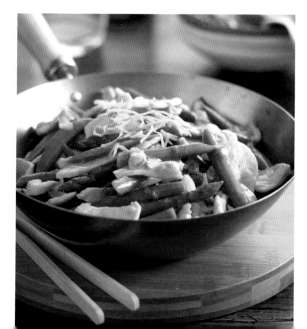

# BRAISED CHICKEN WITH WINTER VEGETABLES

Serves 4
**Prep Time:** 15 minutes plus soaking
**Cook Time:** 35 minutes
**Healing Foods:** mushrooms, chicken, leeks, potatoes, brussels sprouts
**Ailments It Heals:** hepatitis, hives, indigestion and heartburn, migraines and other headaches

½ cup dried shiitake mushrooms
2 cups water
8 skinless bone-in chicken thighs (about 5 oz or 150 g each)
2 Tbsp flour
3 tsp olive oil
2 leeks, halved lengthwise, cut crosswise into 1-in (2.5 cm) lengths, and well washed
1½ lb (750 g) small red-skinned potatoes, cut into ½-in (1 cm) chunks
10 oz (300 g) frozen brussels sprouts
½ tsp salt
½ tsp dried thyme

**1.** Bring 1 cup of water to a boil. In small bowl, combine mushrooms and boiling water. Let stand for 20 minutes, or until softened. With your fingers, remove mushrooms from soaking liquid, reserving liquid. Trim any stems from mushrooms and thinly slice caps. Strain reserved liquid through a fine-meshed sieve or coffee filter and set aside.

**2.** Dredge chicken in flour, shaking off excess. In nonstick Dutch oven, heat 2 tsp oil over medium heat. Add chicken and cook for 3 minutes per side, or until golden brown. Transfer chicken to a plate.

**3.** Add leeks, mushrooms, and remaining 1 tsp oil to Dutch oven. Cook, stirring frequently, for 2 minutes, or until leeks are golden.

**4.** Add reserved soaking liquid, potatoes, brussels sprouts, salt, thyme, and remaining water to Dutch oven. Bring to a boil. Return chicken to pan and reduce to a simmer. Cover and cook, stirring occasionally for 25 minutes, or until chicken is cooked through and brussels sprouts and potatoes are tender.

**Per serving:** 501 calories, 48 g protein, 50 g carbohydrates, 6 g fiber, 12 g total fat, 3 g saturated fat, 172 mg cholesterol, 502 mg sodium

# ORANGE CHICKEN WITH ARTICHOKES AND SUN-DRIED TOMATOES

Serves 4
**Prep Time:** 15 minutes
**Cook Time:** 12 minutes
**Healing Foods:** chicken, artichokes, tomatoes, rosemary
**Ailments It Heals:** diverticulitis, hepatitis, irritable bowel syndrome, memory loss

1 Tbsp extra-virgin olive oil
4 skinless, bone-in chicken breast halves (about 6 oz or 175 g each)
2 Tbsp whole wheat flour
3 cloves garlic, thinly sliced
1 cup low-sodium chicken stock
9 oz (275 g) frozen artichoke hearts, thawed and quartered

⅓ cup dry-pack sun-dried tomatoes, thinly sliced
½ tsp grated orange zest
¼ cup fresh orange juice
½ tsp chopped fresh or dried rosemary
½ tsp fine sea salt
¼ tsp ground black pepper

**1.** In large skillet, heat oil over medium-high heat. Dredge chicken in flour, add to skillet, and cook for 5 minutes, or until golden brown on both sides. Transfer to a plate.

**2.** Reduce heat to medium, add garlic to skillet, and cook for 2 minutes, or until golden brown.

**3.** Add stock, artichokes, tomatoes, orange zest, orange juice, rosemary, salt, and pepper and bring to a boil.

**4.** Return chicken to skillet and reduce heat to a simmer. Cover and cook for 5 minutes, or until chicken is cooked through.

**Per serving:** 237 calories, 28 g protein, 15 g carbohydrates, 5 g fiber, 7 g total fat, 1 g saturated fat, 73 mg cholesterol, 576 mg sodium

# CHICKEN BREASTS WITH PEACHES AND GINGER

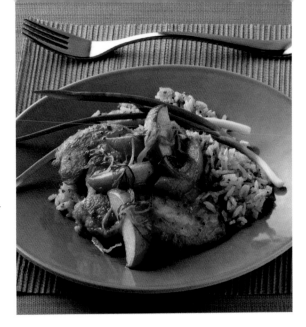

**Serves 4**

**Prep Time:** 25 minutes

**Cook Time:** 15 minutes

**Healing Foods:** onions, chicken, vinegar, ginger, peaches

**Ailments It Heals:** cancer, cholesterol (high), motion sickness

1 bunch scallions, trimmed

1 lb (500 g) boneless, skinless chicken breast halves, trimmed

¼ tsp salt or to taste

Ground black pepper to taste

2 tsp canola oil

3 Tbsp apple cider vinegar

2 Tbsp sugar

½ cup no-sugar-added peach juice or nectar, or apple juice

2 Tbsp grated fresh ginger

1¼ cups reduced-sodium chicken broth

1 large peach, peeled and sliced (½-in or 1 cm wedges)

2 tsp cornstarch

2 tsp water

**1.** Chop scallions, reserving all of white portions and ¼ cup of green portions separately.

**2.** If chicken pieces are large, cut them in half lengthwise so you have at least 4 pieces. Place chicken between 2 pieces of plastic wrap and pound with rolling pin or meat mallet into ½-in (1 cm) thickness. Season with salt and pepper.

**3.** Heat oil in large nonstick skillet over medium-high heat. Add chicken and cook for 3 to 3½ min-utes per side, or until browned and no longer pink in center. Transfer to a plate.

**4.** Add vinegar and sugar to skillet. Stir to dissolve sugar. Cook, swirling skillet, for 30 to 60 seconds, or until syrup turns dark amber. Add scallion whites, peach juice, and ginger. Bring to a boil, stirring to scrape up any caramelized bits in skil-let. Cook for 1 minute. Add broth and peach and return to a boil. Cook, turning peach slices from time to time, for 2 to 4 minutes, or until tender. Mix cornstarch and water and add to sauce. Cook, stirring, for 30 seconds, or until slightly thickened.

**5.** Reduce heat to low and return chicken and any accumulated juices to skillet. Simmer gently for 1 minute, or until chicken is heated through. Gar-nish with reserved scallion greens.

**Per serving:** 223 calories, 28 g protein, 17 g carbohy-drates, 1 g fiber, 4 g total fat, 1 g saturated fat, 67 mg cholesterol, 275 mg sodium

# EARL GREY CHICKEN

Serves 4
**Prep Time:** 15 minutes
**Cook Time:** 25 minutes
**Healing Foods:** tea, chicken, onions
**Ailments It Heals:** bleeding problems, jaundice, varicose veins

- 6 cups water
- 8 Earl Grey tea bags
- 1 Tbsp fresh lemon juice
- 4 boneless, skinless chicken breasts (about 1½ lb or 750 g)
- 2 tsp olive oil
- ½ cup chopped onion
- 1 clove garlic, minced
- 1 cup chicken broth
- ¾ cup heavy cream
- ¼ tsp salt
- ⅛ tsp ground black pepper
- 1 Tbsp chopped fresh oregano or parsley

**1.** Put water in deep sauté pan and bring to a boil. Turn off heat and add tea bags. Let steep for 5 minutes. Remove bags, squeezing to release any liquid.

**2.** Add lemon juice and return to a boil over high heat. Reduce heat to medium-low and barely simmer liquid (keep temperature at 160°F or 71°C). Add chicken, completely submerging it. Cook, uncovered, for 10 minutes, or until chicken is just barely pink in center. Remove from heat and let stand for 5 minutes.

**3.** Meanwhile, in small nonstick skillet, heat oil over medium heat. Add onion and garlic and cook for 4 minutes, or until tender.

**4.** Add broth, cream, and ¼ cup of poaching liquid. Raise heat to high and boil for 5 minutes, or until reduced to about half the original volume. Stir in salt and pepper.

**5.** Transfer chicken to platter or plates, and spoon sauce over top. Sprinkle with oregano (or parsley).

**Per serving:** 410 calories, 39 g protein, 10 g carbohydrates, 3 g fiber, 24 g total fat, 12 g saturated fat, 172 mg cholesterol, 603 mg sodium

# MAPLE-GLAZED CHICKEN WITH ROOT VEGETABLES

Serves 4
**Prep Time:** 30 minutes
**Cook Time:** 58 minutes
**Healing Foods:** carrots, parsnips, celeriac, turnips, chicken
**Ailments It Heals:** acne, Alzheimer's disease, eye problems, hives

- 4 cups assorted diced ½ x ¾-in (1 x 1.5 cm) peeled root vegetables, such as carrots, parsnips, celeriac, rutabaga, and/or turnips (1 lb 3 oz or 590 g)
- 1 Tbsp olive oil
- ½ tsp salt
- ½ tsp ground black pepper
- 2½ lb (1.25 kg) bone-in chicken thighs and/or drumsticks, skin removed and fat trimmed
- 1 Tbsp dijon mustard
- 1 Tbsp maple syrup
- 2 tsp chopped fresh thyme or ¾ tsp dried
- ½ cup apple cider
- ½ cup reduced-sodium chicken broth

**1.** Preheat oven to 400°F (200°C). Coat large roasting pan with cooking spray.

**2.** Place vegetables in pan and toss with oil, ¼ tsp salt, and ¼ tsp pepper. Push vegetables toward sides of pan. Sprinkle chicken with remaining ¼ tsp salt and ¼ tsp pepper and place, skin side down, in center of pan. Bake, uncovered, for 15 minutes.

3. Meanwhile, in small bowl, combine mustard, syrup, and thyme.

4. Stir vegetables and turn chicken pieces. Brush chicken with mustard mixture. Bake, stirring vegetables occasionally, for 30 to 40 minutes, or until vegetables are glazed and tender and chicken is cooked through (an instant-read thermometer should register 165°F or 74°C). If either chicken or vegetables are done first, remove and keep warm. When finished baking, transfer to platter or individual plates.

5. Add apple cider and broth to roasting pan, place over 2 burners, and bring to a boil over medium-high heat. Boil for 2 to 3 minutes. Drizzle sauce over chicken and vegetables.

**Per serving:** 370 calories, 33 g protein, 24 g carbohydrates, 4 g fiber, 16 g total fat, 4 g saturated fat, 108 mg cholesterol, 568 mg sodium

# PINEAPPLE-CHIPOTLE CHICKEN

**Serves 4**
**Prep Time:** 15 minutes
**Cook Time:** 27 minutes
**Healing Foods:** olive oil, chicken, peppers, ginger, pineapples, chiles
**Ailments It Heals:** arthritis, jaundice, motion sickness

- 1 Tbsp plus 2 tsp olive oil
- 4 boneless, skinless chicken breast halves (about 5 oz or 150 g each)

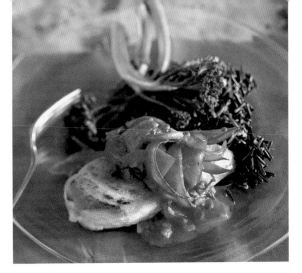

- 2 Tbsp flour
- 1 medium red onion, halved and sliced ½ in (1 cm) thick
- 3 cloves garlic, minced
- 1 red bell pepper, cut into ½-in (1 cm) chunks
- ¼ cup minced fresh ginger
- 2½ cups pineapple juice
- ¼ cup tomato paste
- 2 chipotle peppers in adobo, minced (4 tsp)
- ½ tsp salt

1. In large nonstick skillet, heat 1 Tbsp oil over medium heat. Dredge chicken in flour, shaking off excess. Add chicken to skillet and cook for 2 minutes per side, or until golden brown. Transfer to plate.

2. Add 2 tsp oil to skillet along with onion and garlic. Cook, stirring frequently, for 5 minutes, or until onion is tender.

3. Add bell pepper and ginger and cook for 3 minutes. Stir in pineapple juice, tomato paste, chipotle peppers, and salt. Bring to a boil. Boil for 5 minutes.

4. Return chicken to pan. Reduce heat to a simmer and cook for 10 minutes, or until chicken is cooked through.

**Per serving:** 350 calories, 36 g protein, 34 g carbohydrates, 2 g fiber, 8 g total fat, 1 g saturated fat, 82 mg cholesterol, 564 mg sodium

# WHOLE WHEAT NOODLES WITH PEANUT SAUCE AND CHICKEN

Serves 8
**Prep Time:** 35 minutes
**Cook Time:** 9 minutes
**Healing Foods:** peanut butter, tofu, pasta, chicken, carrots, peppers, herbs and spices
**Ailments It Heals:** cardiovascular disease, cystic fibrosis, diabetes, infertility, multiple sclerosis

### DRESSING

- ½ cup natural-style peanut butter
- ⅓ cup low-fat firm silken tofu
- ¼ cup reduced-sodium soy sauce
- 3 Tbsp lime juice
- 3 cloves garlic, minced
- 2 Tbsp firmly packed light brown sugar
- ¾ tsp crushed red-pepper flakes

### SALAD

- 12 oz (375 g) whole wheat spaghetti
- 2 tsp toasted sesame oil
- 2½ cups shredded cooked skinless chicken breast
- 1 cup grated carrots (2 to 4 medium)
- 1 cup finely diced red bell pepper (1 small)
- ¾ cup grated seedless (English) cucumber (¼ medium)
- ⅓ cup coarsely chopped fresh cilantro leaves
- ¼ cup chopped scallions
- 3 Tbsp unsalted dry-roasted peanuts, chopped

Lime wedges

**1.** Bring a large pot of lightly salted water to a boil for cooking spaghetti.

**2.** To make dressing: In food processor, combine peanut butter, tofu, soy sauce, lime juice, garlic, sugar, and red pepper. Process until smooth and creamy, stopping once or twice to scrape down sides of work bowl.

**3.** To make salad: Cook spaghetti in boiling water, stirring often, for 6 to 9 minutes, or until al dente (or according to package directions). Drain and rinse with cold running water. Transfer to large bowl. Drizzle with oil and toss to coat.

**4.** Add chicken, carrots, and bell pepper to spaghetti. Add dressing and toss to coat. Sprinkle with cucumber, cilantro, scallions, and peanuts. Serve with lime wedges.

**Per serving:** 364 calories, 22 g protein, 43 g carbohydrates, 8 g fiber, 13 g total fat, 2 g saturated fat, 28 g cholesterol, 560 mg sodium

# HERBED TURKEY MEATBALLS AND FUSILLI

Serves 4
**Prep Time:** 20 minutes
**Cook Time:** 22 minutes
**Healing Foods:** turkey, eggs, cheese, tomatoes, wheat
**Ailments It Heals:** atherosclerosis, cardiovascular disease, mood disorders, Parkinson's disease

- 2 Tbsp olive oil
- 1 medium onion, finely chopped
- 3 cloves garlic, minced
- 2 slices firm white sandwich bread, crumbled
- ¼ cup low-fat milk
- 1 lb (500 g) lean ground turkey breast
- ½ cup chopped parsley
- 1 large egg
- ⅓ cup grated parmesan cheese
- ¼ cup dried currants

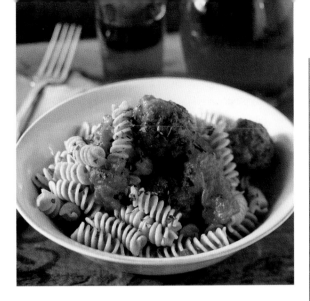

¾ tsp rubbed sage

Pinch of salt

2 Tbsp flour

28 oz (796 g) crushed tomatoes

3 strips (3 x ½-in or 7.5 x 1 cm each) orange zest

8 oz (250 g) whole wheat fusilli

1. In large skillet, heat 1 Tbsp oil over medium heat. Add onion and garlic and cook for 7 minutes, or until golden. Transfer to large bowl. Add bread and milk to bowl and let stand for 1 minute to soften bread.

2. Add turkey, parsley, egg, cheese, currants, sage, and salt to bowl and mix well. Shape mixture into 24 walnut-size meatballs. Dredge meatballs in flour, shaking off excess.

3. In same skillet, heat remaining 1 Tbsp oil over medium heat. Add meatballs and sauté for 3 minutes, or until golden brown. Add tomatoes and orange zest and bring to a boil. Reduce heat to a simmer, cover, and cook for 12 minutes, or until meatballs are cooked through.

4. Meanwhile, in a large pot of boiling water, cook fusilli according to package directions. Drain and toss in large bowl with meatballs and sauce.

**Per serving:** 579 calories, 46 g protein, 74 g carbohydrates, 10 g fiber, 13 g total fat, 3 g saturated fat, 130 mg cholesterol, 611 mg sodium

# JERK TURKEY BREAST WITH GINGER BARBECUE SAUCE

Serves 6

**Prep Time:** 20 minutes plus marinating

**Cook Time:** 1 hour 40 minutes

**Healing Foods:** onions, chiles, allspice, turkey

**Ailments It Heals:** mood disorders, neuralgia, stroke

5 scallions, chopped

4 cloves garlic

1 onion, quartered

2 jalapeño chile peppers, seeded and deveined (wear gloves when handling)

1 piece (½ in or 1 cm) fresh ginger, peeled

¼ cup canola oil

2 Tbsp low-sodium soy sauce

2 tsp allspice

1 tsp dried thyme

1 bone-in turkey breast (6 lbs or 3 kg)

1 tsp salt

1 cup ginger ale

1 cup low-sodium barbecue sauce

1. In blender, combine green onions, garlic, onion, chile peppers, ginger, oil, soy sauce, allspice, and thyme. Blend until thick paste forms, then transfer to large bowl.

2. With tip of sharp knife, make several slits all over turkey breast. Add turkey to green onion mixture, turning to coat. Refrigerate for at least 4 hours, or overnight, turning occasionally.

3. Preheat gas grill on high until thermometer reaches maximum temperature. Turn off one burner and reduce heat on other burner(s) to medium. Remove turkey from marinade and sprinkle with salt. On lightly oiled grill rack, grill turkey

breast, skin side down, over unlit burner (using indirect heat), turning every 20 minutes, for 1 hour 40 minutes, or until an instant-read thermometer inserted into thickest part of breast registers 165°F (74°C). Remove to a cutting board and let rest for 10 minutes before slicing.

**4.** Meanwhile, in small pot, combine ginger ale and barbecue sauce and bring to a boil over medium-high heat. Reduce heat to medium-low and simmer for 18 to 20 minutes, or until thickened and reduced to about 1¾ cups.

**Per serving:** 398 calories, 57 g protein, 26 g carbohydrates, 1 g fiber, 6 g total fat, 1 g saturated fat, 141 mg cholesterol, 657 mg sodium

# TURKEY BRACIOLA STUFFED WITH PROVOLONE AND SPINACH

Serves 4
**Prep Time:** 15 minutes
**Cook Time:** 15 minutes
**Healing Foods:** turkey, cheese, spinach, tomatoes, raisins
**Ailments It Heals:** cancer, diabetes, insomnia

- 8 turkey cutlets (1 lb or 500 g total)
- 1 tsp rubbed sage
- ¼ tsp salt
- 4 slices (4 oz or 25 g each) thinly sliced provolone cheese, halved
- 10 oz (300 g) frozen chopped spinach, thawed and squeezed dry
- 3 Tbsp flour

- 1 Tbsp olive oil
- 1¼ cups canned crushed tomatoes
- 1 tsp grated orange zest
- ¼ cup fresh orange juice
- 2 Tbsp dried currants or chopped raisins

**1.** Sprinkle one side of each cutlet with sage and salt. Lay 1 half-slice of provolone on top of sage. Top with spinach. Roll up cutlets and secure with wooden pick.

**2.** Dredge turkey rolls in flour, shaking off excess. In large nonstick skillet, heat oil over medium heat. Add turkey rolls and sauté for 2 minutes per side, or until golden brown.

**3.** Add tomatoes, orange zest, orange juice, and currants and bring to a boil. Reduce heat to a simmer, cover, and cook for 10 minutes, or until turkey is cooked through.

**4.** To serve, remove wooden picks and spoon sauce over turkey rolls.

**Per serving:** 329 calories, 39 g protein, 16 g carbohydrates, 3 g fiber, 12 g total fat, 6 g saturated fat, 90 mg cholesterol, 622 mg sodium

# GRILLED DUCK BREAST WITH POLENTA

Serves 4
**Prep Time:** 15 minutes
**Cook Time:** 15 minutes
**Healing Foods:** turmeric, ginger, duck, peas, corn
**Ailments It Heals:** depression, mood disorders, nail problems

2 tsp turmeric

1 tsp salt

¾ tsp sugar

½ tsp ground ginger

4 boneless, skinless duck breast halves (about 5 oz or 150 g each)

1 Tbsp olive oil

¾ cup yellow cornmeal

2¼ cups cold water

1½ cups frozen peas

1½ cups frozen corn kernels

3 Tbsp mango chutney, finely chopped

**1.** In small bowl, stir together turmeric, ¼ tsp salt, sugar, and ginger. Rub mixture into both sides of duck breasts.

**2.** Preheat grill to medium-hot. Brush grill pan with oil. Add duck breasts, and cook for 3 minutes per side for medium-rare. (If cooking on stove, add oil to large skillet and cook duck breasts over medium-high heat.)

**3.** In small bowl, combine cornmeal and 1 cup cold water, stirring until smooth. In a medium saucepan, bring remaining 1¼ cups water to a boil over high heat. Stir in cornmeal mixture and remaining ¾ tsp salt. Reduce heat to low and cook, stirring frequently, for 7 minutes, or until polenta is thickened and tender.

**4.** Stir peas, corn, and chutney into saucepan and cook for 2 minutes, or until vegetables are heated through. Slice duck across grain on diagonal and serve alongside polenta.

**Per serving:** 415 calories, 35 g protein, 57 g carbohydrates, 5 g fiber, 5 g fat, 1 g saturated fat, 149 mg cholesterol, 920 mg sodium

# BROILED SALMON WITH AVOCADO-MANGO SALSA

Serves 4

**Prep Time:** 15 minutes

**Cook Time:** 5 minutes

**Healing Foods:** herbs and spices, fish, mangoes, avocados, chickpeas, lettuce

**Ailments It Heals:** atherosclerosis, cardiovascular disease, cholesterol (high), circulatory disease, gallstones

2½ tsp paprika

2 tsp ground coriander

¼ tsp salt

4 4 oz (125 g) boneless, skinless salmon fillets

1 large mango, peeled and cut into ½-in (1 cm) chunks (about 1½ cups)

1 Hass avocado, peeled, pitted, and cut into ½-in (1 cm) chunks

1 cup canned chickpeas, drained and rinsed

⅓ cup chopped cilantro

1 tsp freshly grated lemon zest

2 Tbsp fresh lemon juice

2 tsp olive oil

6 cups mesclun or frisée lettuce, torn into bite-size pieces

**1.** In large bowl, stir together paprika, coriander, and salt. Measure out 2 tsp of mixture and sprinkle it over salmon, rubbing it into fish. Place salmon on broiler pan.

**2.** To remaining spice mixture in bowl, add mango, avocado, chickpeas, cilantro, lemon zest, lemon juice, and oil. Toss to combine.

**3.** Broil salmon 6 in (15 cm) from heat for 5 minutes for medium. Serve salmon and salsa on bed of lettuce.

**Per serving:** 430 calories, 27 g protein, 25 g carbohydrates, 7 g fiber, 26 g total fat, 5 g saturated fat, 60 mg cholesterol, 320 mg sodium

# POACHED SALMON WITH CUCUMBER-DILL SAUCE

**Serves 4**
**Prep Time:** 10 minutes
**Cook Time:** 10 minutes
**Healing Foods:** fish, cucumbers, dill
**Ailments It Heals:** asthma, atherosclerosis, jet lag, obesity, rosacea

1½   cups water
1   cup dry white wine or reduced-sodium chicken broth
2   scallions, sliced
8   black peppercorns
4   salmon fillets (4 oz or 125 g each)
¾   cup nonfat sour cream
⅓   cup diced peeled cucumber
2   Tbsp snipped fresh dill
1   Tbsp fresh lemon juice
¼   tsp salt
⅛   tsp ground black pepper
Fresh dill sprigs

**1.** Pour water into large nonstick skillet. Stir in wine, scallions, and peppercorns. Put salmon in skillet in single layer and bring just to a boil over high heat.

**2.** Reduce heat to medium-low, cover, and simmer for 6 minutes, or until fish flakes when tested with a fork.

**3.** Meanwhile, in medium bowl, stir sour cream, cucumber, dill, lemon juice, salt, and pepper to make sauce. Refrigerate if not serving immediately.

**4.** Carefully transfer fillets with slotted spatula to large platter. Garnish with fresh dill sprigs. Serve hot or chilled with sauce.

**Per serving:** 229 calories, 27 g protein, 5 g carbohydrates, 0 g fiber, 10 g total fat, 2 g saturated fat, 70 mg cholesterol, 229 mg sodium

# GRILLED SALMON WITH SAUTÉED GREENS

**Serves 4**
**Prep Time:** 5 minutes
**Cook Time:** 11 minutes
**Healing Foods:** vinegar, fish, onions, spinach
**Ailments It Heals:** asthma, cardiovascular disease, cholesterol (high), stroke

¼   cup balsamic vinegar
2   Tbsp brown sugar
1   tsp mustard powder
½   tsp salt
1¼   lb (625 g) salmon, cut into 4 pieces
1   Tbsp olive oil
1   large red onion, cut into thin strips
8   oz (250 g) baby spinach

**1.** Preheat grill or broiler. In small bowl, combine vinegar, brown sugar, mustard, and salt. Brush half of mixture over salmon. Grill or broil for 4 to 5 minutes on each side, or until opaque, brushing with vinegar mixture after 2 minutes.

**2.** Meanwhile, heat oil in large skillet over medium heat. Add onion and cook for 2 minutes, or until

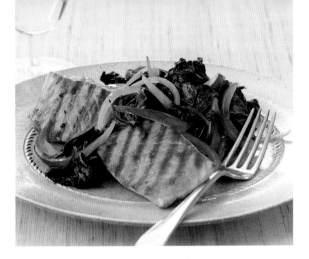

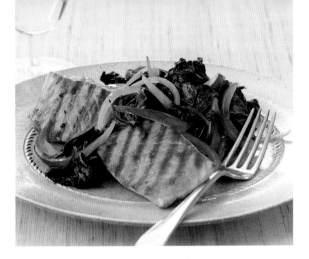

8  oz (250 g) boneless salmon fillet
¼  cup extra-virgin olive oil
¼  cup chopped walnuts
1  clove garlic, minced or crushed
12  oz (375 g) farfalle (bow-tie) or butterfly-shaped pasta
12  oz (375 g) asparagus, trimmed and cut into ½-in (1 cm) diagonals
½  cup crumbled mild goat's milk feta cheese (about 2 oz or 60 g)
2  Tbsp finely slivered fresh basil leaves

lightly browned. Cover and cook for 2 minutes, or until tender. Add spinach and cook, stirring, for 1 minute, or until almost wilted. Add remaining vinegar mixture and cook, stirring, for 1 minute, or until spinach is wilted and sauce thickens slightly.

**3.** Divide spinach mixture equally among 4 dinner plates. Top each serving with a piece of salmon.

**Per serving:** 356 calories, 31 g protein, 13 g carbohydrates, 2 g fiber, 20 g total fat, 4 g saturated fat, 84 mg cholesterol, 428 mg sodium

# SALMON AND ASPARAGUS FARFALLE WITH WALNUT-FETA SAUCE

Serves 4
**Prep Time:** 40 minutes
**Cook Time:** 28 minutes
**Healing Foods:** fish, olive oil, nuts, asparagus, cheese
**Ailments It Heals:** Alzheimer's disease, blood pressure, gallstones, hay fever, psoriasis

**1.** Heat 10-in (25 cm) nonstick skillet over medium-low heat until hot enough that a drop of water sizzles. Add salmon and cook on one side for 5 minutes. Turn with a wide spatula and cook for 3 to 5 minutes, or until center of thickest part of fish is opaque, depending on thickness. When cool enough to handle, remove and discard salmon skin and flake fish apart into ½-in (1 cm) pieces. Set aside.

**2.** Wipe out skillet and add oil, walnuts, and garlic. Cook over medium-low heat for 2 minutes, or until garlic sizzles and turns golden. (Do not leave unattended; walnuts burn quickly.) Remove from heat.

**3.** Bring large pot of water to a boil. Add pasta and cook, stirring occasionally, for 10 to 12 minutes, or until just cooked. Add asparagus and cook for 2 minutes, or until tender. Drain, reserving ½ cup of cooking water. Return pasta and asparagus to pot.

**4.** Reduce heat to medium-low. Add reserved cooking water, walnut mixture, salmon, and ¼ cup cheese to pot. Toss gently for 2 minutes, or until heated through and blended. Spoon into serving bowls and sprinkle the remaining ¼ cup cheese and basil on top.

**Per serving:** 623 calories, 29 g protein, 69 g carbohydrate, 5 g fiber, 27 g total fat, 5 g saturated fat, 38 mg cholesterol, 83 mg sodium

# TUNA AND TOMATO PIZZAS

Serves 4
**Prep Time:** 10 minutes
**Cook Time:** 25 minutes
**Healing Foods:** onions, tomatoes, tuna, olives
**Ailments It Heals:** cancer, cholesterol (high), mood disorders

  3  tsp extra-virgin olive oil
  1  onion, finely chopped
14.5  oz (410 mL) canned chopped tomatoes with juice
  ½  tsp dried oregano
Pinch of sugar
Salt and ground black pepper
  2  ready-made thick pizza crusts (8 oz or 250 g each)
  2  Tbsp tomato paste
  6  oz (170 g) canned tuna in spring water, drained and flaked into chunks
  8  pitted black olives, sliced
Fresh basil leaves

**1.** Preheat oven to 425°F (220°C). In small pan, heat 1 tsp oil over medium heat. Add onion and cook for 4 minutes, or until softened. Add tomatoes (with juice), oregano, and sugar. Season with salt and pepper to taste. Simmer sauce for 10 minutes, stirring occasionally.

**2.** Put pizza crusts on 2 baking trays. Spread 1 Tbsp tomato paste on each. Spoon tomato sauce over each, then add tuna. Sprinkle evenly with capers and olives, and drizzle remaining 2 tsp oil over top.

**3.** Bake for 10 minutes, or until crusts are crisp and golden. Sprinkle with torn basil leaves and serve at once.

**Per serving:** 377 calories, 18 g protein, 58 g carbohydrates, 8 g fiber, 11 g fat, 1 g saturated fat, 25 mg cholesterol, 960 mg sodium

# GRILLED TUNA STEAK WITH CORN AND ZUCCHINI

Serves 4
**Prep Time:** 20 minutes
**Cook Time:** 10 minutes
**Healing Foods:** fish, corn, tomatoes, zucchini, garlic, chiles
**Ailments It Heals:** cancer, cardiovascular disease, cholesterol (high)

  4  tuna steaks (1 in or 2.5 cm thick) (1½ lb or 750 g total)
  ½  tsp salt
  ¼  tsp ground black pepper
  ¼  cup apricot jam
  1  Tbsp dijon mustard
  1  ear corn, husked and cut into 8 equal pieces
  2  tomatoes, cored and each cut into 8 equal wedges
  2  medium zucchini, each quartered lengthwise and cut crosswise into ¼-in-thick (0.5 cm) slices
  2  cloves garlic, minced
  2  serrano chile peppers, seeded and finely chopped
  4  tsp olive oil

**1.** Preheat grill to medium-hot or preheat broiler.

**2.** Season tuna steaks with ¼ tsp salt and ⅛ tsp black pepper. In small cup, stir together jam and mustard. Spread one side of tuna steaks with half of jam mixture.

**3.** In center of each of four 12-in (30 cm) squares of foil, place corn, tomatoes, and zucchini, dividing equally. Sprinkle evenly with garlic, chile peppers, oil, and remaining ¼ tsp salt and ⅛ tsp black pepper. Fold edges of foil over to form tightly sealed packets.

**4.** Grill or broil tuna and foil packets 4 in (10 cm) from heat for 4 minutes. Turn tuna over. Spread with remaining jam mixture. Cook for 4 to 6 minutes, or until tuna is opaque in center and begins to flake when touched with fork. Carefully open vegetable packets and serve with tuna.

**Per serving:** 302 calories, 35 g protein, 27 g carbohydrates, 3 g fiber, 7 g total fat, 1 g saturated fat, 62 mg cholesterol, 458 mg sodium

# COD WITH GREMOLATA CRUST

Serves 4

**Prep Time:** 20 minutes

**Cook Time:** 25 minutes

**Healing Foods:** lemons, fish, tomatoes, zucchini, potatoes

**Ailments It Heals:** cholesterol (high), chronic fatigue syndrome, hepatitis, jaundice

2  lemons
½  cup white bread crumbs
3  Tbsp chopped parsley
2  cloves garlic, crushed
Salt and ground black pepper
4  4 oz (125 g) skinless cod fillets
2  tsp coarse-grain mustard
3  plum tomatoes, quartered
1  large zucchini, thinly sliced diagonally
1  Tbsp olive oil
1  lb (500 g) potatoes, peeled and cut into chunks

1  tsp saffron threads
3  Tbsp low-fat milk

**1.** Preheat oven to 400°F (200°C). Finely grate zest and squeeze juice from one lemon, reserving juice. Mix zest with bread crumbs, parsley, and garlic. Season lightly with salt and pepper.

**2.** Place cod fillets in large ovenproof dish coated with cooking spray. Spread mustard evenly over top of fish, then sprinkle on reserved lemon juice. Arrange tomatoes and zucchini around fish. Cut remaining lemon into 4 wedges and place in dish.

**3.** Spoon bread crumb mixture over fish and press down lightly. Drizzle with oil. Bake for 25 minutes, or until fish flakes easily and topping is crisp.

**4.** Meanwhile, place potatoes in saucepan, cover with boiling water, and add saffron. Cook potatoes for 15 to 20 minutes, or until tender. Drain potatoes and mash with milk. Season lightly with salt and pepper. Serve fish with potatoes, tomatoes, and zucchini.

**Per serving:** 251 calories, 24 g protein, 28 g carbohydrates, 4 g fiber, 5 g total fat, 1 g saturated fat, 49 mg cholesterol, 174 mg sodium

# MACKEREL TANDOORI STYLE

Serves 4

**Prep Time:** 20 minutes plus marinating

**Cook Time:** 39 minutes

**Healing Foods:** yogurt, ginger, fish, olive oil, onions, peppers

**Ailments It Heals:** atherosclerosis, cholesterol (high), nail problems, stroke

1 tsp ground cumin

¼ cup low-fat plain yogurt

1 Tbsp fresh lemon juice

2 tsp minced fresh ginger

1 clove garlic, peeled

2 tsp paprika

½ tsp salt

¼ tsp ground cardamom

¼ tsp cayenne pepper

4 mackerel fillets (about 6 oz or 175 g each), skin on, each cut crosswise in half

1 Tbsp plus 2 tsp olive oil

2 large onions, halved and thinly sliced

1½ tsp sugar

1 large red bell pepper, cut into matchsticks

**1.** In small skillet, toast cumin over low heat for 2 minutes, or until fragrant. Transfer to blender along with yogurt, lemon juice, ginger, garlic, paprika, salt, cardamom, and cayenne. Puree.

**2.** Place mackerel pieces, skin side down, in shallow ovenproof pan and make several diagonal slashes in mackerel flesh. Spread yogurt mixture over fish. Refrigerate for 2 hours or up to overnight.

**3.** About 30 minutes before serving time, remove fish from refrigerator. In large skillet, heat 1 Tbsp oil over medium heat. Add onions and sugar and cook, stirring frequently, for 20 minutes, or until onions are lightly browned. Add bell pepper and cook for 5 minutes, or until crisp-tender. Set aside.

**4.** Meanwhile, preheat oven to 450°F (230°C). Sprinkle mackerel with remaining 2 tsp oil and bake for 12 minutes, or until cooked through. Serve mackerel topped with the caramelized onion mixture.

**Per serving:** 414 calories, 29 g protein, 16 g carbohydrates, 2 g fiber, 26 g total fat, 5 g saturated fat, 100 mg cholesterol, 432 mg sodium

# ROASTED MACKEREL WITH CHERRY TOMATOES AND POTATOES

Serves 4

**Prep Time:** 15 minutes

**Cook Time:** 40 minutes

**Healing Foods:** potatoes, tomatoes, paprika, fish

**Ailments It Heals:** asthma, atherosclerosis, cholesterol (high), eye problems, stroke

1 lb (500 g) small Yukon Gold or red-skinned potatoes, unpeeled, cut into ½-in (1 cm) wedges

1½ cups small cherry tomatoes

½ medium onion, cut into thin slices

1 clove garlic, thinly sliced

1 Tbsp extra-virgin olive oil

1½ tsp smoked paprika

¼ tsp ground black pepper

4 boneless, skinless mackerel fillets (4 oz or 125 g each)

1 Tbsp chopped flat-leaf parsley

1 lemon, cut into wedges

**1.** Preheat oven to 400°F (200°C).

**2.** In large shallow baking dish or roasting pan, toss potatoes, tomatoes, onion, garlic, and oil. Spread in single layer and sprinkle with 1 tsp paprika and ⅛ tsp pepper. Roast vegetables, turning once, for 30 minutes, or until lightly browned.

**3.** Remove pan from oven and increase temperature to 450°F (230°C). Arrange fish in a single layer, redistributing vegetables on top of and around fish. Sprinkle with remaining ½ tsp paprika and ⅛ tsp of pepper. Roast for 10 minutes, or until center of thickest part of fish is opaque, depending on thickness.

4. Sprinkle with parsley and serve with lemon wedges.

**Per serving:** 366 calories, 24 g protein, 23 g carbohydrate, 3 g fiber, 20 g total fat, 4 g saturated fat, 79 mg cholesterol, 114 mg sodium

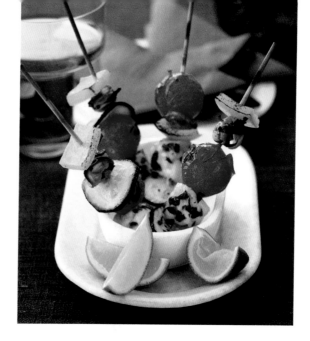

# MONKFISH AND MUSSEL KEBABS

Serves 8
**Prep Time:** 20 minutes plus marinating
**Cook Time:** 10 minutes
**Healing Foods:** limes, fish, peppers, zucchini, tomatoes
**Ailments It Heals:** Alzheimer's disease, asthma, prostate problems, psoriasis, stroke

Finely grated zest and juice of 1 lemon
Juice of 1 lime
  1  Tbsp olive oil
  2  tsp honey
  1  clove garlic, crushed
  1  Tbsp chopped fresh oregano or marjoram
  1  Tbsp chopped parsley
Salt and ground black pepper
  7  oz (210 g) monkfish fillet, cut into 16 small cubes
 16  shelled fresh mussels
  1  small yellow bell pepper, seeded and cut into 16 small chunks
  1  zucchini, cut into 16 thin slices
 16  cherry tomatoes
Lime or lemon wedges

1. In shallow nonmetallic dish, whisk together lemon zest and juice, lime juice, oil, honey, garlic, chopped oregano (or marjoram), parsley, and salt and pepper to taste. Add monkfish and mussels. Turn seafood to coat all over with marinade. Cover and marinate in refrigerator for 1 hour.

2. Meanwhile, put 16 wooden skewers in warm water and leave to soak for 10 minutes. Drain. Preheat grill or oven broiler to medium-high.

3. Onto each skewer, thread 1 monkfish cube, 1 mussel, 1 bell pepper chunk, 1 zucchini slice, and a cherry tomato. (Reserve marinade.) Leave ends of skewers empty so they will be easy to hold.

4. Place kebabs on grill rack or broiler pan, and grill or broil for 8 to 10 minutes, or until monkfish is cooked and vegetables are just tender, turning occasionally and brushing frequently with reserved marinade. Serve hot, garnished with lime or lemon wedges. Each serving is 2 kebabs.

**Per serving:** 90 calories, 9 g protein, 7 g carbohydrates, 1 g fiber, 3 g total fat, 0 g saturated fat, 17 mg cholesterol, 84 mg sodium

# SNAPPER AND SNAPS IN A PACKET

Serves 4
**Prep Time:** 10 minutes
**Cook Time:** 12 minutes
**Healing Foods:** peas, lemons, fish
**Ailments It Heals:** diabetes, eye problems, nail problems

- 3 cups sugar snap peas or snow peas
- 2 Tbsp lemon juice
- 2 tsp olive oil
- Salt and ground black pepper to taste
- 4 red snapper fillets, 6 oz (175 g) each

**1.** Preheat oven to 400ºF (200°C) or prepare gas or charcoal grill.

**2.** In a large bowl, toss together peas, lemon juice, oil, salt, and pepper.

**3.** Coat four 15-in (38 cm) lengths of parchment paper (or foil) with cooking spray. Place each fillet on one half of the paper. Top with about 3/4 cup of pea mixture. Fold paper over fish and peas, and seal by folding over all edges.

**4.** Place packets on baking sheet and bake in oven, or place directly onto grill, and cook for 10 to 12 minutes.

**Per serving:** 233 calories, 37 g protein, 10 g carbohydrates, 2 g fiber, 5 g total fat, 1 g saturated fat, 63 mg cholesterol, 109 mg sodium

# TROUT WITH LEMON-MUSHROOM STUFFING

Serves 4
**Prep Time:** 15 minutes
**Cook Time:** 52 minutes
**Healing Foods:** mushrooms, garlic, rice, fish, lemons
**Ailments It Heals:** Alzheimer's disease, cardiovascular disease, prostate problems

- 1 tsp olive oil
- ½ cup coarsely chopped carrots
- 8 oz (250 g) mushrooms, coarsely chopped
- 3 cloves garlic, minced
- ½ cup Texmati or jasmine rice
- 2 tsp grated lemon zest
- ¾ tsp salt
- ¼ tsp rosemary, minced
- 1¼ cups water
- 4 skin-on brook trout fillets (3 oz or 90 g each)
- 2 lemons, cut into 6 wedges each

**1.** In large nonstick skillet, heat oil over medium heat. Add carrots and cook for 4 minutes, or until crisp-tender. Add mushrooms and garlic and cook for 5 minutes, or until mixture is almost dry.

**2.** Stir in rice, lemon zest, ½ tsp salt, rosemary, and water and bring to a boil. Reduce heat to a simmer, cover, and cook for 17 minutes, or until rice is tender. Let stuffing cool to room temperature.

**3.** Preheat oven to 400°F (200°C). Coat 11 x 7-in (28 x 18 cm) baking pan with cooking spray. Spoon half of stuffing into pan. Place fillets skin side down on work surface. Place remaining stuffing on one half of each fillet and fold fillets over.

**4.** Place fillets on top of stuffing. Squeeze a wedge of lemon over each fillet and sprinkle with remaining ¼ tsp salt. Bake for 25 minutes, or until cooked through. Serve with remaining lemon wedges and additional stuffing from pan.

**Per serving:** 270 calories, 25 g protein, 24 g carbohydrates, 2 g fiber, 8 g total fat, 2 g saturated fat, 58 mg cholesterol, 478 mg sodium

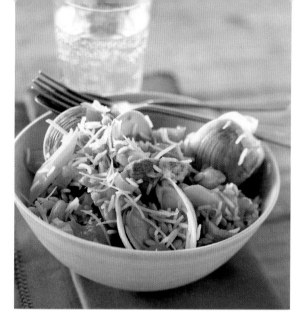

# LENTIL AND RICE PAELLA WITH CLAMS

Serves 4

**Prep Time:** 20 minutes

**Cook Time:** 45 minutes

**Healing Foods:** leeks, garlic, carrots, lentils, clams

**Ailments It Heals:** constipation, eczema, hypoglycemia, sex drive (diminished)

| | |
|---|---|
| 1 | Tbsp olive oil |
| 2 | large leeks, quartered lengthwise, thinly sliced crosswise, and well washed |
| 5 | cloves garlic, minced |
| 3 | large carrots, cut crosswise into ½-in (1 cm) slices |
| 1 | pickled jalapeño chile pepper, minced (wear gloves when handling) |
| ⅔ | cup lentils, picked over and rinsed |
| 3 | cups water |
| ½ | tsp salt |
| ⅔ | cup rice |
| 1⅓ | cups frozen lima beans |
| 1 | large tomato, coarsely chopped |
| 2 | tsp finely slivered lemon zest |
| 18 | littleneck clams, well scrubbed |

**1.** In nonstick Dutch oven or flameproof casserole, heat oil over medium heat. Add leeks and garlic and cook, stirring frequently, for 7 minutes, or until leeks are tender.

**2.** Add carrots and chile pepper and cook for 5 minutes, or until carrots are crisp-tender.

**3.** Add lentils, stirring to coat. Add water and salt and bring to a boil over high heat. Reduce heat to a simmer, cover, and cook for 10 minutes.

**4.** Add rice, cover, and simmer for 10 minutes. Stir in lima beans, tomato, and lemon zest and cook for 2 minutes. Place clams on top of lentil-rice mixture. Cover and cook for 5 to 7 minutes, or until clams open (check after 3 minutes as some will open before others; discard any that do not open).

**Per serving:** 457 calories, 25 g protein, 79 g carbohydrates, 11 g fiber, 5 g total fat, 1 g saturated fat, 21 mg cholesterol, 464 mg sodium

# LINGUINE WITH CLAMS

Serves 4
**Prep Time:** 15 minutes
**Cook Time:** 15 minutes
**Healing Foods:** carrots, garlic, clams, pasta
**Ailments It Heals:** cancer, cholesterol (high), diabetes

- 2 tsp olive oil
- 1 small onion, finely chopped
- 3 carrots, quartered lengthwise and thinly sliced crosswise
- 4 cloves garlic, minced
- 1 cup carrot juice
- 2 dozen littleneck clams, well scrubbed
- 8 oz (250 g) whole wheat linguine
- ¼ tsp salt
- ¼ cup chopped parsley
- 2 tsp unsalted butter

**1.** In large skillet, heat oil over low heat. Add onion, carrots, and garlic. Cook, stirring frequently, for 5 minutes, or until onion is tender.

**2.** Add carrot juice and bring to a boil. Add clams, cover, and cook for 5 minutes, or until clams open (check after 3 minutes as some will open before others). Remove clams as they open (discard any that do not open). Set skillet aside. When clams are cool enough to handle, remove clam meat and discard shells.

**3.** Meanwhile, in large pot of boiling water, cook linguine according to package directions. Drain.

**4.** Return carrot mixture to a boil and boil for 3 minutes. Stir in salt. Transfer to large bowl, add pasta, clam meat, parsley, and butter and toss well.

**Per serving:** 371 calories, 18 g protein, 60 g carbohydrates, 8 g fiber, 7 g total fat, 2 g saturated fat, 45 mg cholesterol, 291 mg sodium

# PAN-SEARED SCALLOPS WITH ORANGES AND SUN-DRIED TOMATOES

Serves 6
**Prep Time:** 10 minutes
**Cook Time:** 20 minutes
**Healing Foods:** shellfish, tomatoes, oranges, basil
**Ailments It Heals:** cancer, urinary tract infections, varicose veins

- 2 tsp olive oil
- 1 lb (500 g) sea scallops
- 3 cloves garlic, sliced
- ¼ cup sliced oil-packed sun-dried tomatoes
- 1 cup dry white wine or sherry
- 1 cup vegetable broth
- 2 tsp fresh lemon juice
- 3 Tbsp fresh orange juice
- 2 Tbsp butter, cut into pieces
- 1 large navel orange, peeled, segmented, segments chopped
- 1½ Tbsp chopped fresh basil

**1.** In large, deep skillet, heat oil over medium-high heat. When very hot, add scallops and cook for 2 minutes per side, or just until lightly browned and barely translucent in center. Remove to a plate.

**2.** Add garlic, sun-dried tomatoes, and wine (or sherry) to skillet. Boil, scraping pan bottom occasionally, for 5 minutes, or until liquid is reduced by about half. Add broth and boil for 8 minutes, or until liquid is again reduced by about half.

**3.** Reduce heat to low and stir in lemon juice, orange juice, butter, orange segments, and 1 Tbsp basil. Simmer for 1 minute.

**4.** Divide sauce among bottoms of 6 small plates. Arrange scallops over sauce and sprinkle with remaining ½ Tbsp basil.

**Per serving:** 182 calories, 14 g protein, 10 g carbohydrates, 1 g fiber, 7 g total fat, 3 g saturated fat, 35 mg cholesterol, 214 mg sodium

# SCALLOPS FLORENTINE

Serves 4
**Prep Time:** 10 minutes
**Cook Time:** 12 minutes
**Healing Foods:** spinach, olive oil, shellfish, garlic, peas
**Ailments It Heals:** cholesterol (high), hives, PCOS, shingles

- ¾ lb (375 g) fresh spinach
- 2 Tbsp olive oil
- 1½ lb (750 g) sea scallops
- 2 cloves garlic, minced
- 1 tsp grated lemon zest
- 1 cup reduced-sodium, fat-free chicken broth
- 1 cup frozen peas, thawed
- 1 Tbsp fresh-squeezed lemon juice
- ¼ tsp salt
- ¼ tsp ground black pepper

**1.** In steamer set over a pan of boiling water, steam spinach for 3 minutes, or just until wilted. Cool under cold running water. Squeeze dry.

**2.** In large nonstick skillet, heat oil over high heat. Add scallops. Sauté for 2 minutes per side, or until still slightly uncooked in center. Transfer to plate.

**3.** Lower heat to medium. Add garlic and lemon zest to skillet. Cook 30 seconds. Add chicken broth and peas. Simmer 3 minutes. Add spinach, scallops, lemon juice, salt, and pepper. Cook just until heated through. Serve in shallow bowls.

**Per serving:** 286 calories, 31 g protein, 13 g carbohydrates, 13 g total fat, 2 g saturated fat, 52 mg cholesterol, 4 g fiber, 550 mg sodium

# SHRIMP AND VEGETABLE STIR-FRY

Serves 4
**Prep Time:** 20 minutes
**Cook Time:** 9 minutes
**Healing Foods:** ginger, shrimp, broccoli, peppers, peas, corn
**Ailments It Heals:** cancer, cystic fibrosis, prostate problems

- ⅔ cup water
- ⅓ cup light soy sauce
- 3 Tbsp white wine or orange juice
- 2 Tbsp cornstarch
- 1½ tsp grated peeled fresh ginger
- 1 Tbsp vegetable oil
- 2 cloves garlic, minced
- 1 lb (500 g) large shrimp, peeled and deveined
- 4 cups fresh broccoli florets
- 1 large red bell pepper, cut into strips
- 1 large yellow bell pepper, cut into strips
- 4 oz (125 g) snow peas
- ½ cup drained whole baby corn
- ½ cup sliced water chestnuts
- 4 scallions, cut diagonally into 2-in (5 cm) pieces

**1.** In small bowl, blend water, soy sauce, wine (or orange juice), cornstarch, and ginger until smooth. Set aside.

**2.** In large wok or large deep skillet, heat oil over medium-high heat until hot. Stir-fry garlic for 2 minutes, or until soft. Add shrimp and stir-fry for 3 minutes, or until pink. Remove shrimp with slotted spoon and set aside.

**3.** Add broccoli to wok and stir-fry for 2 minutes, or until bright green. Add bell peppers and snow peas and stir-fry for 1 minute, or until crisp-tender.

**4.** Return shrimp to wok. Add corn, water chestnuts, and scallions. Pour in reserved sauce mixture and stir-fry for 1 minute, or until sauce thickens and boils.

**Per serving:** 266 calories, 29 g protein, 23 g carbohydrates, 4 g fiber, 6 g total fat, 1 g saturated fat, 172 mg cholesterol, 992 mg sodium

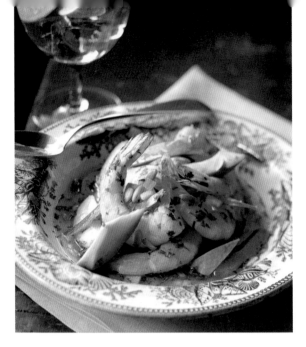

# SHRIMP SEVICHE WITH AVOCADO AND PUMPKIN SEEDS

### Serves 4
**Prep Time:** 15 minutes plus cooling
**Cook Time:** 3 minutes
**Healing Foods:** shrimp, oranges, peppers, avocados, seeds
**Ailments It Heals:** burns, chronic fatigue syndrome, diabetes

- 1½ tsp ground coriander
- ¾ tsp salt
- 1½ lb (750 g) medium shrimp, shelled and deveined
- 2 tsp grated orange zest
- 2 cups orange juice
- 3 Tbsp fresh lime juice
- ¼ tsp cayenne pepper
- 1 red bell pepper, cut into matchsticks
- ¼ cup diced red onion
- ½ cup chopped cilantro
- 1 Hass avocado, peeled and cut into ½-in (1 cm) chunks
- 3 Tbsp hulled roasted pumpkin seeds

**1.** In large bowl, combine 1 tsp coriander and ¼ tsp salt. Add shrimp, tossing to coat.

**2.** In separate bowl, stir together orange zest, orange juice, lime juice, cayenne, and remaining ½ tsp salt and ½ tsp coriander. Stir in bell pepper, onion, and cilantro.

**3.** Preheat broiler. Broil shrimp 6 in (15 cm) from heat, turning once halfway through, for 3 minutes, or until cooked through. Transfer shrimp to bowl with orange mixture and toss to coat. Refrigerate for at least 2 hours, or until well chilled.

**4.** Serve chilled seviche topped with avocado and pumpkin seeds.

**Per serving:** 335 calories, 33 g protein, 23 g carbohydrates, 3 g fiber, 13 g total fat, 2 g saturated fat, 211 mg cholesterol, 650 mg sodium

# THAI ROASTED SHRIMP

Serves 4
**Prep Time:** 5 minutes
**Cook Time:** 8 minutes
**Healing Foods:** coconuts, shrimp, tomatoes, rice
**Ailments It Heals:** cancer, celiac disease, respiratory disorders

14 oz (398 mL) light coconut milk
1 cup reduced-sodium vegetable or chicken broth
2 Tbsp reduced-sodium soy sauce
¼ to ½ tsp green curry paste
1 lb (500 g) shrimp, peeled and deveined
8 scallions, thinly sliced
1 large tomato, seeded and chopped
1 Tbsp lime juice
2 cups cooked brown rice or quinoa

**1.** In large saucepan, whisk together coconut milk, broth, soy sauce, and curry paste. Bring to a boil over medium-high heat. Add shrimp and scallions and cook for 5 minutes, or until shrimp is opaque.

**2.** Remove from heat and stir in tomato and lime juice. Serve over rice (or quinoa).

**Per serving:** 311 calories, 23 g protein, 31 g carbohydrates, 3 g fiber, 9 g total fat, 6 g saturated fat, 168 mg cholesterol, 516 mg sodium

# BLACK BEAN AND SWEET POTATO BURRITOS

Serves 8
**Prep Time:** 25 minutes
**Cook Time:** 20 minutes
**Healing Foods:** sweet potatoes, tomatoes, beans, wheat, cheese
**Ailments It Heals:** constipation, diverticulitis, hemorrhoids

2 tsp canola oil
1 cup chopped onion (1 medium)
2 cloves garlic, minced
4 tsp ground cumin
½ tsp dried oregano
¾ cup vegetable broth or reduced-sodium chicken broth
1 medium sweet potato, peeled and diced (3 cups)
14.5 oz (410 mL) mild green chile–seasoned diced tomatoes with juice
15.5 oz (440 mL) black beans, drained and rinsed
¾ cup frozen corn
¼ cup chopped fresh cilantro
1 Tbsp fresh lime juice
⅛ tsp ground black pepper
8 whole wheat wraps or tortillas, (8-in or 20 cm each)
1 cup shredded pepper jack or monterey jack cheese
½ cup reduced-fat sour cream

**1.** Preheat oven to 325°F (160°C).

**2.** In large nonstick skillet, heat oil over medium heat. Add onion and cook, stirring often, for 2 to 3 minutes, or until softened. Add garlic, cumin, and oregano. Cook, stirring, for 10 to 20 seconds, or until fragrant. Add broth and sweet potato. Bring to a simmer. Cover and cook for 5 minutes. Add tomatoes (with juice), beans, and corn. Return to a simmer. Cover and cook for 5 to 10 minutes, or until sweet potato is tender. Mash about one-quarter of vegetable mixture with potato masher. Stir mashed and unmashed portions together. Stir in cilantro, lime juice, and pepper.

**3.** Meanwhile, enclose wraps (or tortillas) in foil and heat in oven for 10 to 15 minutes.

**4.** To serve, spoon about ⅔ cup of sweet potato filling down center of each tortilla. Sprinkle with about 2 Tbsp cheese. Fold in edges of wrap, then fold one side over filling and wrap up burrito. Serve with sour cream for dipping.

**Per serving:** 349 calories, 12 g protein, 47 g carbohydrates, 15 g fiber, 11 g total fat, 4 g saturated fat, 23 mg cholesterol, 562 mg sodium

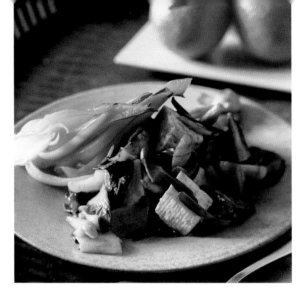

# BOK CHOY, TOFU, AND MUSHROOM STIR-FRY

Serves 4

**Prep Time:** 15 minutes

**Cook Time:** 13 minutes

**Healing Foods:** tofu, ginger, garlic, mushrooms, cooking greens

**Ailments It Heals:** diabetes, menopause, osteoporosis, stroke

15  oz (450 g) extra-firm tofu
 3  Tbsp reduced-sodium soy sauce
 4  tsp dark brown sugar
1½  tsp cornstarch
 1  cup water
 4  tsp olive oil
 4  scallions, thinly sliced
 2  Tbsp minced fresh ginger
 3  cloves garlic, minced
 8  oz (250 g) fresh shiitake mushrooms, stems removed and caps quartered
 8  oz (250 g) button mushrooms, halved
 ¼  tsp salt
 1  large head bok choy, sliced crosswise into 1-in-wide (2.5 cm) strips

**1.** Halve tofu horizontally, then cut each piece into 12 squares or triangles. In small bowl, stir together soy sauce, brown sugar, cornstarch, and ½ cup water.

**2.** In large nonstick skillet, heat 2 tsp oil over medium heat. Add scallions, ginger, and garlic and cook for 1 minute, or until tender.

**3.** Stir in mushrooms. Add salt and remaining ½ cup water. Cover and cook, stirring occasionally, for 5 minutes, or until mushrooms are tender. Transfer to a bowl.

**4.** Add bok choy and remaining 2 tsp oil to skillet. Cook, stirring frequently for 5 minutes, or until bok choy is tender.

**5.** Return mushroom-scallion mixture to skillet and add tofu. Stir soy sauce mixture to recombine and add to skillet. Cook for 2 minutes, or until tofu is heated through and vegetables are coated with sauce.

**Per serving:** 240 calories, 20 g protein, 20 g carbohydrates, 4 g fiber, 11 g total fat, 1 g saturated fat, 0 mg cholesterol, 760 mg sodium

# VEGETABLE POT PIE

**Serves 6**
**Prep Time:** 20 minutes
**Cook Time:** 55 minutes
**Healing Foods:** celery, onions, carrots, peppers, broccoli, cauliflower
**Ailments It Heals:** kidney disease, obesity, prostate problems

2   Tbsp butter
2   celery stalks, coarsely chopped
1   yellow onion, coarsely chopped
1   large carrot, peeled and cut into small chunks
1   small red bell pepper, seeded and coarsely chopped
¾   tsp dried thyme, crumbled
3   Tbsp all-purpose flour
1   cup vegetable broth or bouillon
1   cup broccoli florets
1   cup cauliflower florets
1   cup frozen pearl onions
2   oz (60 g) cheddar cheese, cut into small cubes
Pastry dough for one-crust 9-in (23 cm) pie

**1.** In large nonstick saucepan, melt butter over medium heat. Add celery, yellow onion, carrot, pepper, and thyme. Sauté for 10 minutes, or until vegetables are tender.

**2.** Stir in flour until well blended. Stir in broth. Increase heat to medium-high. Add broccoli, cauliflower, and pearl onions. Bring to boil, then lower heat and simmer, uncovered, for 15 minutes. Remove saucepan from heat. (If making filling ahead, let cool to room temperature, then cover and refrigerate.)

**3.** Preheat oven to 400°F (200°C).

**4.** Spread vegetable mixture in 9-in (23 cm) glass or ceramic pie plate. Top with cheese. Cover filling with pastry. Trim edges. (If crust is not lattice, cut

6 long slits in it, to vent steam.) Place dish on baking sheet.

**6.** Bake for 25 to 30 minutes, or until pastry is golden and filling is bubbly. Let stand for 10 minutes before serving.

**Per serving:** 296 calories, 7 g protein, 32 g carbohydrates, 4 g fiber, 17 g total fat, 8 g saturated fat, 27 mg cholesterol, 408 mg sodium

# BAKED PASTA WITH GARLIC AND GREENS

**Serves 8**
**Prep Time:** 15 minutes
**Cook Time:** 50 minutes
**Healing Foods:** pasta, kale, tomatoes, cheese, olives
**Ailments It Heals:** Alzheimer's disease, arthritis, jet lag, osteoporosis

1   lb (500 g) penne or rigatoni pasta
1   Tbsp olive oil
6   cloves garlic, thinly sliced
10  oz (300 g) frozen kale or collard greens, thawed and well drained
3   cups prepared tomato sauce
1   cup part-skim ricotta cheese
1   cup shredded part-skim mozzarella cheese
Kalamata olives

**1.** Preheat oven to 350°F (180°C). Lightly coat 2-quart (2 L) baking dish with cooking spray.

**2.** In large pot of lightly salted boiling water, cook penne until tender, following package directions, and drain.

**3.** Meanwhile, in medium nonstick skillet, heat oil over medium-low heat. Add garlic. Sauté for 5 minutes, or until golden. Add kale and cook for 5 minutes. Transfer to large bowl. Stir in tomato sauce and ricotta cheese.

**4.** Add penne to bowl. Mix well. Scrape into baking dish. Top with mozzarella cheese. Cover with foil.

**5.** Bake for 25 minutes. Remove foil and bake for 10 minutes, or until lightly golden. Garnish with olives.

**Per serving:** 341 calories, 17 g protein, 53 g carbohydrates, 4 g fiber, 8 g total fat, 4 g saturated fat, 18 mg cholesterol, 810 mg sodium

# FARFALLE WITH WINTER SQUASH SAUCE

**Serves 4**
**Prep Time:** 15 minutes
**Cook Time:** 15 minutes
**Healing Foods:** raisins, pasta, peppers, garlic, squash
**Ailments It Heals:** constipation, eye problems, Parkinson's disease

⅓ cup raisins
1 cup boiling water
8 oz (250 g) farfalle (bow-tie) pasta
1 Tbsp olive oil
1 large red bell pepper, diced
4 cloves garlic, minced
18 oz (510 g) winter squash puree, thawed
1 tsp rubbed sage
½ tsp salt
½ tsp ground black pepper
3 Tbsp reduced-fat cream cheese (Neufchâtel)
⅓ cup grated parmesan cheese

**1.** In small bowl, soak raisins in boiling water for 5 minutes, or until plump. In large pot of boiling water, cook pasta according to package directions. Drain, reserving ⅓ cup of cooking liquid.

**2.** Meanwhile, in large skillet, heat oil over medium heat. Add bell pepper and garlic. Cook, stirring frequently, for 5 minutes, or until pepper is tender. Add squash puree, sage, salt, and black pepper and cook until heated through.

**3.** Stir in raisins and their soaking liquid and cream cheese. Cook until cream cheese has melted. Transfer mixture to large bowl. Add pasta, reserved cooking liquid, and parmesan and toss to combine.

**Per serving:** 418 calories, 14 g protein, 73 g carbohydrates, 7 g fiber, 9 g total fat, 3 g saturated fat, 13 mg cholesterol, 469 mg sodium

# FUSILLI WITH PAN-ROASTED VEGETABLES

**Serves 4**
**Prep Time:** 20 minutes
**Cook Time:** 25 minutes
**Healing Foods:** peppers, butternut squash, garlic, tomatoes, spinach, pasta
**Ailments It Heals:** cancer, cardiovascular disease, eye problems

2 Tbsp olive oil
1 large sweet onion, cut into thin wedges
1 yellow bell pepper, seeded and chopped
1 small butternut squash, 1¼ lb (625 g), peeled, seeded, and cut into 1-in (2.5 cm) chunks
½ tsp salt
¼ cup minced fresh basil
5 cloves garlic, minced

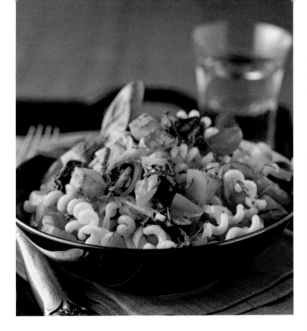

Per serving: 372 calories, 12 g protein, 66 g carbohydrates, 9 g fiber, 9 g total fat, 1 g saturated fat, 1 mg cholesterol, 485 mg sodium

# MACARONI AND CHEESE WITH SPINACH

**Serves 6**
**Prep Time:** 15 minutes
**Cook Time:** 55 minutes
**Healing Foods:** milk, cheese, spinach, pasta, wheat germ
**Ailments It Heals:** ADHD, cystic fibrosis, interstitial cystitis, jet lag, Parkinson's disease

- 1 cup grape or cherry tomatoes, each cut in half
- 4 cups fresh baby spinach, tough stems removed
- 4 cups reduced-sodium, fat-free chicken broth
- 2 cups water
- 8 oz (250 g) fusilli whole wheat pasta

1. In large nonstick skillet, heat 1 Tbsp oil over medium heat. Add onion and bell pepper. Sauté for 5 minutes, or until softened. Add squash, ¼ tsp salt, basil, and half of garlic. Cover and cook, stirring occasionally, for 8 minutes. Increase heat to high. Cook, uncovered, stirring occasionally, for 5 to 7 minutes, or until vegetables brown slightly and squash is just tender. Transfer mixture to large bowl. Add tomatoes to bowl.

2. In same skillet, heat remaining 1 Tbsp oil over medium heat. Add spinach, remaining garlic, and ¼ tsp salt. Cook, stirring occasionally, for 2 minutes, or until spinach wilts. Add spinach to squash mixture.

3. Meanwhile, in large pot, bring broth and water to a boil. Add fusilli. Cook until tender, following package directions. Reserve ½ cup cooking liquid. Drain fusilli. Combine fusilli, squash mixture, and reserved cooking liquid and serve.

- 1 ¾ cups cold low-fat milk
- 3 Tbsp all-purpose flour
- 2 cups (6 oz or 170 g) grated extra-sharp cheddar cheese
- 1 cup 1% cottage cheese
- ⅛ tsp ground nutmeg
- ½ tsp salt, or to taste
- Ground black pepper to taste
- 10 oz (300 g) frozen spinach or 4 cups individually quick-frozen spinach
- 8 oz (250 g) whole wheat macaroni
- ¼ cup toasted wheat germ

1. Preheat oven to 400°F (200°C). Coat 8-in (20 cm) square baking dish (2-qt or 2 L capacity) with cooking spray. Bring large pot of lightly salted water to a boil for cooking macaroni.

2. Whisk ¼ cup milk with flour in small bowl until smooth. Set aside. In heavy medium saucepan, heat remaining 1½ cups milk over medium heat until steaming. Add flour mixture and cook, whisking constantly, for 2 to 3 minutes, or until sauce boils and thickens. Remove from heat. Add

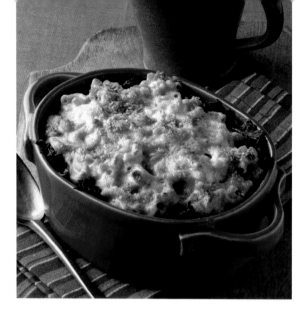

cheddar cheese, stirring until melted. Stir in cottage cheese, nutmeg, salt, and pepper.

**3.** Cook spinach according to package directions. Drain, refresh under cold water, and press out excess moisture.

**4.** Cook macaroni in boiling water, stirring often, for 4 to 5 minutes, or until not quite tender. (The macaroni will continue to cook during baking.) Drain, rinse with cold running water, then drain again.

**5.** In large bowl, mix macaroni with cheese sauce. Spread half of macaroni mixture in baking dish. Spoon spinach on top. Spread remaining macaroni mixture over spinach layer. Sprinkle with wheat germ.

**6.** Bake for 35 to 45 minutes, or until bubbly and golden.

**Per serving:** 357 calories, 22 g protein, 40 g carbohydrates, 6 g fiber, 12 g total fat, 7 g saturated fat, 35 mg cholesterol, 606 mg sodium

# PASTA PRIMAVERA

**Serves 4**
**Prep Time:** 20 minutes
**Cook Time:** 18 minutes
**Healing Foods:** cauliflower, broccoli, pasta, mushrooms, tomatoes, milk
**Ailments It Heals:** alcoholism, hyperthyroidism, interstitial cystitis, jaundice

1⅓   cups small cauliflower florets
1⅓   cups small broccoli florets
  7   oz (200 g) plain or spinach fettuccine
  2   tsp olive oil
  1   small red onion, diced
  2   cloves garlic, minced
  ½   lb (250 g) mushrooms, thinly sliced
  ½   tsp salt
  ½   tsp dried rosemary, crumbled
  1   medium tomato, cut into ½-in (1 cm) cubes
  2   tsp flour
  1   cup skim or low-fat milk
  ¼   cup grated parmesan cheese
  ¼   cup parsley

**1.** In large pot of boiling water, cook cauliflower and broccoli for 2 minutes to blanch. With slotted spoon, transfer vegetables to a plate.

**2.** Add fettuccine to boiling water and cook according to package directions. Drain and transfer to large serving bowl.

**3.** While fettuccine cooks, heat 1 tsp oil in large nonstick skillet over medium heat. Add onion and garlic and sauté for 5 minutes, or until tender. Add mushrooms and sauté for 3 minutes or until softened.

**4.** Add remaining 1 tsp oil to skillet and add cauliflower and broccoli, sprinkle with salt and rosemary, and sauté for 1 minute, or until vegetables are heated through. Add tomato and cook for 3 minutes, or until softened.

**5.** Sprinkle flour over vegetables, stirring to coat. Add milk and bring to a boil. Reduce to a simmer and cook, stirring, for 3 minutes, or until slightly thickened. Stir in cheese and parsley. Add to hot pasta, tossing until combined.

**Per serving:** 302 calories, 15 g protein, 49 g carbohydrates, 5 g fiber, 6 g total fat, 2 g saturated fat, 11 mg cholesterol, 467 mg sodium

# PASTA WITH CABBAGE, APPLES, AND LEEKS

Serves 4
**Prep Time:** 20 minutes
**Cook Time:** 15 minutes
**Healing Foods:** leeks, cabbage, apples, vinegar, pasta
**Ailments It Heals:** cholesterol (high), lupus, osteoporosis

2  Tbsp olive oil
2  leeks, halved lengthwise, thinly sliced crosswise, and well washed
3  cups packed shredded green cabbage (about 12 oz or 340 g)
3  cloves garlic, minced
2  large red apples (unpeeled), cut into ½-in (1 cm) chunks
½  tsp salt
½  tsp ground black pepper
2  Tbsp cider vinegar
1  Tbsp dijon mustard
8  oz (250 g) farfalle (bow-tie) pasta

**1.** In large skillet, heat oil over medium heat. Add leeks, and cook, stirring frequently, for 5 minutes, or until tender. Add cabbage and garlic and increase heat to high. Cook, stirring frequently, for 5 minutes, or until cabbage is golden brown.

**2.** Add apples, salt, and pepper and cook for 2 minutes, or until apple is crisp-tender. Stir in vinegar and mustard and cook for 30 seconds to blend flavors.

**3.** Meanwhile, in large pot of boiling water, cook pasta according to package directions. Drain, reserving ½ cup of pasta cooking water. Transfer drained pasta to large bowl. Add cabbage-apple mixture and reserved pasta cooking water and toss to combine.

**Per serving:** 385 calories, 9 g protein, 70 g carbohydrates, 6 g fiber, 8 g total fat, 1 g saturated fat, 0 mg cholesterol, 411 mg sodium

# PASTA WITH WALNUT CREAM SAUCE

Serves 4
**Prep Time:** 10 minutes
**Cook Time:** 10 minutes
**Healing Foods:** pasta, nuts, garlic, olive oil
**Ailments It Heals:** arthritis, cystic fibrosis, stress

8  oz (250 g) whole grain penne, fusilli, or farfalle (bow-tie) pasta
1  cup walnuts, toasted
1 to 3  cloves garlic, mashed
¼  cup basil leaves
2  Tbsp olive oil
½  cup low-fat evaporated milk
¼  cup grated parmesan cheese

**1.** Cook pasta according to package directions. Drain and place in large bowl.

**2.** Meanwhile, in food processor or blender, combine nuts, garlic, and basil. Process or blend until nuts are finely chopped. Add oil and milk and pulse until well blended.

**3.** Add sauce to bowl with hot pasta and sprinkle with cheese.

**Per serving:** 479 calories, 16 g protein, 49 g carbohydrates, 4 g fiber, 26 g total fat, 4 g saturated fat, 9 mg cholesterol, 115 mg sodium

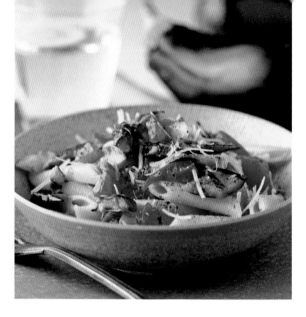

# PENNE WITH FRESH TOMATO SAUCE AND GRILLED EGGPLANT

**Serves 4**
**Prep Time:** 15 minutes plus standing
**Cook Time:** 18 minutes
**Healing Foods:** eggplants, garlic, tomatoes, pasta
**Ailments It Heals:** Alzheimer's disease, prostate problems, urinary tract infections

| | |
|---|---|
| 1 | lb (500 g) eggplant, cut lengthwise into ¾-in-thick (2 cm) slices |
| ½ | tsp salt |
| 2 | Tbsp olive oil |
| 4 | cloves garlic, thinly sliced |
| 1½ | lb (750 g) ripe plum tomatoes, halved, seeded, and coarsely chopped |
| 1 | tsp chopped fresh oregano or ½ tsp dried, crumbled |
| 2 | tsp balsamic vinegar |
| ½ | tsp sugar |
| 8 | oz (250 g) penne pasta |
| ¼ | cup shaved or shredded parmesan cheese |

**1.** Sprinkle eggplant slices with ¼ tsp salt. Let stand at least 30 minutes to draw out liquid.

**2.** Meanwhile, in large nonstick skillet, heat oil over medium-low heat. Add garlic. Cook, stirring, for 1 minute. Add tomatoes, oregano, and remaining ¼ tsp salt. Increase heat to medium and cook for 6 minutes, or just until tomatoes are softened. Stir in vinegar and sugar. Cook for 30 seconds longer.

**3.** Preheat grill or broiler. Rinse eggplant slices and pat dry. Lightly coat both sides of eggplant with olive oil cooking spray. Grill or broil eggplant 4 in (10 cm) from heat for 5 minutes on each side, or until softened and, if grilling, dark grill marks appear. Set aside to cool slightly.

**4.** Meanwhile, in large pot of lightly salted boiling water, cook penne until tender, following package directions. Drain. Toss with tomato mixture. Coarsely chop eggplant. Add to pasta mixture. Stir in parmesan. Serve hot or at room temperature.

**Per serving:** 362 calories, 13 g protein, 59 g carbohydrates, 7 g fiber, 10 g total fat, 2 g saturated fat, 4 mg cholesterol, 406 mg sodium

# BULGUR WITH DRIED CHERRIES AND CORN

Serves 4
**Prep Time:** 20 minutes plus standing
**Healing Foods:** bulgur, tangerines, corn, cherries, peanuts
**Ailments It Heals:** acne, multiple sclerosis, varicose veins

1 cup medium-grain bulgur
2½ cups boiling water
1 tsp grated tangerine or orange zest
1 cup fresh tangerine or orange juice
2 Tbsp tomato paste
2 Tbsp pomegranate molasses
2 Tbsp olive oil
¾ tsp salt
1½ cups corn kernels
⅔ cup dried cherries
⅔ cup thinly sliced scallions
⅓ cup roasted peanuts, coarsely chopped

**1.** In large bowl, combine bulgur and boiling water. Let stand for 30 minutes at room temperature. Drain well.

**2.** Meanwhile, in large bowl, whisk together tangerine zest, tangerine juice, tomato paste, molasses, oil, and salt.

**3.** Add drained bulgur to bowl and fluff with a fork. Add corn, cherries, scallions, and peanuts, tossing to combine. Serve at room temperature or chilled.

**Per serving:** 433 calories, 10 g protein, 69 g carbohydrates, 10 g fiber, 14 g total fat, 2 g saturated fat, 0 mg cholesterol, 511 mg sodium

# BULGUR WITH SPRING VEGETABLES

Serves 6
**Prep Time:** 15 minutes plus standing
**Cook Time:** 10 minutes
**Healing Foods:** bulgur, leeks, asparagus, peas
**Ailments It Heals:** circulatory disorders, depression, diabetes, respiratory disorders

1¼ cups bulgur
3½ cups boiling water
2 Tbsp olive oil
3 Tbsp fresh lemon juice
1 tsp salt
½ tsp ground black pepper
2 leeks, halved lengthwise, cut crosswise into 1-in (2.5 cm) pieces, and well washed
2 cloves garlic, minced
12 asparagus spears, cut into 2-in (5 cm) lengths
1 cup frozen peas
¼ cup chopped fresh mint

**1.** In large heatproof bowl, combine bulgur and boiling water. Let stand for 30 minutes, stirring after 15 minutes, until bulgur is tender. Drain well in large fine-meshed sieve.

**2.** In large bowl, whisk together 1 Tbsp oil, lemon juice, salt, and pepper. Add drained bulgur and fluff with a fork.

**3.** In medium skillet, heat remaining 1 Tbsp oil over low heat. Add leeks and garlic to skillet and cook for 5 minutes, or until leeks are tender. Transfer to bowl with bulgur.

**4.** In steamer set over a pan of boiling water, steam asparagus for 4 minutes, or until tender. Add peas during final 30 seconds of steaming. Add to bowl of bulgur along with mint and toss to combine. Serve at room temperature or chilled.

**Per serving:** 188 calories, 6 g protein, 32 g carbohydrates, 8 g fiber, 5 g total fat, 1 g saturated fat, 0 mg cholesterol, 330 mg sodium

# QUINOA WITH CHILES AND CILANTRO

Serves 6
**Prep Time:** 15 minutes
**Cook Time:** 35 minutes
**Healing Foods:** quinoa, chiles, cilantro, seeds, limes
**Ailments It Heals:** AIDS and HIV infections, celiac disease, jaundice

| | |
|---|---|
| 1 | cup quinoa |
| 2 | tsp canola oil |
| 1 | cup chopped onion (1 medium) |
| 4 | oz (125 g) chopped green chiles |
| 2 | cloves garlic, minced |
| 1¾ | cups reduced-sodium chicken broth or vegetable broth |
| ¾ | cup coarsely chopped fresh cilantro |
| ½ | cup chopped scallions |
| ¼ | cup pepitas (pumpkin seeds), toasted |
| 2 | Tbsp lime juice |
| ¼ | tsp salt, or to taste |

**1.** In large dry skillet, toast quinoa over medium heat, stirring often, for 3 to 5 minutes, or until it crackles and becomes aromatic. Transfer to a fine sieve and rinse thoroughly.

**2.** Heat oil in large saucepan over medium heat. Add onion and cook, stirring often, for 2 to 3 minutes, or until softened. Add chiles and garlic. Cook, stirring, for 30 seconds. Add broth and quinoa and bring to a simmer. Reduce heat to low, cover, and cook for 20 to 25 minutes, or until quinoa is tender and most of liquid has been absorbed.

**3.** Add cilantro, scallions, pepitas, lime juice, and salt to quinoa. Mix gently and fluff with a fork.

**Per serving:** 182 calories, 7 g protein, 27 g carbohydrates, 4 g fiber, 6 g total fat, 1 g saturated fat, 0 mg cholesterol, 145 mg sodium

# SPRINGTIME QUINOA

Serves 6
**Prep Time:** 10 minutes
**Cook Time:** 25 minutes
**Healing Foods:** quinoa, asparagus, peas
**Ailments It Heals:** bleeding problems, jaundice, migraines and other headaches, PCOS

| | |
|---|---|
| 1 | cup quinoa, rinsed and drained |
| ½ | tsp salt |
| 2 | cups water |
| 1 | Tbsp olive oil |
| 1 | small red onion, halved and cut into thin slices |
| ½ | cup vegetable or chicken broth |
| 1 | lb (500 g) asparagus, cut into 2-in (5 cm) pieces |
| 1 | cup fresh peas |

**1.** In small saucepan over high heat, bring quinoa, salt, and water to a boil. Reduce heat to low, cover, and simmer for 15 minutes, or until water is absorbed.

**2.** Meanwhile, in large nonstick skillet, heat oil over medium heat. Add onion and cook for 4 minutes, or until lightly browned. Add broth, asparagus, and peas and cook for 5 minutes, or until crisp-tender. Stir in quinoa.

**Per serving:** 171 calories, 8 g protein, 28 g carbohydrates, 5 g fiber, 4 g total fat, 1 g saturated fat, 0 mg cholesterol, 262 mg sodium

# BAKED RICE WITH WILD MUSHROOMS AND CHEESE

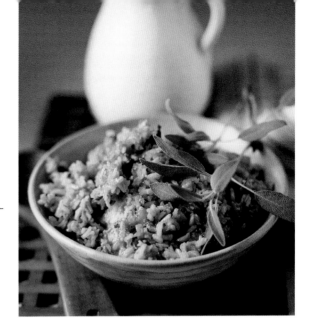

**Serves 6**

**Prep Time:** 20 minutes plus standing

**Cook Time:** 55 minutes

**Healing Foods:** mushrooms, tomatoes, rice, cheese

**Ailments It Heals:** cancer, cystic fibrosis, diverticulitis

⅓ cup dried porcini mushrooms

2½ cups hot water

⅓ cup sun-dried tomatoes (not oil-packed)

1 tsp olive oil

1 large onion, finely chopped

3 cloves garlic, minced

1 cup brown rice

1 tsp salt

½ tsp rubbed sage

½ tsp ground black pepper

½ cup shredded reduced-fat sharp cheddar cheese

2 Tbsp grated parmesan cheese

**1.** Place porcini in small bowl and pour 1 ½ cups hot water over them. Place sun-dried tomatoes in separate small bowl and pour remaining 1 cup hot water over them. Let both stand for 20 minutes, or until softened.

**2.** Scoop mushrooms out of soaking liquid. Finely chop mushrooms. Strain soaking liquid through fine-meshed sieve into bowl. Strain sun-dried tomato soaking liquid into same bowl and set aside. Coarsely chop tomatoes.

**3.** Preheat oven to 350°F (180°C). In medium saucepan, heat oil and 3 Tbsp mushroom-tomato soaking liquid over medium heat. Add onion and garlic and cook for 7 minutes, or until onion is golden. Add rice, stirring to coat. Add mushrooms, tomatoes, salt, sage, and pepper. Stir until well combined.

**4.** Transfer mixture to 8-in (2 L) square glass baking dish. Pour remaining soaking liquid on top and stir to combine. Cover with foil and bake for 45 minutes, or until rice is tender and liquid is absorbed. Sprinkle with cheeses.

**Per serving:** 199 calories, 9 g protein, 33 g carbohydrates, 3 g fiber, 4 g total fat, 2 g saturated fat, 5 mg cholesterol, 518 mg sodium

# BROWN RICE WITH CABBAGE AND CHICKPEAS

Serves 4

**Prep Time:** 15 minutes

**Cook Time:** 47 minutes

**Healing Foods:** garlic, cabbage, rice, chickpeas, tomatoes, raisins

**Ailments It Heals:** depression, gallstones, infertility, obesity, psoriasis

1   Tbsp olive oil

1   large red onion, finely chopped

5   cloves garlic, thinly sliced

12   oz (375 g) green cabbage, cut into 1-in (2.5 cm) chunks (about 6 cups)

¾   cup brown rice

2   cups water

¾   tsp salt

19   oz (540 mL) canned chickpeas, drained and rinsed

1   cup canned tomatoes, chopped, with their juice

¾   cup raisins

**1.** In large saucepan, heat oil over medium heat. Add onion and garlic and cook, stirring frequently, for 7 minutes, or until onion is tender.

**2.** Stir in cabbage. Cover and cook for 5 minutes, or until cabbage begins to wilt.

**3.** Stir in brown rice, water, and salt and bring to a boil. Reduce to a simmer, cover, and cook for 25 minutes, or until rice is almost done.

**4.** Stir in chickpeas, tomatoes, and raisins and bring to a boil. Reduce to a simmer, cover, and cook for 10 minutes, or until rice is tender.

**Per serving:** 392 calories, 11 g protein, 75 g carbohydrates, 10 g fiber, 7 g total fat, 1 g saturated fat, 0 mg cholesterol, 710 mg sodium

# FRIED RICE WITH TOFU AND VEGETABLES

Serves 4

**Prep Time:** 20 minutes plus marinating

**Cook Time:** 20 minutes

**Healing Foods:** ginger, tofu, rice

**Ailments It Heals:** cystic fibrosis, menopause, osteoporosis, stroke

1   cup dry white wine or chicken broth

¼   cup light soy sauce

2   Tbsp honey

1   Tbsp grated peeled fresh ginger

12   oz (375 g) extra-firm tofu, cut into 1-in (2.5 cm) cubes

1   cup long-grain white or brown rice

2   cloves garlic, minced

16   oz (480 g) frozen mixed Chinese vegetables, slightly thawed

¼   tsp ground black pepper

5   scallions, cut into 2-in (5 cm) pieces

1   large egg, lightly beaten

**1.** In large resealable plastic bag, combine wine, 1 Tbsp soy sauce, honey, and 1 tsp ginger. Add tofu, press out excess air, close bag, and shake gently to coat. Marinate in refrigerator for 1 hour, turning occasionally.

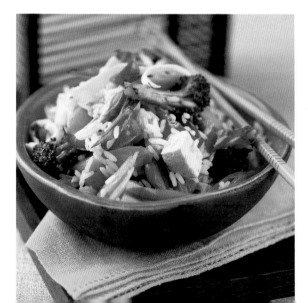

**2.** Cook rice according to package directions. Keep warm.

**3.** Meanwhile, lightly coat wok or large deep skillet with cooking spray and set over high heat until hot but not smoking. Stir-fry garlic and remaining ginger for 1 minute, or until fragrant. Add rice, mixed vegetables, pepper, half of scallions, and remaining soy sauce. Stir-fry for 4 minutes, or until mixed vegetables are heated through. Push ingredients to one side of wok, then pour in beaten egg. Cook egg until almost set, cutting into strips with heatproof spatula.

**4.** Pour marinade into small saucepan. Boil over high heat for 2 minutes. Add tofu and marinade to wok. Stir-fry for 4 minutes, or until tofu is heated. Sprinkle with remaining scallions.

**Per serving:** 442 calories, 21 g protein, 61 g carbohydrates, 3 g fiber, 9 g total fat, 2 g saturated fat, 53 mg cholesterol, 668 mg sodium

# RICE SALAD WITH CHICKEN AND GRAPES

Serves 8
**Prep Time:** 15 minutes
**Cook Time:** 25 minutes
**Healing Foods:** onions, rice, vinegar, chicken, grapes
**Ailments It Heals:** celiac disease, insomnia, peptic ulcers

⅓ cup olive oil
2 onions, finely chopped
1 tsp sugar
2 cups jasmine rice (Thai fragrant rice) or basmati rice
1½ cups salt-reduced chicken stock
¾ tsp salt
1½ cups water
½ cup rice vinegar
4 cups shredded cooked chicken breasts, leftover or poached
2 cups seedless grapes
4 Tbsp chopped fresh cilantro
½ cup pine nuts, toasted

**1.** In large saucepan, heat 2 Tbsp oil over medium-low heat. Add onions and sugar and cook, stirring frequently, for 7 minutes, or until onions are tender. Stir in rice, stock, ½ tsp salt, and water. Bring to a boil, reduce to a simmer, cover, and cook for 17 minutes, or until rice is tender. Drain off any excess liquid.

**2.** In large bowl, whisk together vinegar and remaining oil and ¼ tsp salt. Add rice mixture to bowl and toss with a fork to combine.

**3.** Add chicken, grapes, coriander, and pine nuts and toss with a fork. Serve immediately, or chilled.

**Per serving:** 441 calories, 25 g protein, 45 g carbohydrates, 2 g fiber, 17 g total fat, 2 g saturated fat, 54 mg cholesterol, 276 mg sodium

# RICE-STUFFED SQUASH

Serves 4
**Prep Time:** 25 minutes
**Cook Time:** 1 hour 5 minutes
**Healing Foods:** rice, acorn squash, cranberries, cheese
**Ailments It Heals:** blood pressure, eczema, gallstones

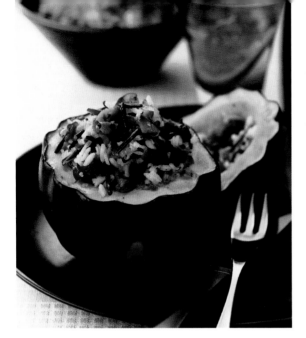

4. Spoon rice stuffing into squashes, pressing it down, and mounding it up neatly on top. Replace reserved hats on top. Bake for 45 minutes, or until flesh of squash is tender when pierced with a small sharp knife. Serve hot.

**Per serving:** 415 calories, 12 g protein, 89 g carbohydrates, 12 g fiber, 4 g total fat, 2 g saturated fat, 8 mg cholesterol, 85 mg sodium

- 1 cup mixed basmati and wild rice
- 3 cups water
- 4 small acorn squashes

Salt and ground black pepper

- ¾ cup cooked chestnuts (canned or vacuum packed), roughly chopped
- ¾ cup dried cranberries
- 1 small red onion, finely chopped
- 2 Tbsp chopped fresh thyme
- 2 Tbsp chopped parsley
- ¾ cup grated mozzarella cheese

1. Put rice and water in saucepan and bring to a boil. Cover and simmer very gently for 20 minutes, or until rice is just tender. Drain off any excess water.

2. Meanwhile, preheat oven to 350°F (180°C). Using a large, sharp knife, slice off top quarter (stalk end) of each squash. Set aside these little "hats," then scoop out seeds and fiber from center of squashes using a small spoon. Trim bases to make them level, if necessary. Season cavity of each squash lightly with salt and pepper, then place in large ovenproof dish or roasting pan.

3. In large bowl, mix together rice, chestnuts, cranberries, onion, thyme, parsley, and cheese. Season lightly with salt and pepper.

# THAI COCONUT RICE

Serves 6

**Prep Time:** 5 minutes plus standing
**Cook Time:** 20 minutes
**Healing Foods:** coconuts, rice, cilantro
**Ailments It Heals:** celiac disease, insomnia

- 1¼ cups water
- ¾ cup canned light coconut milk
- ½ tsp salt

Pinch of allspice

- 1 cup jasmine rice, rinsed
- ¼ tsp coconut extract
- 1 Tbsp chopped fresh cilantro (optional)

1. In medium saucepan, bring water, coconut milk, salt, and allspice to a boil. Stir in rice and coconut extract, cover, and reduce heat to low. Simmer for 15 to 20 minutes, or until liquid is absorbed and rice is tender.

2. Remove pan from heat and let stand, covered, for 10 minutes. Fluff rice with a fork and scatter on the cilantro, if using.

**Per serving:** 75 calories, 2 g protein, 12 g carbohydrates, 1 g fiber, 2 g total fat, 2 g saturated fat, 0 mg cholesterol, 200 mg sodium

# ARTICHOKES WITH LENTILS AND LIMA BEANS

**Serves 4**
**Prep Time:** 25 minutes
**Cook Time:** 45 minutes
**Healing Foods:** artichokes, lemons, garlic, lentils, lima beans
**Ailments It Heals:** constipation, irritable bowel syndrome, multiple sclerosis

- 4 large artichokes
- 3 Tbsp fresh lemon juice
- 1 Tbsp olive oil
- 1 small onion, finely chopped
- 3 cloves garlic, minced
- 1 large carrot, diced
- ¾ cup lentils, picked over and rinsed
- 1½ cups carrot juice
- ¾ tsp salt
- ½ tsp dried thyme
- 1 cup water
- 10 oz (300 g) frozen lima beans
- 3 oz (90 g) feta cheese

**1.** To trim artichokes: Remove tough outer leaves. Trim tough end of stem. Then, with a paring knife, peel tough skin off remaining stem. Cut off top of artichoke to just about 1 in (2.5 cm) above base. Halve artichokes lengthwise, then scoop out and discard chokes. Halve artichokes again. Place cleaned artichokes in a bowl with cold water to cover. Add 1 Tbsp lemon juice and set aside.

**2.** In Dutch oven, heat oil over medium heat. Add onion and garlic and cook, stirring frequently for 5 minutes, or until onion is golden brown. Stir in carrot and cook for 4 minutes.

**3.** Remove artichokes from water and place in Dutch oven. Stir in lentils, carrot juice, salt, thyme, water, and remaining 2 Tbsp lemon juice. Bring to a boil. Reduce to a simmer, cover, and cook for 25 minutes.

**4.** Stir in lima beans and cook for 10 minutes, or until artichokes, lima beans, and lentils are tender. Serve topped with crumbled feta cheese.

**Per serving:** 423 calories, 25 g protein, 68 g carbohydrates, 16 g fiber, 9 g total fat, 4 g saturated fat, 19 mg cholesterol, 907 mg sodium

# BALSAMIC BEETS WITH TOASTED PECANS

**Serves 4**
**Prep Time:** 5 minutes
**Cook Time:** 10 minutes
**Healing Foods:** pecans, vinegar, beets
**Ailments It Heals:** cardiovascular disease, eye problems, menstrual problems

- 3 Tbsp chopped pecans
- 2 Tbsp balsamic vinegar
- 1 tsp sugar
- 2 tsp butter or margarine
- 3 medium beets, steamed, peeled, and sliced or 1 jar (15 oz or 450 g) sliced beets, drained

**1.** In medium nonstick skillet over medium heat, toast pecans, stirring often, for 4 minutes, or until browned. Transfer to plate.

**2.** In same skillet over medium-low heat, add vinegar, sugar, butter, and beets. Cook, stirring often, for 5 minutes, or until beets are heated through and liquid is absorbed. Top with pecans. Serve at once.

**Per serving:** 86 calories, 1 g protein, 8 g carbohydrates, 2 g fiber, 6 g total fat, 2 g saturated fat, 5 mg cholesterol, 140 mg sodium

# ORANGE BEETS

Serves 6
**Prep Time:** 15 minutes
**Cook Time:** 50 minutes plus cooling
**Healing Foods:** beets, olive oil, vinegar
**Ailments It Heals:** cancer, circulatory
  disorders, psoriasis

4 medium beets with greens
1 Tbsp olive oil
1 clove garlic, minced
½ tsp salt
3 Tbsp orange marmalade
1 Tbsp white wine vinegar
¼ tsp ground black pepper

**1.** Preheat oven to 350°F (180°C). Trim greens
from beets and set aside. Fold a 36-in (90 cm)
piece of foil in half crosswise. Scrub beets and
place in center of foil. Sprinkle with 1 tsp water
and seal foil around beets. Roast for 45 minutes, or
until tender. Let cool for 15 minutes, then remove
skins and cut each beet into eight wedges.

**2.** Meanwhile, trim stems from beet greens, wash
greens, and cut into 1-in (2.5 cm) strips. While beets
are cooling, heat oil in skillet over medium-high
heat. Add garlic and cook for 1 minute. Add greens
and ¼ tsp salt and cook, stirring constantly, for 2
minutes, or until wilted. Transfer to a serving dish.

**3.** Add marmalade, vinegar, pepper, and remaining ¼ tsp salt to skillet over medium-high heat and
cook for 5 minutes, or until hot and bubbling. Add
beets and toss to coat well. Transfer to serving dish
with greens and toss.

**Per serving:** 75 calories, 1 g protein, 13 g carbohydrates,
2 g fiber, 2 g total fat, 0 g saturated fat, 0 mg cholesterol,
253 mg sodium

# SESAME GREENS AND BEAN SPROUTS

Serves 6
**Prep Time:** 10 minutes
**Cook Time:** 8 minutes
**Healing Foods:** seeds, cabbage, bean sprouts
**Ailments It Heals:** arthritis, bleeding
  problems, chronic fatigue syndrome,
  eczema, fibroids

1 Tbsp sesame seeds
2 tsp canola oil
1 onion, chopped
2 cloves garlic, chopped
1 small Savoy cabbage, finely shredded
1 small head bok choy, finely shredded
1 cup bean sprouts
4 Tbsp oyster sauce
2 Tbsp water

**1.** Salt and ground black pepper

**2.** Heat small saucepan over medium heat and dry-
roast sesame seeds, shaking pan frequently, until
they are just beginning to brown. Pour seeds into
small bowl and set aside.

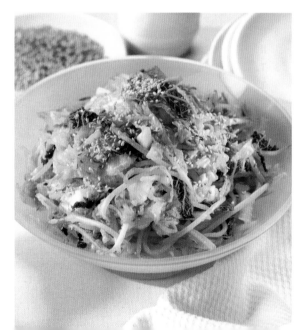

3. Heat oil in wok or large frying pan. Add onion and garlic and stir-fry for 2 to 3 minutes, or until softened slightly. Add cabbage and bok choy and stir-fry over high heat for 2 to 3 minutes, or until vegetables are just beginning to soften. Add bean sprouts and continue cooking for a few seconds.

4. Make a space in center of pan. Add oyster sauce and water and stir until hot, then toss vegetables into sauce. Taste and add salt if necessary (depending on the saltiness of the oyster sauce) and pepper. Serve immediately, sprinkled with toasted sesame seeds.

**Per serving:** 68 calories, 3 g protein, 10 g carbohydrates, 4 g fiber, 3 g total fat, 0 g saturated fat, 0 mg cholesterol, 336 mg sodium

# ORANGE-WALNUT BROCCOLI

Serves 6
**Prep Time:** 5 minutes
**Cook Time:** 11 minutes
**Healing Foods:** nuts, broccoli, oranges
**Ailments It Heals:** gout, halitosis, infertility, varicose veins

  6  large walnut halves
  1  lb (500 g) broccoli florets
  3  Tbsp orange juice
1½  Tbsp extra-virgin olive oil
  1  Tbsp chopped fresh basil
  1  tsp grated orange zest
  ¼  tsp salt
  ⅛  tsp ground black pepper

1. Heat large nonstick skillet over medium-high heat. When hot, add walnuts and toast for 2 to 3 minutes, or until fragrant. Remove to cutting board, cool, and chop.

2. Add broccoli and orange juice to same skillet, cover, and cook for 3 minutes. Uncover and cook until liquid evaporates.

3. Add oil and sauté for 5 to 6 minutes, or until broccoli is tender.

4. Add basil, orange zest, salt, and pepper and remove from heat. Sprinkle with walnuts.

**Per serving:** 70 calories, 3 g protein, 5 g carbohydrates, 2 g fiber, 5 g total fat, 1 g saturated fat, 0 mg cholesterol, 117 mg sodium

# BROCCOLI AND CAULIFLOWER WITH CREAM SAUCE

Serves 4
**Prep Time:** 10 minutes
**Cook Time:** 13 minutes
**Healing Foods:** carrots, broccoli, cauliflower
**Ailments It Heals:** dental problems, lupus, memory loss, prostate problems

  ½  cup carrot juice
  3  Tbsp reduced-fat sour cream
  2  cups broccoli florets
  2  cups cauliflower florets

1. In small saucepan over high heat, boil carrot juice for 8 minutes, or until reduced to ¼ cup. Remove from heat. Whisk in sour cream.

2. In steamer set over a pan of boiling water, steam broccoli and cauliflower for 5 minutes, or until crisp-tender. Transfer to serving dish. Serve with sour cream sauce.

**Per serving:** 44 calories, 3 g protein, 6 g carbohydrates, 2 g fiber, 2 g total fat, 1 g saturated fat, 4 mg cholesterol, 45 mg sodium

# BASIL-SCENTED SAUTÉED VEGETABLES

Serves 4
**Prep Time:** 10 minutes
**Cook Time:** 8 minutes
**Healing Foods:** broccoli, garlic, peppers, turnips
**Ailments It Heals:** acne, burns, gout, varicose veins

- 1 lb (500 g) broccoli
- 2 tsp olive oil
- 3 or 4 large cloves garlic, thinly sliced
- 1 large or 2 small red bell peppers, seeded and cut into 1-in (2.5 cm) squares
- 1 small turnip, cut into ½-in (1 cm) cubes
Pinch of sugar
Salt
- 6 Tbsp water
- 8 sprigs fresh basil, stems discarded, leaves finely shredded

**1.** Cut broccoli into small florets, then trim and thinly slice stalks. In large nonstick skillet or wok, heat oil over medium-high heat. Add garlic, bell pepper, turnip, and broccoli stalks. Sprinkle in sugar and salt to taste. Cook for 2 to 3 minutes, stirring frequently.

**2.** Add broccoli florets and stir. Add water to provide a thin covering on bottom of pan. Cover and cook over high heat for 3 to 4 minutes, or until just tender and bright green.

**3.** Stir in basil, cover, and heat for a few more seconds. Serve immediately.

**Per serving:** 74 calories, 4 g protein, 11 g carbohydrates, 5 g fiber, 3 g total fat, 0 g saturated fat, 0 mg cholesterol, 43 mg sodium

# FRUITY BRUSSELS SPROUTS

Serves 4
**Prep Time:** 25 minutes
**Healing Foods:** brussels sprouts, apples, carrots, celery, dates
**Ailments It Heals:** colds and flu, fibroids, infertility, interstitial cystitis

- 3 tsp créme fraîche
- 1½ Tbsp low-fat mayonnaise
- 2 tsp olive oil
Grated zest and juice of 1 orange
- 2 tsp white wine vinegar
Salt and ground black pepper
- 8 oz (250 g) brussels sprouts
- 1 apple
- 1 carrot, grated
- 3 celery stalks, chopped
- 2 Tbsp chopped fresh cilantro
- 1 oz (30 g) fresh dates, stoned and chopped

**1.** In a small bowl, whisk together crème fraîche, mayonnaise, oil, orange zest and juice, and vinegar. Season to taste with salt and pepper. Set dressing aside.

**2.** Trim off and discard bases and outer leaves of sprouts, then shred finely and put into a large bowl. Cut unpeeled apple into quarters, remove core, and chop into small chunks. Add to bowl along with carrot and celery.

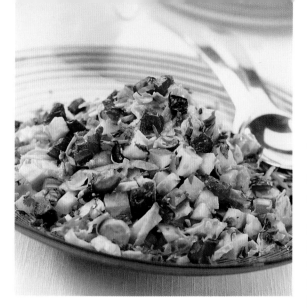

**3.** Stir in enough dressing to coat salad, saving any left over to serve on the side. Scatter cilantro and dates over salad and serve.

**Per serving:** 122 calories, 2 g protein, 18 g carbohydrates, 4 g fiber, 5 g total fat, 1 g saturated fat, 5 mg cholesterol, 104 mg sodium

½ cup reduced-sodium chicken broth or
  vegetable broth
3 Tbsp cider vinegar
¼ tsp salt, or to taste

**1.** Ground black pepper to taste

**2.** Quarter brussels sprouts with sharp knife or shred in food processor fitted with a slicing disk.

**3.** In large nonstick skillet, heat oil over medium-high heat. Add onion and bell pepper. Cook, stirring often, for 3 to 4 minutes, or until softened. Add caraway seeds and cook, stirring, for 30 seconds. Add brussels sprouts and cook, stirring, for 2 minutes.

**4.** Add broth, cover, and cook for 2 to 3 minutes, or until sprouts are crisp-tender. Stir in vinegar, salt, and pepper.

**Per serving:** 75 calories, 3 g protein, 11 g carbohydrates, 4 g fiber, 3 g total fat, 0 g saturated fat, 0 mg cholesterol, 233 mg sodium

# BRUSSELS SPROUTS WITH CARAWAY SEEDS

Serves 4
**Prep Time:** 15 minutes
**Cook Time:** 10 minutes
**Healing Foods:** brussels sprouts, onions, peppers, seeds, vinegar
**Ailments It Heals:** Alzheimer's disease, bleeding disorders, fibroids

3 cups brussels sprouts, trimmed and cored
2 tsp canola oil
1 cup sliced onion (1 medium)
1 medium red bell pepper, cored, seeded, and cut into 2-in-long (5 cm) slivers
1½ tsp caraway seeds

# NAPA CABBAGE SLAW WITH PEANUT DRESSING

Serves 6
**Prep Time:** 20 minutes
**Healing Foods:** peanut butter, tea, vinegar, chiles, cabbage
**Ailments It Heals:** blood pressure, cancer, osteoporosis

⅓ cup natural peanut butter
¼ cup hot brewed black or green tea
4 tsp reduced-sodium soy sauce
4 tsp rice vinegar
1½ tsp brown sugar
1 tsp hot sauce, such as sriracha, chile-garlic sauce, or Tabasco

1   clove garlic, minced
4   cups thinly sliced napa cabbage
1   cup shredded carrots
½   cup chopped scallions
⅓   cup unsalted roasted peanuts

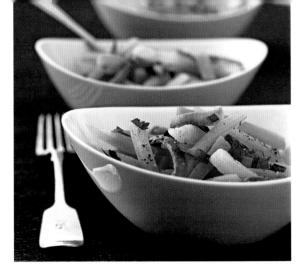

**1.** Place peanut butter in large bowl and gradually whisk in hot tea. Add soy sauce, vinegar, brown sugar, hot sauce, and garlic and whisk until smooth.

**2.** Add cabbage, carrots, and scallions and toss to coat well. Sprinkle with peanuts.

**Per serving:** 158 calories, 7 g protein, 11 g carbohydrates, 3 g fiber, 11 g total fat, 2 g saturated fat, 0 mg cholesterol, 226 mg sodium

boil, then reduce heat and simmer, covered, for 15 minutes, or until vegetables are tender.

**2.** Uncover saucepan. Boil for 2 to 3 minutes, or until liquid reduces slightly. Season to taste with salt and pepper. Stir in butter and serve.

**Per serving:** 77 calories, 3 g protein, 13 g carbohydrates, 4 g fiber, 2 g total fat, 1 g saturated fat, 5 mg cholesterol, 616 mg sodium

# BRAISED CARROT, CELERY, AND FENNEL

Serves 4
**Prep Time:** 10 minutes
**Cook Time:** 18 minutes
**Healing Foods:** carrots, celery, onions, fennel
**Ailments It Heals:** blood pressure, eye problems, obesity

4   carrots, peeled, halved lengthwise, and cut into 2½ × ¼-in (6 × 0.5 cm) pieces
3   celery ribs, peeled and cut into 2½ × ¼-in (6 × 0.5 cm) pieces
1   small red onion, thinly sliced
½   fennel bulb, cored and thinly sliced
14.5   oz (440 mL) reduced-sodium, fat-free chicken broth
Salt and ground black pepper
2   tsp butter

**1.** In large saucepan over medium-high heat, add carrots, celery, onion, fennel, and broth. Bring to

# CARROT AND PARSNIP PUREE

Serves 4
**Prep Time:** 10 minutes
**Cook Time:** 20 minutes
**Healing Foods:** carrots, parsnips
**Ailments It Heals:** dental problems, multiple sclerosis, Parkinson's disease, PCOS

3   large carrots, peeled and chopped
1   large parsnip, peeled and chopped
½   tsp salt
1   Tbsp butter or vegetable oil
1   tsp grated orange zest

**1.** In medium saucepan, combine carrots, parsnip, salt, and enough water to barely cover vegetables.

Simmer, uncovered, for 20 minutes, or until vegetables are very tender and most of liquid has evaporated.

**2.** Drain vegetables. Transfer to food processor or blender. Add butter and orange zest. Process until vegetables form a smooth puree.

**Per serving:** 82 calories, 1 g protein, 13 g carbohydrates, 3 g fiber, 3 g total fat, 2 g saturated fat, 8 mg cholesterol, 408 mg sodium

# ROASTED ROOT VEGETABLES

Serves 4
**Prep Time:** 10 minutes
**Cook Time:** 40 minutes
**Healing Foods:** carrots, parsnips, ginger, cinnamon
**Ailments It Heals:** AIDS and HIV infections, migraines and other headaches, stroke, respiratory disorders

1   lb (500 g) carrots, peeled and sliced diagonally into ½-in (1 cm) pieces
1   lb (500 g) parsnips, peeled and sliced diagonally into ½-in (1 cm) pieces
2   Tbsp olive oil
1   Tbsp grated fresh ginger
1   tsp ground cinnamon
½   tsp salt

**1.** Preheat oven to 400°F (200°C). Place carrots, parsnips, oil, ginger, cinnamon, and salt in large roasting pan and toss to coat well. Roast, turning occasionally, for 40 minutes, or until tender and browned.

**Per serving:** 199 calories, 3 g protein, 33 g carbohydrates, 9 g fiber, 7 g total fat, 1 g saturated fat, 0 mg cholesterol, 361 mg sodium

# CAULIFLOWER AND SPINACH CASSEROLE

Serves 6
**Prep Time:** 20 minutes
**Cook Time:** 50 minutes
**Healing Foods:** paprika, cauliflower, spinach, milk, cheese
**Ailments It Heals:** Alzheimer's disease, chronic fatigue syndrome, lupus, prostate problems

3   Tbsp plain dry bread crumbs
1   tsp olive oil
¼   tsp paprika
1   medium cauliflower (about 2½ lb or 1.25 kg), cored and cut into 1½-in (3.5 cm) florets (about 7 cups)
10   oz (300 g) fresh spinach or kale (12 cups), stems trimmed, washed
1¾   cups cold low-fat milk
3   Tbsp all-purpose flour
1⅓   cups grated extra-sharp cheddar cheese
1½   tsp dry mustard
½   tsp salt, or to taste
Ground black pepper to taste

**1.** Preheat oven to 425°F (220°C). Coat a 12 × 8-in (30 × 20 cm) shallow baking dish (2½-qt or 2½ L capacity) with cooking spray.

**2.** In small bowl, mix bread crumbs, oil, and paprika.

**3.** In large pot of lightly salted boiling water, cook cauliflower, uncovered, for 6 minutes, or until tender. Stir in spinach and cook for 1 minute, or until spinach has wilted. Drain and rinse vegetables with cold water to stop further cooking. Drain thoroughly and spread in baking dish.

**4.** In small bowl, whisk ¼ cup milk with flour until smooth. In heavy medium saucepan, heat remaining

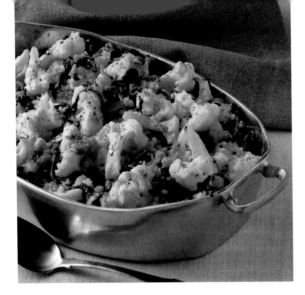

1 Tbsp canola oil

1 tsp cumin seeds

2 medium onions, thinly sliced (2 cups)

2 jalapeño chile peppers, seeded and minced
   (wear gloves when handling; they burn)

4 cloves garlic, minced

1 Tbsp grated fresh ginger

1 Tbsp ground coriander

1 tsp ground cumin

½ tsp turmeric

1 cup water

1 medium head cauliflower, cut into florets
   (7 to 8 cups)

¾ tsp salt, or to taste

1 medium tomato, diced (1 cup)

1 cup frozen green peas, rinsed under cold
   water to thaw

⅓ cup chopped fresh cilantro

Lime wedges

1½ cups milk over medium heat until steaming. Remove from heat and whisk in flour mixture. Return to medium heat and cook, whisking constantly, for 2 to 3 minutes, or until sauce bubbles and thickens. Remove from heat. Stir in cheese, mustard, salt, and pepper. Pour sauce over vegetables in baking dish, spreading evenly. Sprinkle with bread crumb mixture.

**5.** Bake, uncovered, for 30 to 35 minutes, or until golden and bubbly.

**Per serving:** 224 calories, 14 g protein, 21 g carbohydrates, 14 g fiber, 11 g total fat, 6 g saturated fat, 31 mg cholesterol, 530 mg sodium

**1.** In Dutch oven, heat oil over medium-high heat. Add cumin seeds and cook, stirring, for 10 to 20 seconds, or until they sizzle. Add onions, chile peppers, garlic, and ginger. Cook, stirring often, for 2 to 3 minutes, or until softened. Add coriander, ground cumin, and turmeric. Stir for 10 to 20 seconds, or until fragrant. Add water, cauliflower, and salt. Stir to coat well. Cover and cook for 8 minutes, or until cauliflower is almost tender.

**2.** Stir in tomato and peas. Cover and cook for 2 to 3 minutes, or until cauliflower is tender and peas are heated through. Sprinkle with cilantro and serve with lime wedges. Leftovers will keep, covered, in refrigerator for up to 2 days. Reheat in microwave.

**Per serving:** 85 calories, 4 g protein, 13 g carbohydrates, 4 g fiber, 3 g total fat, 0 g saturated fat, 0 mg cholesterol, 349 mg sodium

# SPICED CAULIFLOWER WITH PEAS

Serves 6

**Prep Time:** 25 minutes

**Cook Time:** 15 minutes

**Healing Foods:** cumin, cauliflower, tomatoes, peas, cilantro

**Ailments It Heals:** diabetes, fibroids, neuralgia

# GREEN BEANS WITH TOMATOES AND OLIVES

Serves 4
**Prep Time:** 5 minutes
**Cook Time:** 25 minutes
**Healing Foods:** onions, green beans, tomatoes, olives
**Ailments It Heals:** Alzheimer's disease, prostate problems, urinary tract infections

1 Tbsp olive oil
1 cup chopped onions
1 small clove garlic, minced
1 lb (500 g) green beans, trimmed
15 oz (425 mL) petite-cut diced tomatoes, with juice
½ tsp dried oregano
1 tsp red wine vinegar
1 Tbsp chopped pitted kalamata olives
⅛ tsp ground black pepper

**1.** In large nonstick skillet, heat oil over medium-high heat. Add onions and cook for 4 minutes, or until soft. Add garlic and green beans and cook for 1 minute.

**2.** Stir in tomatoes (with juice) and oregano. Reduce heat to medium-low, cover, and simmer gently for 15 to 20 minutes, or until green beans are tender.

**3.** Stir in vinegar, olives, and pepper.

**Per serving:** 107 calories, 3 g protein, 17 g carbohydrates, 4 g fiber, 4 g total fat, 1 g saturated fat, 0 mg cholesterol, 343 mg sodium

# BRAISED MIXED GREENS WITH DRIED CURRANTS

Serves 4 to 6
**Prep Time:** 10 minutes
**Cook Time:** 16 minutes
**Healing Foods:** garlic, cooking greens
**Ailments It Heals:** hyperthyroidism, hypothyroidism, mood disorders, sex drive (diminished)

1 Tbsp extra-virgin olive oil
3 cloves garlic, thinly sliced
1 lb (500 g) mixed cooking greens (collards, kale, turnip greens, and mustard), rinsed and slightly drained
1 Tbsp dried currants

**1.** In small skillet, heat oil and garlic over low heat, stirring, until garlic begins to sizzle. Watch carefully and remove from heat when garlic begins to turn golden, after about 5 minutes. Set aside.

**2.** In large wide pan, cook greens and currants over medium heat, covered, turning once or twice with tongs, for 10 minutes, or until wilted and tender. Raise heat to high. Cook, uncovered, to evaporate any excess moisture.

**3.** Add garlic and reheat, stirring, for 1 minute.

**Per serving:** 81 calories, 3 g protein, 10 g carbohydrates, 4 g fiber, 4 g total fat, 1 g saturated fat, 0 mg cholesterol, 24 mg sodium

# SWEET AND SOUR GREENS WITH BACON

Serves 4
**Prep Time:** 15 minutes
**Cook Time:** 15 minutes
**Healing Foods:** garlic, mustard greens, prunes, honey
**Ailments It Heals:** blood pressure, constipation, hyperthyroidism

1 Tbsp extra-virgin olive oil
3 slices turkey bacon, cut into thin strips
3 cloves garlic, thinly sliced
24 cups (loosely packed) cleaned mustard greens, shredded
¼ cup water
3 small pitted prunes, diced
¼ tsp salt
2 tsp red wine vinegar
1 tsp honey
¼ tsp hot sauce, or more to taste

**1.** In Dutch oven, heat oil over medium-low heat. Add turkey bacon and cook for 5 minutes, or until lightly crisped. Remove with slotted spoon. Add garlic to pan and cook for 3 minutes, or until golden brown.

**2.** Add mustard greens and toss to coat. Add water, prunes, and salt and cook, stirring occasionally, for 5 minutes, or until soft and tender.

**3.** Return bacon to pan along with vinegar, honey, and hot sauce and stir to combine. Serve hot.

**Per serving:** 163 calories, 10 g protein, 22 g carbohydrates, 10 g fiber, 6 g fat, 1 g saturated fat, 9 mg cholesterol, 464 mg sodium

# NEW POTATOES WITH NORI

Serves 4
**Prep Time:** 5 minutes
**Cook Time:** 15 minutes
**Healing Foods:** potatoes, lemons, seaweed, chives
**Ailments It Heals:** celiac disease, mood disorders, neuralgia, stroke

1 lb (500 g) unpeeled small new potatoes
1 oz (30 g) butter
Grated zest and juice of ½ small lemon
1 sheet toasted sushi nori, about 8 x 7 in (20 x 18 cm)
Salt and ground black pepper
2 Tbsp snipped fresh chives

**1.** Cook potatoes in saucepan of boiling water for 12 minutes, or until just tender.

**2.** Reserve 3 Tbsp of cooking water, then drain potatoes and return them to saucepan with reserved water. Add butter and lemon zest and juice, and toss potatoes to coat with liquid.

**3.** Use scissors to snip sushi nori into fine strips. Sprinkle nori over potatoes and cover pan. Cook over low heat for 1 to 2 minutes, or until nori has softened. Add salt and pepper to taste, sprinkle with chives, and serve.

**Per serving:** 134 calories, 2 g protein, 19 g carbohydrates, 2 g fiber, 6 g total fat, 4 g saturated fat, 15 mg cholesterol, 22 mg sodium

# SWEET POTATO AND CELERIAC PUREE

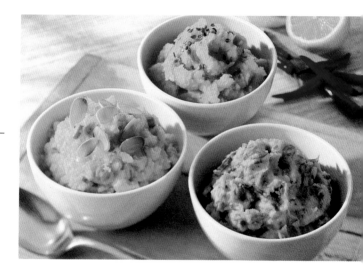

Serves 6
**Prep Time:** 15 minutes
**Cook Time:** 20 minutes
**Healing Foods:** sweet potatoes, celeriac, ginger, apples, coriander
**Ailments It Heals:** arthritis, cancer, cardiovascular disease

1 lb (500 g) sweet potato, peeled and cut into 1-in (2.5 cm) cubes
1 medium celeriac, peeled and cut into 1-in (2.5 cm) cubes
Juice of 1 lemon
1 Tbsp olive oil
2 cloves garlic, finely chopped
1 Tbsp coarsely grated fresh ginger
1 tsp ground cumin
1 Golden Delicious apple, peeled, cored, and finely chopped
1 Tbsp coriander seeds, roughly crushed

**1.** Cut sweet potato and celeriac into similar-size chunks and place in large saucepan. Add half of lemon juice and enough water to cover vegetables and bring to a boil. Reduce heat and simmer gently for 15 to 20 minutes, or until vegetables are tender.

**2.** Meanwhile, heat oil in small saucepan. Add garlic, ginger, and cumin and cook for 30 seconds. Stir in apple and remaining lemon juice and cook for 5 minutes, or until apple begins to soften.

**3.** In small, dry pan, toast crushed coriander seeds, stirring occasionally, for a few minutes or until fragrant.

**4.** Drain vegetables well, place in large bowl, and mash them. Stir in apple mixture and sprinkle with toasted coriander seeds. Serve hot.

**Per serving:** 113 calories, 2 g protein, 22 g carbohydrates, 3 g fiber, 3 g total fat, 0 g saturated fat, 0 mg cholesterol, 46 mg sodium

# TWICE-BAKED STUFFED SWEET POTATOES

Serves 4
**Prep Time:** 10 minutes
**Cook Time:** 1 hour 10 minutes
**Healing Foods:** sweet potatoes, pineapples, pecans
**Ailments It Heals:** hypothyroidism, interstitial cystitis, memory loss

2 large sweet potatoes (1½ lb or 750 g)
8 oz (225 mL) crushed pineapple, drained
1 Tbsp vegetable oil
1 Tbsp butter
1 Tbsp light or dark brown sugar
1 tsp grated orange zest
½ tsp salt
2 Tbsp chopped pecans

1. Preheat oven to 350°F (180°C). Pierce each sweet potato twice with tip of knife.

2. Bake for 50 minutes, or until soft. Set aside until cool enough to handle but still very warm. Reduce oven heat to 325°F (160°C).

3. Cut potatoes in half lengthwise. Scoop out flesh and place in medium bowl, being careful not to tear skin. Reserve skins. Add pineapple, oil, butter, brown sugar, orange zest, and salt to potato flesh. Whip with electric mixer or whisk until slightly fluffy.

4. Place skin shells on baking sheet. Fill with potato mixture, mounding each. Bake for 15 minutes. Sprinkle with pecans and bake for 5 minutes.

**Per serving:** 236 calories, 2 g protein, 38 g carbohydrates, 4 g fiber, 9 g total fat, 2 g saturated fat, 8 mg cholesterol, 303 mg sodium

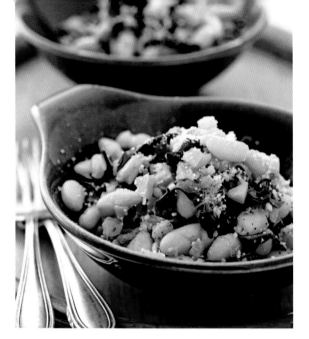

# WHITE BEANS STEWED WITH SWISS CHARD

Serves 8
**Prep Time:** 10 minutes
**Cook Time:** 26 minutes
**Healing Foods:** cooking greens, carrots, beans, cheese
**Ailments It Heals:** diabetes, eye problems, fibroids, menstrual problems

1   small bunch Swiss chard (½ lb or 250 g)
2   Tbsp olive oil
1   small onion, finely chopped
1   carrot, peeled and finely chopped
1   tsp dried oregano, crumbled
1   bay leaf
2   cloves garlic, minced
1   cup reduced-sodium, fat-free chicken broth
38  oz (1,080 mL) cannellini beans, drained and rinsed
½   tsp salt
⅛   tsp ground black pepper
½   cup grated parmesan cheese

1. Remove tough stems from chard and finely chop. Coarsely chop leaves.

2. In large nonstick skillet, heat oil over medium heat. Add onion, carrot, oregano, and bay leaf. Sauté for 8 minutes, or until onion and carrot are very soft. Add garlic. Sauté 30 seconds.

3. Add chard and broth to skillet. Cook, stirring occasionally, for 2 minutes, or until chard just begins to wilt. Stir in beans. Simmer, covered, for 10 minutes. Uncover and cook for 5 minutes, or until chard is tender. Add salt and pepper. Remove bay leaf. Sprinkle with cheese and serve.

**Per serving:** 139 calories, 7 g protein, 16 g carbohydrates, 5 g fiber, 5 g total fat, 1 g saturated fat, 4 mg cholesterol, 482 mg sodium

# ROASTED TOMATOES WITH GARLIC AND HERBS

Serves 4
**Prep Time:** 10 minutes
**Cook Time:** 3 hours
**Healing Foods:** tomatoes, garlic, basil, rosemary
**Ailments It Heals:** Alzheimer's disease, cancer, circulatory disorders, gallstones, prostate problems

3  lb (1.5 kg) plum tomatoes, halved lengthwise
2  Tbsp olive oil
5  cloves garlic, finely chopped
½  cup finely chopped fresh basil
2  Tbsp minced fresh rosemary
1  tsp sugar
¾  tsp salt

**1.** Preheat oven to 250°F (120°C). Line a jelly-roll pan with foil.

**2.** In large bowl, toss tomatoes with oil, garlic, basil, rosemary, sugar, and salt. Place tomatoes, cut side up, in prepared pan. Bake for 3 hours, or until tomatoes have collapsed and their skins have wrinkled.

**3.** Serve at room temperature, or refrigerate and serve chilled.

**Per serving:** 148 calories, 4 g protein, 19 g carbohydrates, 5 g fiber, 8 g total fat, 1 g saturated fat, 0 mg cholesterol, 468 mg sodium

# HERB-BUTTERED TURNIPS

Serves 4
**Prep Time:** 5 minutes
**Cook Time:** 15 minutes
**Healing Foods:** turnips, chives, mint, parsley
**Ailments It Heals:** infertility, mood disorders, nail problems

10  tiny young turnips with leaves reserved and shredded (leaves optional)
3½  Tbsp butter
Rosemary sprig
Salt and ground black pepper
1  Tbsp snipped chives
1  Tbsp shredded mint
2  Tbsp chopped parsley

**1.** Wash turnips gently and cut off leaves, leaving ½ in (1 cm) green stalk attached. Put turnips in saucepan of salted water and bring to a boil. Cook for 10 minutes, or until just tender, then drain thoroughly.

**2.** In wide frying pan, heat butter and rosemary, then add turnips. Cook for 2 to 3 minutes, or until shiny and just beginning to show patches of color.

**3.** Remove rosemary, add salt and pepper to taste, and scatter on chives, mint, parsley, and turnip leaves, if using. Shake pan to coat turnips evenly. Serve warm.

**Per serving:** 124 calories, 1 g protein, 8 g carbohydrates, 2 g fiber, 10 g total fat, 6 g saturated fat, 27 mg cholesterol, 83 mg sodium

# MASHED TURNIPS WITH CARROTS AND POTATOES

Serves 4

**Prep Time:** 15 minutes

**Cook Time:** 20 minutes

**Healing Foods:** turnips, potatoes, carrots, garlic, thyme

**Ailments It Heals:** cirrhosis, menstrual problems, sore throat

1¾ lb (875 g) turnips, peeled, quartered and thinly sliced

9 oz (275 g) potatoes (about 2 medium), peeled and thinly sliced

9 oz (275 g) carrots (about 4 medium), peeled and thinly sliced

5 cloves garlic, peeled

1 bay leaf

1 tsp fresh thyme leaves

4 cups water

Salt and ground black pepper

2 tsp olive oil

¼ cup grated parmesan cheese

**1.** In large saucepan, combine turnips, potatoes, carrots, garlic, bay leaf, thyme, water, and a pinch each of salt and pepper. Bring to a boil over medium heat, reduce to a simmer, cover, and cook for 15 minutes, or until tender. Drain, reserving ½ cup of cooking liquid. Discard bay leaf.

**2.** Mash vegetables and garlic with a potato masher, adding reserved cooking liquid and oil. Stir in cheese just before serving.

**Per serving:** 211 calories, 7 g protein, 36 g carbohydrates, 6 g fiber, 5 g total fat, 2 g saturated fat, 10 mg cholesterol, 292 mg sodium

# CIDER-BAKED ACORN SQUASH WITH APPLE STUFFING

Serves 4

**Prep Time:** 15 minutes

**Cook Time:** 1 hour

**Healing Foods:** acorn squash, apples, cinnamon, nutmeg

**Ailments It Heals:** cardiovascular disease, indigestion and heartburn, interstitial cystitis

2 small acorn squash (about 1 lb or 500 g each), halved lengthwise and seeded

½ cup apple cider or apple juice

½ tsp salt

1 apple pared, cored, and chopped

1 Tbsp light brown sugar

¼ tsp ground cinnamon

⅛ tsp ground nutmeg

**1.** Preheat oven to 350°F (180°C).

**2.** Place squash halves, cut side down, in 13 × 9-in (33 x 23 cm) baking dish. Add cider to the dish.

**3.** Bake for 30 minutes. Remove from oven and leave oven on. Carefully turn squash cut side up and sprinkle with salt.

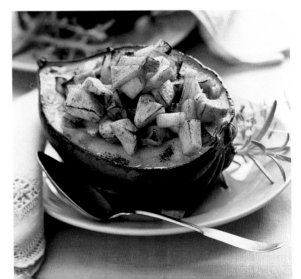

4. In small bowl, combine apple, brown sugar, cinnamon, and nutmeg. Spoon evenly into squash halves. Drizzle cider from baking dish over mixture, using a baster if you have one. Add a couple spoonfuls of water to dish.

5. Bake, stuffed side up, for 30 minutes or until tender.

**Per serving:** 123 calories, 2 g protein, 32 g carbohydrates, 7 g fiber, 0 g total fat, 0 g saturated fat, 0 mg cholesterol, 298 mg sodium

# FRUITY BUTTERNUT SQUASH CASSEROLE WITH PAPAYA

**Serves 4**
**Prep Time:** 15 minutes
**Cook Time:** 10 minutes
**Healing Foods:** butternut squash, papayas, sage, oranges, beans
**Ailments It Heals:** eczema, memory loss, multiple sclerosis

½ butternut squash (about 1¼ lb or 625 g)
1 papaya (about 10 oz or 300g)
1 red onion
1 Tbsp vegetable oil
4 to 6 large fresh sage leaves
1 tsp ground cinnamon
1 Juice of 1 large orange (about 7 Tbsp)
14 oz (398 mL) canned borlotti, kidney, or pinto beans, drained

1. Peel and seed butternut squash and dice flesh into 1-in (2.5 cm) chunks. Seed and peel papaya, then slice it and set aside. Thinly slice onion.

2. Heat oil in large pan with lid. Add onion and squash and cook over high heat, stirring occasionally, for 1 minute. Reduce heat to medium or medium-low, cover, and cook for 2 minutes.

3. Shred sage leaves. Stir leaves, cinnamon, and orange juice into pan. Bring to a boil, reduce heat to low, and cover again. Simmer for 5 minutes, stirring once, or until squash is tender but not soft.

4. Stir in beans, cover, and heat gently for 2 minutes. Top with papaya and serve immediately.

**Per serving:** 215 calories, 7 g protein, 42 g carbohydrates, 10 g fiber, 4 g total fat, 1 g saturated fat, 0 mg cholesterol, 295 mg sodium

# BAKED YUCCA CHIPS

**Serves 10**
**Prep Time:** 10 minutes
**Cook Time:** 10 minutes
**Healing Foods:** yucca, cilantro, limes
**Ailments It Heals:** circulatory disorders, osteoporosis, varicose veins

1 large yucca root
2 Tbsp olive oil
½ cup chopped cilantro
2 tsp ground ginger
Pinch of salt
Pinch of ground black pepper
3 Tbsp fresh lime juice

1. Preheat oven to 375°F (190°C).

2. Peel yucca with vegetable peeler, removing all waxy brown skin and pinkish layer underneath. Then cut into ⅛ in (0.3 cm) slices.

3. Toss yucca and oil in bowl. Mix in cilantro, ginger, salt, pepper, and lime juice. Mix to coat.

**4.** Spread slices on nonstick baking sheet. Bake for 4 to 5 minutes on each side, or until golden brown.

**Per serving:** 93 calories, 1 g protein, 16 g carbohydrates, 1 g fiber, 3 g total fat, 0 g saturated fat, 0 mg cholesterol, 43 mg sodium

# SAVORY CRANBERRY CHUTNEY

Serves 6
**Prep Time:** 10 minutes
**Cook Time:** 17 minutes
**Healing Foods:** onions, cranberries, cherries, oranges, allspice
**Ailments It Heals:** acne, urinary tract infections, varicose veins

2 tsp olive oil
1 large red onion, finely chopped
3 cloves garlic, minced
12 oz (375 g) fresh or frozen cranberries
½ cup firmly packed light brown sugar
½ cup dried cherries
2 tsp grated orange zest
½ cup orange juice
½ tsp ground black pepper
¼ tsp salt
⅛ tsp allspice

**1.** In large saucepan, heat oil over medium-low heat. Add onion and garlic and cook, stirring frequently, for 7 minutes, or until onion is tender.

**2.** Stir in cranberries, brown sugar, dried cherries, orange zest, orange juice, pepper, salt, and allspice. Cook, stirring occasionally, for 10 minutes, or until berries have popped. Cool to room temperature. Serve at room temperature or chilled.

**Per serving:** 174 calories, 1 g protein, 42 g carbohydrates, 3 g fiber, 2 g total fat, 0 saturated fat, 0 mg cholesterol, 108 mg sodium

# TOMATO BISCUITS

Makes 12
**Prep Time:** 12 minutes
**Cook Time:** 12 minutes
**Healing Foods:** tomatoes, yogurt, olive oil
**Ailments It Heals:** Alzheimer's disease, colds and flu, gallstones

1 medium tomato, seeded and finely chopped
1 cup all-purpose flour
1 cup whole wheat flour
1 Tbsp baking powder
½ tsp salt
1 cup low-fat plain yogurt
⅓ cup olive oil
2 Tbsp finely chopped scallions
1 Tbsp finely chopped sun-dried tomatoes

**1.** Preheat oven to 450°F (230°C). Lightly coat baking sheet with cooking spray. Drain chopped fresh tomato on paper towels.

**2.** In medium bowl, combine flour, baking powder, and salt. In small bowl, combine yogurt and oil. Stir into flour mixture until evenly moistened.

**3.** Stir fresh tomato, scallions, and sun-dried tomatoes into flour mixture. Drop dough, ¼ cup at a time, onto prepared baking sheet, for a total of 12 biscuits.

**4.** Bake for 12 minutes, or until tops are golden brown. Serve warm.

**Per serving:** 145 calories, 4 g protein, 18 g carbohydrates, 1 g fiber, 7 g total fat, 1 g saturated fat, 1 mg cholesterol, 255 mg sodium

# WHOLE WHEAT PUMPKIN ROLLS

**Per serving:** 177 calories, 6 g protein, 27 g carbohydrates, 2 g fiber, 6 g total fat, 1 g saturated fat, 0 mg cholesterol, 197 mg sodium

Makes 24
**Prep Time:** 25 minutes plus rising
**Cook Time:** 12 minutes
**Healing Foods:** pumpkins, wheat, seeds
**Ailments It Heals:** arthritis, depression, diabetes

 1  envelope active dry yeast
 ½  cup warm water (105° to 115°F or 40° to 46°C)
 ¼  cup honey
 15  oz (450 g) solid-pack unsweetened pumpkin
 2  Tbsp olive oil
 4½  cups all-purpose flour
 1  cup whole wheat flour
 2  tsp salt
 1½  cups unsalted, shelled pumpkin seeds, lightly toasted

**1.** In large bowl, sprinkle yeast over warm water. Let stand for 5 minutes, or until foamy. Stir in honey until dissolved. Stir in pumpkin and oil. Stir in 4 cups all-purpose flour, whole wheat flour, and salt until dough forms.

**2.** Turn dough out onto floured surface. Knead for 10 minutes, or until smooth and elastic, adding more flour as needed to prevent sticking. Work in pumpkin seeds. Place dough in lightly oiled bowl. Turn to coat. Cover loosely with plastic wrap. Let rise in warm place until doubled in volume, about 1½ hours.

**3.** Line 2 baking sheets with foil. Punch dough down. Form dough into 24 equal-size rolls. Place on prepared baking sheets. Cover loosely with plastic wrap. Let rise in warm place for 1 hour, or until doubled in volume.

**4.** Preheat oven to 400°F (200°C). Uncover rolls.

**5.** Bake for 12 minutes, or until puffed and golden and sounds hollow when tapped on bottom. Serve warm or at room temperature.

# MULTIGRAIN SEEDED LOAF

Serves 8
**Prep Time:** 25 minutes plus rising
**Cook Time:** 35 minutes
**Healing Foods:** wheat, buckwheat, seeds, flax
**Ailments It Heals:** chronic fatigue syndrome, circulatory disorders, menstrual problems, neuralgia, prostate problems

 2  cups white flour
 1⅓  cups whole wheat flour
 ¾  cup buckwheat flour
 ½  cup coarse polenta (cornmeal)
 2  tsp instant or rapid rise yeast
 1  tsp brown sugar
 3  Tbsp sunflower seeds
 2  Tbsp pumpkin seeds
 2  Tbsp flaxseed
 2  Tbsp sunflower oil
 2  cups tepid water
Low-fat milk to glaze

**1.** Sift flours into large bowl, tipping in any bran left in sieve. Stir in polenta, yeast, and brown sugar.

**2.** Mix seeds together, reserving 1 Tbsp for the topping. Stir remainder into flour mixture.

**3.** Make a well in dry ingredients and pour in oil and water. Mix with your hands to make a soft dough, adding more water if dough is too dry. Turn out onto lightly floured work surface and knead for 10 minutes, or until smooth and elastic. Place in large, lightly oiled bowl and cover with damp tea towel. Set aside in warm, draft-free place for 1½ hours, or until doubled in size.

**4.** Punch the dough and knead firmly for a few minutes. Shape into 8-in (20 cm) round and place on lightly greased baking sheet. Cover with oiled plastic wrap and leave for 20 to 30 minutes, or until well risen and springy to the touch.

**5.** Preheat oven to 450°F (230°C). Use a sharp knife to make slashes on top of loaf to mark eight wedges. Brush top with a little milk and sprinkle with reserved mixed seeds.

**6.** Bake for 15 minutes, then reduce oven temperature to 400°F (200°C). Bake for 15 to 20 minutes, or until golden brown and sounds hollow when tapped on bottom. Cool for 5 minutes on baking sheet, then transfer to wire rack to cool completely.

**Per serving:** 391 calories, 12 g protein, 62 g carbohydrates, 8 g fiber, 11 g total fat, 1 g saturated fat, 0 mg cholesterol, 10 mg sodium

# WHOLE WHEAT FLAXSEED BREAD

**Serves 8**
**Prep Time:** 20 minutes plus rising
**Cook Time:** 30 minutes
**Healing Foods:** wheat, flax, olive oil
**Ailments It Heals:** chronic fatigue syndrome, hemorrhoids, menopause, osteoporosis, stress

1⅓ cups whole wheat flour
⅔ cup bread flour or all-purpose flour
3 Tbsp whole flaxseed, ground, or ¼ cup flaxseed meal
2 Tbsp nonfat dry milk
1½ tsp instant or rapid rise yeast
¾ tsp salt
¾ cup water, at room temperature
1 Tbsp molasses or honey
1 Tbsp olive oil
1 egg white, lightly beaten with 1 Tbsp water
1 Tbsp whole flaxseed

**1.** In food processor fitted with a metal chopping blade, combine flours, ground flaxseed (or flaxseed meal), dry milk, yeast, and salt. Pulse several times to blend. In a measuring cup, stir together water, molasses (or honey), and oil until molasses is fully dissolved. With motor running, slowly pour enough liquid through feeder tube to make a smooth dough that pulls away from the work bowl sides. Consistency should be smooth yet soft to the touch; adjust if necessary by adding flour 1 Tbsp at a time or water 1 tsp at a time. Process for 1 minute to knead. Transfer dough to a bowl coated with cooking spray and turn to coat. Cover with plastic wrap and let rise at room temperature until doubled in bulk, 1½ to 1¾ hours.

**2.** Coat a baking sheet with cooking spray. When dough has doubled, turn it out onto a lightly floured surface. Punch it down and shape into a round or oval loaf (or make 2 small loaves). Place loaf on baking sheet. Coat a sheet of plastic wrap with cooking spray and cover loaf with it. Let rise until almost doubled in bulk, about 1 hour.

**3.** Meanwhile, place a small metal baking pan on bottom oven rack. Preheat oven to 400°F (200°C).

**4.** When loaf has risen, brush it with egg white mixture and sprinkle with whole flaxseed. Pour 1 cup water into baking pan in oven to create steam. Use a serrated knife to score four ¼-in-deep (0.5 cm) slashes in loaf. Bake for 20 to 30 minutes, or until bread is golden and sounds hollow when tapped. Transfer to wire rack to cool.

**Per serving:** 155 calories, 5 g protein, 27 g carbohydrates, 3 g fiber, 4 g total fat, 1 g saturated fat, 0 mg cholesterol, 229 mg sodium

# BANANA-PEANUT BREAD

Serves 10
**Prep Time:** 10 minutes
**Cook Time:** 50 minutes plus cooling
**Healing Foods:** bananas, peanut butter, wheat, oats, flax
**Ailments It Heals:** hypoglycemia, infertility, insomnia, muscle cramps, stress

3 very ripe medium bananas, mashed (about 1 cup)
½ cup natural peanut butter
2 eggs
1 Tbsp canola oil
1½ cups whole wheat pastry flour
½ cup whole oats, ground
¼ cup sugar
2 Tbsp ground flaxseed
2 tsp baking powder
½ tsp baking soda
½ tsp salt

**1.** Preheat oven to 350°F (180°C). Lightly coat a 9 x 5-in (23 x 12 cm) loaf pan with cooking spray.

**2.** In medium bowl, stir together bananas, peanut butter, eggs, and oil. In large bowl, mix together flour, oats, sugar, flaxseed, baking powder, baking soda, and salt.

**3.** Make a well in center of flour mixture, add banana mixture, and stir just until moistened. Place in pan.

**4.** Bake for 40 to 50 minutes, or until a wooden pick inserted in center comes out clean. Transfer to a rack and let cool for 5 minutes, then remove from pan and let cool completely.

**Per serving:** 234 calories, 7 g protein, 31 g carbohydrates, 4 g fiber, 9 g total fat, 1 g saturated fat, 42 mg cholesterol, 351 mg sodium

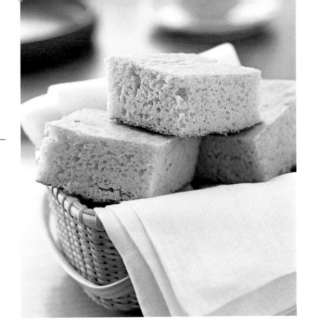

# CARROT-FLECKED CORN BREAD

Serves 9
**Prep Time:** 10 minutes
**Cook Time:** 25 minutes plus cooling
**Healing Foods:** flour, eggs, carrots
**Ailments It Heals:** cirrhosis, indigestion and heartburn, migraines and other headaches, rosacea

2 Tbsp vegetable oil
2 cups white or yellow cornmeal
⅓ cup all-purpose flour
2 tsp baking powder
1 tsp baking soda
2 Tbsp sugar
1 tsp salt
1¾ cups low-fat buttermilk
1 large egg, lightly beaten
2 medium carrots, peeled and finely shredded

**1.** Preheat oven to 400°F (200°C). Swirl oil in 8 × 8 × 2-in (20 x 20 x 5 cm) baking pan. Place pan in oven for 5 minutes while preheating.

**2.** Meanwhile, in large bowl, combine cornmeal, flour, baking powder, baking soda, sugar, and salt. Stir in buttermilk, egg, and carrots. Carefully pour in oil from baking pan. Mix well. Pour batter into hot pan.

**3.** Bake for 25 minutes, or until wooden pick inserted in center comes out clean,. Let cool in pan 10 minutes. Turn out onto wire rack. Let cool slightly before cutting. Serve warm.

**Per serving:** 202 calories, 6 g protein, 34 g carbohydrates, 3 g fiber, 5 g total fat, 1 g saturated fat, 26 mg cholesterol, 550 mg sodium

# TOASTED OAT-RAISIN BREAD

Serves 12
**Prep Time:** 15 minutes
**Cook Time:** 1 hour 29 minutes plus cooling
**Healing Foods:** oats, flax, bran, yogurt, raisins
**Ailments It Heals:** cholesterol (high), diverticulitis, stroke,

1½  cups old-fashioned rolled oats
 ½  cup flaxseed
 ½  cup wheat bran
 1  cup all-purpose flour
 ½  cup firmly packed light brown sugar
 2  tsp baking powder
 ¾  tsp salt
1½  cups low-fat plain yogurt
 ⅔  cup honey
 1  large egg
 1  cup raisins

**1.** Preheat oven to 350°F (180°C). Lightly grease a 9 x 5-in (23 x 12 cm) metal loaf pan.

**2.** Place oats, flaxseed, and wheat bran on a baking sheet. Bake for 7 to 9 minutes, or until oats are golden brown. Transfer to food processor and process until finely ground.

**3.** Transfer oat mixture to large bowl. Stir in flour, brown sugar, baking powder, and salt.

**4.** In separate bowl, whisk together yogurt, honey, and egg. Make a well in center of dry ingredients and fold in yogurt mixture until just combined. Fold in raisins.

**5.** Spoon batter into prepared pan, smoothing the top. Bake for 1 hour 20 minutes, or until a wooden pick inserted in center of loaf comes out clean. Cool for 5 minutes in pan, then invert loaf onto wire rack to cool completely.

**Per serving:** 276 calories, 7 g protein, 57 g carbohydrates, 5 g fiber, 4 g total fat, 1 g saturated fat, 20 mg cholesterol, 261 mg sodium

# WALNUT SHORTBREAD

Serves 8
**Prep Time:** 15 minutes
**Cook Time:** 37 minutes
**Healing Foods:** nuts, wheat
**Ailments It Heals:** AIDS and HIV infection, cystic fibrosis, gallstones, hay fever, stroke

 ⅔  cup walnuts
 ¾  cup all-purpose flour
 ½  cup whole wheat flour
 ½  cup confectioners' sugar
 ¼  tsp salt
 ¼  cup walnut oil
 ¼  cup light olive oil
1½  tsp grated lemon zest
 1  tsp vanilla extract

1. Preheat oven to 325°F (160°C). Place walnuts on baking sheet and toast for 7 minutes, or until crisp and fragrant. Leave oven on. Cool walnuts, then transfer to food processor with all-purpose flour, and process until nuts are finely ground.

2. Transfer flour-walnut mixture to large bowl. Stir in whole wheat flour, confectioners' sugar, and salt. Add walnut oil, olive oil, lemon zest, and vanilla and stir until well combined.

3. Press dough onto bottom of 9-in (23 cm) tart pan with removable bottom. With tines of a fork, prick dough. With a sharp knife, score dough into 16 wedges, cutting almost to bottom.

4. Bake for 30 minutes, or until crisp and light golden. Check shortbread after 20 minutes. If it is overbrowning, decrease oven temperature to 300°F (150°C). Remove from oven and, while shortbread is still warm, cut wedges through to bottom. Cool in pan on wire rack.

**Per serving:** 273 calories, 3 g protein, 24 g carbohydrates, 2 g fiber, 19 g total fat, 2 g saturated fat, 0 mg cholesterol, 73 mg sodium

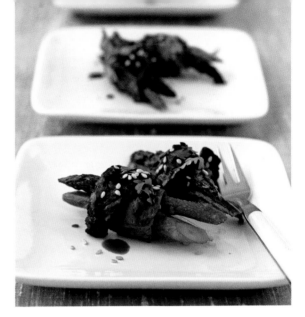

## SNACKS

# BEEF, SCALLION, AND ASPARAGUS ROLL-UPS

**Serves 4**
**Prep Time:** 15 minutes
**Cook Time:** 6 minutes
**Healing Foods:** asparagus, beef, onions, seeds, cilantro
**Ailments It Heals:** mood disorders, PCOS, peptic ulcers

8   asparagus stalks, trimmed to 6-in (15 cm) lengths
8   thin slices sirloin steak (¼ lb or 125 g total)
4   scallions, trimmed to 6-in (15 cm) lengths
2   tsp vegetable oil
3   Tbsp bottled teriyaki sauce
1   Tbsp sesame seeds, toasted
1   Tbsp chopped cilantro

1. Heat saucepan of water to a boil. Cut each asparagus stalk in half. Blanch in boiling water for 1 minute, then drain. Meanwhile, pound sirloin slices to ⅛-in (0.3 cm) thickness. Cut each scallion into two 3-in (7.5 cm) pieces.

2. Place 2 pieces of asparagus and 1 piece of scallion near one end of each beef strip. Roll beef around middle of vegetables to form eight bundles.

3. In large nonstick skillet, heat oil over medium-high heat. Add rolls. Brown for 2 minutes, turning frequently. Add teriyaki sauce, lower heat to medium, and boil for 3 minutes.

4. Transfer rolls to serving platter. Sprinkle with sesame seeds and cilantro.

**Per serving:** 91 calories, 7 g protein, 4 g carbohydrates, 1 g fiber, 5 g total fat, 1 g saturated fat, 16 mg cholesterol, 533 mg sodium

# BUFFALO CHICKEN FINGERS

Serves 4
**Prep Time:** 15 minutes
**Cook Time:** 4 minutes
**Healing Foods:** chicken, vinegar, cheese
**Ailments It Heals:** anorexia, cystic fibrosis, iron overload, PCOS

1 lb (500 g) boneless, skinless chicken breast halves
½ tsp celery salt
¼ tsp garlic powder
2 tsp margarine
2 Tbsp red wine vinegar
¼ tsp ground red pepper
¼ cup nonfat sour cream
1 Tbsp nonfat mayonnaise
¼ cup crumbled blue cheese
1 Tbsp Worcestershire sauce

**1.** Cut chicken into sixteen 4 x 1-in (10 x 2.5-cm) fingers. Mix celery salt and garlic powder. Sprinkle chicken with half of this mixture. Coat large nonstick skillet with cooking spray and set over medium-high heat. Pan-fry chicken for 2 minutes on each side, or until cooked through.

**2.** Remove skillet from heat and stir in margarine, vinegar, and red pepper. Toss with spatula to coat chicken evenly. Transfer to serving platter and keep warm.

**3.** In medium bowl, combine sour cream, mayonnaise, blue cheese, Worcestershire sauce, and remaining celery salt mixture to make dipping sauce.

**Per serving:** 188 calories, 29 g protein, 3 g carbohydrates, 0 g fiber, 6 g total fat, 2 g saturated fat, 72 mg cholesterol, 620 mg sodium

# PESTO CHICKEN SPIRALS WITH ROASTED PEPPERS

Serves 4
**Prep Time:** 15 minutes
**Cook Time:** 15 minutes
**Healing Foods:** chicken, cheese, salad greens, peppers, basil
**Ailments It Heals:** bleeding problems, depression, hepatitis

4 boneless, skinless chicken breast halves (about 1½ lb or 750 g)
¼ tsp ground black pepper
4 oz (125 g) soft goat cheese
1 packed cup watercress leaves, thick stems removed
¾ cup jarred roasted red peppers
1 small scallion, finely chopped
¼ cup prepared reduced-fat basil pesto

**1.** Put chicken breasts one at a time, with smooth side down, between sheets of waxed paper or plastic wrap. Working from the center to the edges, pound lightly with flat side of a meat mallet or small skillet to make chicken an even ¼-in (0.5 cm) thickness. Remove waxed paper or plastic.

**2.** Sprinkle chicken with pepper, then spread on goat cheese, leaving a ¼-in (0.5 cm) border around edges. Top with watercress, roasted peppers, and scallion. Roll up jelly-roll style from short side, pushing in sides as you roll, to enclose filling. Secure with wooden picks.

**3.** Brush pesto over surface of chicken. If making ahead, bundles can be covered and refrigerated for up to 8 hours; bring to room temperature before cooking.

**4.** Heat large nonstick skillet or griddle over medium heat. When hot, coat with cooking spray and add chicken bundles. Cook for 10 to 15 minutes, or until chicken is no longer pink and filling is hot, turning now and then and covering pan for the last 5 to 7 minutes of cooking.

**5.** Cool slightly, then slice crosswise on a slight diagonal to reveal the filling.

**Per serving:** 338 calories, 47 g protein, 5 g carbohydrates, 1 g fiber, 13 g total fat, 6 g saturated fat, 115 mg cholesterol, 421 mg sodium

# TURKEY BACON AND APRICOT BITES

Makes 24
**Prep Time:** 15 minutes
**Cook Time:** 2 minutes
**Healing Foods:** apricots, oranges, turkey
**Ailments It Heals:** blood pressure, hepatitis, yeast infections

**Bites**
24   dried apricots
Juice of 1 orange
 2   tsp no-sugar-added orange marmalade
 2   tsp dijon mustard
 6   slices lean turkey bacon
 1   tsp olive oil
Chopped fresh parsley (optional)

**1.** Place apricots in small bowl, pour orange juice over, and toss so that apricots are moistened all over (this will prevent them from burning when grilled).

**2.** Mix marmalade with mustard. Spread each slice of turkey bacon with a little mustard mixture. Using scissors, cut bacon in half lengthwise. Cut each piece in half again, this time across the middle, to make a total of 24 strips of bacon.

**3.** Preheat a ridged grill pan or oven broiler to medium. Drain apricots. Wrap a strip of turkey bacon around each apricot and secure it with a wooden pick.

**4.** Arrange turkey bites on grill pan, then brush each with a little oil. Grill on each side for 1 minute, or until bacon is just cooked.

**5.** Pile bites in small, shallow bowl and sprinkle with chopped parsley, if using. Serve hot.

**Per serving:** 29 calories, 1 g protein, 5 g carbohydrates, 1 g fiber, 1 g total fat, 0 g saturated fat, 3 mg cholesterol, 54 mg sodium

# GRILLED OYSTERS WITH FENNEL AND SPINACH

Serves 4
**Prep Time:** 10 minutes
**Cook Time:** 17 minutes
**Healing Foods:** oysters, potatoes, fennel, spinach
**Ailments It Heals:** fibroids, flatulence, infertility, sex drive (diminished)

16   oysters in the shell, opened and top shell discarded
Salt and ground black pepper
1½   Tbsp butter
 1   shallot, finely chopped
 1   small potato, peeled and finely diced
 ½   cup fennel bulb, finely diced
 2   cups spinach, coarsely chopped
 1   Tbsp lemon juice
 2   Tbsp chopped fresh parsley
Lemon wedges

1. Check oysters to make sure there are no bits of shattered shell on them. Arrange them, on their half shells, in four individual flameproof dishes, or on one large dish. Season with salt and pepper to taste. (Propping shells with crumpled foil will prevent them from tipping.)

2. Preheat grill to medium. Heat butter in frying pan, add shallot, and cook over low heat for 2 minutes, or until shallot begins to soften. Add potato and fennel and cook gently, stirring occasionally, for 10 minutes, or until tender.

3. Stir in spinach and cook for 1 to 2 minutes, or until spinach has just wilted. Add lemon juice and parsley and season to taste with salt and pepper. Spoon 1 Tbsp of mixture over each oyster.

4. Grill oysters for 3 minutes, or until topping is tinged brown. Serve immediately, with lemon wedges.

**Per serving:** 98 calories, 4 g protein, 11 g carbohydrates, 2 g fiber, 5 g total fat, 3 g saturated fat, 29 mg cholesterol, 91 mg sodium

# OYSTERS WITH TOMATO SALSA

Serves 4
**Prep Time:** 7 minutes
**Healing Foods:** tomatoes, onions, parsley, limes, oysters
**Ailments It Heals:** acne, chronic fatigue syndrome, respiratory disease

 1  large ripe tomato, seeded and diced
 ½  red onion, finely chopped
 2  Tbsp chopped fresh parsley
 2  Tbsp lime juice
Salt and ground black pepper
 2  dozen oysters, freshly opened

To make salsa: In medium bowl, combine tomato, onion, parsley, lime juice, a pinch of salt, and a good grinding of pepper. To serve, top each oyster with 1 tsp salsa.

**Per serving:** 80 calories, 7 g protein, 7 g carbohydrates, 1 g fiber, 3 g total fat, 1 g saturated fat, 53 mg cholesterol, 110 mg sodium

# PITA PIZZAS

Serves 4
**Prep Time:** 10 minutes
**Cook Time:** 3 minutes
**Healing Foods:** peppers, seeds, cheese, wheat
**Ailments It Heals:** circulatory disorders, diabetes, jaundice, stroke

 ½  cup thinly sliced roasted red peppers
 ¼  tsp crushed fennel seeds or dried oregano, crumbled
 ¼  tsp salt
 ⅛  tsp ground black pepper
 ¼  cup shredded, reduced-fat mozzarella cheese
 2  Tbsp shredded, gruyère or jarlsberg cheese
 2  whole wheat pita breads (4 in or 10 cm)
 8  tsp bottled tomato sauce or pizza sauce
 ½  small red onion, thinly sliced

1. Preheat broiler.

2. In small bowl, combine red peppers, fennel or oregano, salt, and pepper. In another small bowl, combine cheeses.

3. Separate each pita bread into 2 flat rounds. Place rounds, rough side up, on baking sheet. Broil 4 in (10 cm) from heat for 1 minute, or until golden brown around edges. Remove from broiler.

4. Spread 2 tsp sauce over each pita, covering edges. Spoon 2 Tbsp red pepper mixture over each pita. Sprinkle with cheese, dividing equally, then add onion in rings.

5. Broil for 2 minutes, or until cheese is melted and pizzas are hot.

**Per serving:** 137 calories, 7 g protein, 23 g carbohydrates, 3 g fiber, 3 g total fat, 2 g saturated fat, 7 mg cholesterol, 475 mg sodium

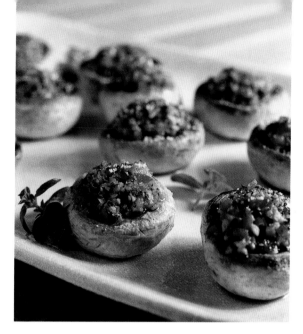

# VEGETABLE-STUFFED MUSHROOMS

Serves 4
**Prep Time:** 20 minutes
**Cook Time:** 25 minutes
**Healing Foods:** mushrooms, onions, carrots, peppers, cheese
**Ailments It Heals:** anorexia, diabetes, diverticulitis

24 large or 12 extra-large mushrooms, stems removed
2 tsp vegetable oil
1 onion, finely chopped
3 cloves garlic, minced
1 carrot, finely chopped
1 red bell pepper, finely chopped
½ cup chicken broth
½ tsp dried oregano
3 Tbsp grated parmesan cheese
2 Tbsp chopped parsley

1. Preheat oven to 400°F (200°C). In a medium pot of boiling water, cook mushroom caps for 2 minutes to blanch. Drain on paper towels.

2. In large skillet, heat oil over medium heat. Add onion and garlic and sauté for 5 minutes. Add carrot and pepper and cook for 4 minutes. Add broth and oregano and cook for 4 minutes, or until vegetables are very soft. Remove from heat and stir in cheese and parsley.

3. Spoon mixture into mushroom caps and place on baking sheet. Bake for 10 minutes, or until piping hot.

**Per serving:** 90 calories, 6 g protein, 9 g carbohydrates, 2 g fiber, 5 g total fat, 1 g saturated fat, 5 mg cholesterol, 120 mg sodium

# ASIAN PEANUT DIP

Serves 8
**Prep Time:** 10 minutes
**Healing Foods:** peanut butter, tofu, limes
**Ailments It Heals:** anorexia, cardiovascular disease, hypoglycemia, infertility

½ cup natural-style peanut butter
⅓ cup low-fat firm silken tofu
3 Tbsp firmly packed light brown sugar
2 Tbsp reduced-sodium soy sauce
2 Tbsp lime juice
½ to ¾ tsp crushed red-pepper flakes
2 cloves garlic, crushed

1. In a food processor, combine peanut butter, tofu, brown sugar, soy sauce, lime juice, red pepper, and garlic. Process until smooth and creamy, stopping once or twice to scrape down sides of work bowl. The dip will keep, covered, in refrigerator for up to 2 days.

**Per serving:** 120 calories, 5 g protein, 10 g carbohydrates, 1 g fiber, 7 g total fat, 2 g saturated fat, 0 mg cholesterol, 216 mg sodium

Stir in cumin and coriander. Remove from heat and transfer to food processor.

2. Add chickpeas, yogurt, lime juice, salt, and black pepper to taste. Process until smooth. Transfer to medium bowl and stir in cilantro (or parsley).

**Per serving:** 65 calories, 2 g protein, 7 g carbohydrates, 2 g fiber, 3 g total fat, 0 g saturated fat, 0 mg cholesterol, 108 mg sodium

# INDIAN CHICKPEA SPREAD

Serves 12
**Prep Time:** 10 minutes
**Cook Time:** 1 minute
**Healing Foods:** ginger, spices, chickpeas, yogurt, limes
**Ailments It Heals:** anemia, obesity, osteoporosis, psoriasis

2 Tbsp canola oil
2 jalapeño chile peppers, seeded and minced (wear gloves when handling; they burn)
1 Tbsp minced fresh ginger
2 cloves garlic, minced
2 tsp ground cumin
1 tsp ground coriander
19 oz (540 mL) canned chickpeas, drained and rinsed
⅓ cup nonfat plain yogurt
2 Tbsp lime juice
⅛ tsp salt
Ground black pepper
2 Tbsp chopped fresh cilantro or parsley

1. In small skillet, heat canola oil over medium-high heat. Add chile peppers, ginger, and garlic. Cook, stirring, until fragrant, about 30 seconds.

# ITALIAN WHITE BEAN SPREAD

Serves 12
**Prep Time:** 10 minutes
**Healing Foods:** beans, lemons, rosemary
**Ailments It Heals:** arthritis, cancer, cirrhosis, shingles

19 oz (540 mL) cannellini beans, drained and rinsed
2 Tbsp extra-virgin olive oil
2 Tbsp lemon juice
1 clove garlic, minced
Pinch of cayenne pepper
Pinch of salt
Ground black pepper
1½ tsp chopped fresh rosemary

In a food processor, combine beans, oil, lemon juice, garlic, cayenne, and salt and black pepper to taste. Pulse into a chunky puree. Transfer to a medium bowl and stir in rosemary.

**Per serving:** 55 calories, 2 g protein, 6 g carbohydrates, 2 g fiber, 3 g total fat, 0 g saturated fat, 0 mg cholesterol, 66 mg sodium

# WARM ARTICHOKE AND BEAN DIP

**Serves 8**

Prep Time: **10 minutes**
Cook Time: **25 minutes**
Healing Foods: **beans, artichokes, garlic, cheese, parsley**
Ailments It Heals: **diverticulitis, irritable bowel syndrome, multiple sclerosis**

- 19 oz (540 mL) cannellini beans, drained and rinsed
- 14 oz (398 mL) artichoke hearts, drained and rinsed
- 3 cloves garlic, minced
- 1 Tbsp reduced-fat mayonnaise
- Pinch of cayenne pepper
- Ground black pepper to taste
- ⅔ cup plus 2 Tbsp grated parmesan cheese
- ¼ cup chopped fresh parsley
- 1 tsp freshly grated lemon zest

1. Preheat oven to 400°F (200°C). Coat 2- to 3-cup baking dish with cooking spray.

2. In food processor, place beans, artichoke hearts, garlic, mayonnaise, cayenne, and black pepper. Process until almost smooth, stopping to scrape down sides of work bowl once or twice. Transfer to medium bowl. Stir in ⅔ cup cheese, parsley, and lemon zest. Scrape into baking dish and smooth with spatula. Sprinkle with remaining 2 Tbsp cheese.

3. Bake, uncovered, for 20 to 25 minutes, or until heated through.

**Per serving:** 116 calories, 7 g protein, 16 g carbohydrates, 5 g fiber, 3 g total fat, 2 g saturated fat, 7 mg cholesterol, 517 mg sodium

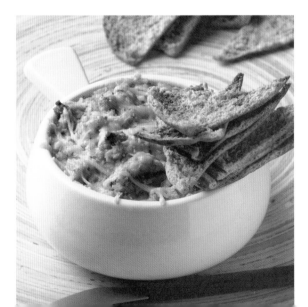

# EDAMAME HUMMUS WITH PITA CRISPS

**Serves 8**

Prep Time: **20 minutes**
Cook Time: **10 minutes**
Healing Foods: **edamame, lemons, garlic, olive oil**
Ailments It Heals: **constipation, dental problems, menopause**

- 4 whole wheat pita breads (8 in or 20 cm), halved crosswise
- ½ tsp ground cumin
- 2 cups shelled edamame
- ⅓ cup water
- ¼ cup sesame tahini
- 3 Tbsp lemon juice
- 2 cloves garlic, mashed
- ½ tsp salt
- 2 Tbsp extra-virgin olive oil

1. Preheat oven to 350°F (180°C). Place pita halves on cutting board and lightly coat with cooking spray. Sprinkle with cumin and cut each into eight wedges. Place on baking sheet and bake for 10 minutes, or until lightly browned. Transfer to a rack and let cool.

**2.** Meanwhile, place edamame in medium saucepan, add enough water to cover, and bring to a boil over medium-high heat. Cook for 10 minutes, or until very tender. Drain and rinse under cold water. Let cool slightly.

**3.** In food processor, combine edamame, ⅓ cup water, tahini, lemon juice, garlic, and salt. Process until smooth. With motor running, gradually add oil and blend until combined. Serve with pita wedges.

**Per serving:** 212 calories, 9 g protein, 24 g carbohydrates, 5 g fiber, 10 g total fat, 1 g saturated fat, 0 mg cholesterol, 333 mg sodium

# SPICED ALMONDS

**Serves 8**
**Prep Time:** 5 minutes
**Cook Time:** 30 minutes
**Healing Foods:** almonds, olive oil, cumin
**Ailments It Heals:** cardiovascular disease, lupus, sex drive (diminished), stress

1 cup unpeeled whole almonds
1 tsp olive oil
¾ tsp ground cumin
¼ tsp salt
⅛ tsp cayenne pepper

**1.** Preheat oven to 350°F (180°C). In pie plate or shallow baking dish, toss almonds with olive oil, cumin, salt, and cayenne.

**2.** Bake, stirring occasionally, for 25 to 30 minutes, or until fragrant. Let cool. Almonds will keep, enclosed in an airtight container, for up to 1 week.

**Per serving:** 112 calories, 4 g protein, 4 g carbohydrates, 2 g fiber, 10 g total fat, 1 g saturated fat, 0 mg cholesterol, 73 mg sodium

# SWEET AND SPICY SNACK MIX

**Serves 16**
**Prep Time:** 15 minutes
**Cook Time:** 15 minutes
**Healing Foods:** nuts and seeds, corn, spices
**Ailments It Heals:** atherosclerosis, memory loss, respiratory disease

1 cup walnut halves
10 cups air-popped popcorn
3 cups unsalted fat-free mini pretzel twists
1⅓ cups sugar
2 Tbsp lemon juice
⅓ cup hulled pumpkin seeds
1 Tbsp ground cumin
1 tsp salt
¾ tsp cayenne pepper

**1.** Preheat oven to 350°F (180°C). Bake walnuts for 7 minutes, or until lightly crisp and fragrant. Coarsely chop.

**2.** Coat large heatproof bowl with cooking spray. Add popcorn and pretzels and toss to combine.

**3.** In large heavy skillet, stir together sugar and lemon juice. Cook over medium heat, stirring, for 5 minutes, or until sugar has dissolved and just starts to color. Add walnuts, pumpkin seeds, cumin, salt, and cayenne. Stir quickly to thoroughly coat nuts in caramel. Cook, stirring constantly, until nuts are well coated.

**4.** Transfer to bowl with popcorn and pretzels. Stir quickly to combine. Let cool to room temperature. Store in an airtight container in the refrigerator.

**Per serving:** 178 calories, 4 g protein, 28 g carbohydrates, 2 g fiber, 7 g total fat, 1 g saturated fat, 0 mg cholesterol, 280 mg sodium

# FRUITY GRANOLA MIX

**Serves 12**
**Prep Time:** 10 minutes
**Cook Time:** 55 minutes
**Healing Foods:** oats, nuts, cinnamon, cranberries, cherries
**Ailments It Heals:** anorexia, cholesterol (high), varicose veins

4 cups old-fashioned rolled oats
1 cup coarsely chopped walnuts
1 tsp ground cinnamon
⅛ tsp ground nutmeg
¼ tsp salt
½ cup maple syrup
¼ cup honey
¼ cup canola oil
2 tsp vanilla extract
1 cup dried cranberries
1 cup dried cherries

**1.** Preheat oven to 300°F (150°C). Coat large baking sheet with cooking spray.

**2.** In large bowl, combine oats, walnuts, cinnamon, nutmeg, and salt.

**3.** In small bowl, whisk together syrup, honey, oil, and vanilla. Pour over oats mixture and mix well to combine.

**4.** Spread mixture evenly onto baking sheet. Bake, stirring every 10 minutes, for 45 to 55 minutes, or until lightly golden and toasted.

**5.** Remove from oven and stir in cranberries and cherries. Cool completely on baking sheet. Store in an airtight container for up to 2 weeks.

**Per serving:** 353 calories, 6 g protein, 53 g carbohydrates, 5 g fiber, 13 g total fat, 1 g saturated fat, 0 mg cholesterol, 50 mg sodium

# CHEWY DATE-WALNUT BARS

**Makes 16**
**Prep Time:** 15 minutes
**Cook Time:** 20 minutes
**Healing Foods:** oranges, dates, nuts and seeds, oats
**Ailments It Heals:** chronic fatigue syndrome, circulatory disorders, menstrual problems

2 Tbsp reduced-fat margarine spread
1 Tbsp canola oil
¼ cup light brown sugar
2 Tbsp honey
Zest of 1 orange
2 Tbsp orange juice
⅓ cup dried pitted dates, chopped
¼ cup walnuts, chopped
2 cups old-fashioned oats
2 Tbsp sunflower seeds

**1.** Preheat oven to 350°F (180°). Coat a 9-in (2.5 L) square baking pan with cooking spray and set aside.

**2.** In medium saucepan, place margarine, oil, brown sugar, honey, orange zest, and orange juice. Cook over low heat, stirring until butter has melted. Remove pan from heat and stir in dates and walnuts. Add oats, making sure they are evenly coated with butter mixture.

**3.** Spread mixture in prepared pan, pressing it down firmly and evenly. Sprinkle sunflower seeds over top and press down lightly to embed seeds.

**4.** Bake for 20 minutes, or until golden brown around edges. Remove from oven and allow to cool completely in pan. When cool, turn bars out onto cutting board and slice into 16 bars. They can be kept in an airtight container for up to 1 week.

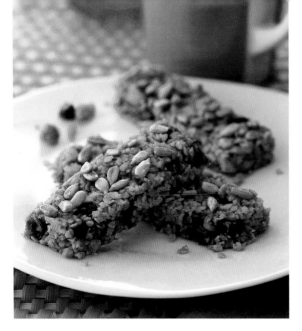

1. Preheat oven to 350°F (180°C). Coat an 8-in (20 cm) square metal baking pan with cooking spray.

2. In large bowl, stir together cereal, peanuts, cranberries, and flaxseed.

3. In small saucepan over low heat, stir together peanut butter and agave syrup for 1 minute, or until mixture boils. Stir into cereal mixture until well-blended. Scrape into prepared pan and press down firmly with back of spatula to compact.

4. Bake for 15 minutes, or until edges are golden. Cool thoroughly before cutting into 24 squares.

**Per serving:** 112 calories, 3 g protein, 19 g carbohydrates, 2 g fiber, 4 g total fat, 1 g saturated fat, 0 mg cholesterol, 78 mg sodium

**Per serving:** 103 calories, 2 g protein, 12 g carbohydrates, 2 g fiber, 4 g total fat, 0 g saturated fat, 0 mg cholesterol, 12 mg sodium

# CRANBERRY-PEANUT CEREAL BARS

Makes 24
**Prep Time:** 10 minutes
**Cook Time:** 16 minutes
**Healing Foods:** grains, peanuts and peanut butter, cranberries, flax
**Ailments It Heals:** cardiovascular disease, stroke, menopause

- 3 cups puffed whole grain cereal, like Kashi
- ½ cup chopped dry-roasted unsalted peanuts
- ¼ cup chopped unsweetened dried cranberries
- 2 Tbsp ground flaxseed
- ⅓ cup creamy peanut butter
- ½ cup agave syrup

# SESAME-FIG BARS

Makes 32
**Prep Time:** 15 minutes
**Cook Time:** 47 minutes
**Healing Foods:** almonds, seeds, figs, carrots, cardamom
**Ailments It Heals:** Alzheimer's disease, atherosclerosis, menstrual problems

- ½ cup raw (unblanched) almonds
- 1 Tbsp sesame seeds
- 1 cup all-purpose flour
- ⅓ cup confectioners' sugar
- ½ tsp salt
- ⅓ cup dark sesame oil
- 1½ tsp grated orange zest
- 1 cup dried figs, coarsely chopped
- 2 carrots, very thinly sliced
- ¾ cup orange juice
- 2 Tbsp fresh lemon juice
- ¾ tsp ground cardamom
- 1 tsp vanilla extract

**1.** Preheat oven to 350°F (180°C). Place almonds and sesame seeds on baking sheet and toast for 5 to 7 minutes, or until almonds are fragrant and seeds are golden.

**2.** Transfer almonds and sesame seeds to food processor. Add flour, confectioners' sugar, and salt and process until powdery. Add sesame oil and orange zest and process until evenly moistened.

**3.** Press into 9-in (23 cm) square metal baking pan. Prick dough all over with fork and bake for 20 minutes. Remove crust from oven and cool on wire rack. Keep oven on.

**4.** While crust bakes, in a medium saucepan, combine figs, carrots, orange juice, lemon juice, and cardamom. Bring to a boil over medium heat. Reduce to a simmer, cover, and cook for 20 minutes, or until figs and carrots are soft and most liquid has been absorbed. Cool to room temperature.

**5.** Transfer fig-carrot mixture to food processor. Add vanilla and process to a coarse puree. Spread mixture over crust and bake for 20 minutes. Cool in pan on wire rack before slicing into 32 pieces.

**Per serving:** 75 calories, 1 g protein, 10 g carbohydrates, 1 g fiber, 4 g total fat, 0 g saturated fat, 0 mg cholesterol, 39 mg sodium

# NO-BAKE FLAXSEED-NUT BARS

Makes 24
**Prep Time:** 25 minutes plus cooling
**Cook Time:** 8 minutes
**Healing Foods:** oats, flax, blueberries, nuts, peanut butter
**Ailments It Heals:** cardiovascular disease, depression, hypoglycemia

1   cup old-fashioned rolled oats
¼   cup whole flaxseed
1   cup whole grain puffed rice, puffed wheat, or toasted oat cereal
1   cup dried blueberries or cranberries
½   cup unsalted roasted peanuts
½   cup almonds, coarsely chopped
½   cup nonfat dry milk
¼   tsp salt
¾   cup natural peanut butter, almond butter, or cashew butter
⅔   cup honey
1   tsp vanilla extract

**1.** Line a 11 x 7-in (28 x 18-cm) or 9-in (23 cm) square baking dish with foil, leaving a 1-in (2.5 cm) overhang on opposite sides. Coat with cooking spray.

**2.** In medium skillet over medium-low heat, toast oats, stirring constantly, for 3 to 4 minutes, or until aromatic and golden. Transfer to large bowl. In small skillet over medium-low heat, toast flaxseed for 2 to 3 minutes, or until aromatic and starting to pop. Transfer to small bowl and let cool. In spice grinder (such as a clean coffee grinder) or blender, grind flaxseed into coarse meal. Add to oats. Add cereal, blueberries, peanuts, almonds, dry milk, and salt and stir to mix.

3. In small saucepan, combine peanut butter and honey. Cook, stirring, over low heat until blended and smooth about 1 minute. Stir in vanilla. Add to oat mixture, mix well, and transfer to baking dish. Use a piece of plastic wrap to press mixture firmly into an even layer. Cover with plastic wrap and refrigerate for 30 minutes, or until firm. Using foil overhang, lift bars and transfer to cutting board. Cut into 24 bars. Store, covered or individually wrapped, in refrigerator for up to 2 weeks.

**Per serving:** 171 calories, 5 g protein, 20 g carbohydrates, 3 g fiber, 8 g total fat, 1 g saturated fat, 1 mg cholesterol, 78 mg sodium

## DESSERTS

# CHEWY OATMEAL RAISIN COOKIES

Makes 3 dozen
**Prep Time:** 15 minutes
**Cook Time:** 12 minutes
**Healing Foods:** wheat, oats, raisins
**Ailments It Heals:** atherosclerosis, cholesterol (high), diverticulitis, inflammatory bowel disease

½ cup whole wheat pastry flour
½ cup all-purpose flour
1 tsp baking powder
½ tsp baking soda
½ tsp salt
¼ tsp ground cinnamon
2 Tbsp unsalted butter, softened
½ cup turbinado sugar
½ cup light brown sugar
1 large egg
¼ cup unsweetened applesauce
1 tsp vanilla extract
1⅓ cups old-fashioned rolled oats
½ cup raisins

1. Preheat oven to 375°F (190°C). Position oven racks in upper and lower thirds of oven. Line two cookie sheets with foil.

2. In medium bowl, stir together flours, baking powder, baking soda, salt, and cinnamon.

3. In large bowl, beat butter and turbinado sugar together with large rubber spatula. One at a time, beat in brown sugar, egg, applesauce, and vanilla, incorporating the ingredients thoroughly. Gently stir in flour mixture, oats, and raisins, one at a time.

4. Drop dough by teaspoonfuls about 2 in (5 cm) apart on prepared sheets. Use fork to gently flatten mounds of dough.

5. Bake both cookie sheets for 10 to 12 minutes, or until cookies look dull but are moist and soft.

6. Grab foil and slide each sheet of cookies from pans onto racks to cool.

**Per cookie:** 59 calories, 1 g protein, 12 g carbohydrates, 1 g fiber, 1 g total fat, 0 g saturated fat, 7 mg cholesterol, 86 mg sodium

# NUTTY CHOCOLATE CHIP COOKIES

Makes 5 dozen
**Prep Time:** 15 minutes
**Cook Time:** 50 minutes
**Healing Foods:** wheat, oats, eggs, chocolate, raisins, nuts
**Ailments It Heals:** cystic fibrosis, hemorrhoids, stroke

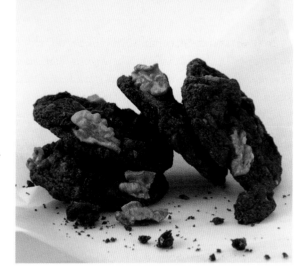

**Per cookie:** 97 calories, 1 g protein, 12 g carbohydrates, 1 g fiber, 5 g total fat, 2 g saturated fat, 7 mg cholesterol, 77 mg sodium

1½ cups whole wheat pastry flour
1 cup rolled oats, ground
⅓ cup cocoa powder
1 tsp baking soda
½ tsp salt
1 cup nonhydrogenated stick margarine
½ cup granulated sugar
1 cup packed light brown sugar
2 eggs
1 Tbsp vanilla extract
1 cup bittersweet chocolate chips
   (60% or higher cocoa content)
1 cup raisins
1 cup walnuts, coarsely chopped

**1.** Preheat oven to 350°F (180°C). Line baking sheet with parchment paper. In medium bowl, whisk together flour, oats, cocoa, baking soda, and salt.

**2.** In large bowl with an electric mixer at medium speed, beat margarine and sugars for 2 minutes, or until light and fluffy. Add eggs and vanilla and beat until smooth. Beat in flour mixture until combined. Stir in chocolate chips, raisins, and walnuts. Drop by teaspoonful onto baking sheet.

**3.** Bake for 10 minutes, or until browned. Let cool on the baking sheet for 2 minutes, then transfer to a rack and let cool completely.

# CHOCOLATE-ALMOND BISCOTTI

Makes 4 dozen
**Prep Time:** 20 minutes plus cooling
**Cook Time:** 1 hour
**Healing Foods:** wheat, almonds, chocolate, eggs
**Ailments It Heals:** atherosclerosis, depression

2½ cups whole wheat pastry flour
¾ cup sugar
2 tsp baking powder
1 tsp ground cinnamon
1 tsp salt
1½ cups whole almonds
6 oz (175 g) bittersweet chocolate (60% or higher cocoa content), chopped
4 large eggs

1. Preheat oven to 350°F (180°C). Line baking sheet with parchment paper. In large bowl, whisk together flour, sugar, baking powder, cinnamon, and salt. Stir in almonds and two-thirds of chocolate. In small bowl, beat eggs, then stir into flour mixture.

2. Place dough on lightly floured surface and knead until smooth. Cut in half and shape each piece into a log 12 in (30 cm) long and 3 in (7.5 cm) thick. Place on baking sheet and bake for 30 minutes, or until outside seems firm and puffed. Transfer to a rack and let cool for 2 hours.

3. With a serrated knife, cut logs crosswise into slices about ½ in (1 cm) thick. Place the slices on their sides on a parchment-lined baking sheet and bake, turning once, for 30 minutes, or until crisp and lightly browned. Transfer to a rack and let cool for 30 minutes.

4. Meanwhile, place remaining chocolate in small bowl and microwave on low for 1 minute, or until almost melted. Stir until melted completely. Drizzle over biscotti.

**Per cookie:** 80 calories, 2 g protein, 10 g carbohydrates, 1 g fiber, 4 g total fat, 1 g saturated fat, 18 mg cholesterol, 75 mg sodium

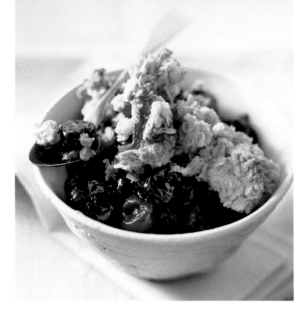

- ⅛ tsp allspice
- 2 tsp grated lime zest
- 24 oz (750 g) frozen pitted sweet cherries, thawed
- 1 Tbsp fresh lime juice
- ¾ cup old-fashioned rolled oats
- ⅓ cup all-purpose flour
- ⅓ cup firmly packed light brown sugar
- 3 Tbsp cold unsalted butter, cut up

1. Preheat oven to 400°F (200°C). In large bowl, stir together granulated sugar, cornstarch, cinnamon, pepper, ¼ tsp salt, allspice, and lime zest. Add cherries and lime juice, tossing to coat. Pour into 9-in (23 cm) square glass baking dish and set aside.

2. In medium bowl, stir together oats, flour, brown sugar, and remaining ¼ tsp salt. With a pastry blender or two knives, cut in butter until mixture resembles coarse crumbs. Sprinkle mixture over fruit.

3. Bake for 25 minutes, or until fruit is bubbly and piping hot and topping is golden brown and crisp.

**Per serving:** 257 calories, 4 g protein, 48 g carbohydrates, 1 g fiber, 7 g total fat, 4 saturated fat, 16 mg cholesterol, 201 mg sodium

# CHERRY CRISP

**Serves 6**
**Prep Time:** 15 minutes
**Cook Time:** 25 minutes
**Healing Foods:** cherries, oats, flour
**Ailments It Heals:** diabetes, peptic ulcers

- ¼ cup granulated sugar
- 2 Tbsp cornstarch
- 1 tsp ground cinnamon
- ½ tsp ground black pepper
- ½ tsp salt

# PEACH AND BLACKBERRY PHYLLO PIZZAS

Makes 6
**Prep Time:** 30 minutes
**Cook Time:** 15 minutes
**Healing Foods:** almonds, peaches, blackberries
**Ailments It Heals:** cancer, hemorrhoids, indigestion and heartburn

Butter-flavored cooking spray
5   sheets phyllo pastry (14 x 18 in or 36 x 46 cm)
2   Tbsp ground almonds
3   large ripe peaches
1   cup fresh blackberries
2   Tbsp sugar
1   cup reduced-fat sour cream (optional)
1   Tbsp light brown sugar (optional)

**1.** Preheat oven to 400°F (200°C) and coat baking sheet with cooking spray. Lay out phyllo sheets and immediately cover with plastic wrap, then a damp towel (phyllo dries out in a couple of minutes if left uncovered). Work fast!

**2.** Place a sheet of phyllo on work surface and spray with cooking spray. Layer four more phyllo sheets, spraying with cooking spray each time, and finally spray top sheet with cooking spray. Using a 5-in (13 cm) saucer as a guide, cut out 6 circles from the layered phyllo. Transfer each layered circle to baking sheet and sprinkle with ground almonds.

**3.** To decorate, cut peaches in half (do not peel), twist apart, and remove pits. Slice peaches very thin. Place slices on phyllo pastry circles in a pinwheel design. Divide blackberries among pizzas. Sprinkle 1 tsp sugar on top of each pizza.

**4.** Bake for 15 minutes, or until pastry is golden brown and peaches are very tender and light

brown. These pizzas are best served within 15 minutes, as pastry can lose its crispness quickly if fruit is juicy. If desired, serve with sour cream mixed with brown sugar. Each serving is 1 pizza.

**Per serving:** 107 calories, 2 g protein, 22 g carbohydrates, 3 g fiber, 2 g total fat, 0 g saturated fat, 0 mg cholesterol, 50 mg sodium

# RHUBARB-BLACKBERRY CRUMBLE

Serves 8
**Prep Time:** 20 minutes
**Cook Time:** 50 minutes plus cooling
**Healing Foods:** rhubarb, blackberries, wheat, oats, almonds
**Ailments It Heals:** hemorrhoids, irritable bowel syndrome, lactose intolerance, stroke

5   cups diced (½-in or 1 cm pieces) rhubarb
1   cup blackberries
½   cup granulated sugar
1   Tbsp cornstarch
⅔   cup whole wheat flour
½   cup old-fashioned rolled oats
½   cup firmly packed light brown sugar
1   tsp ground cinnamon
Pinch of salt
1   Tbsp unsalted butter, cut into small pieces
1   Tbsp canola oil
3   Tbsp frozen orange juice concentrate
1   Tbsp chopped slivered almonds

**1.** Preheat oven to 375°F (190°C). Coat 8-in (20 cm) square baking dish with cooking spray.

**2.** Combine rhubarb, blackberries, granulated sugar, and cornstarch in baking dish. Toss to mix. Cover with foil and bake for 20 minutes.

3. Meanwhile, in medium bowl, mix flour, oats, brown sugar, cinnamon, and salt with fork. Add butter and crumble with pastry blender or your fingertips until well blended. Add oil and stir to coat. Add orange juice concentrate and stir until dry ingredients are moistened.

4. When crumble has baked for 20 minutes, sprinkle flour mixture evenly over fruit. Top with almonds. Bake, uncovered, for 20 to 30 minutes, or until fruit is bubbly and tender and topping is lightly browned. Let cool for at least 10 minutes before serving warm or at room temperature.

**Per serving:** 227 calories, 4 g protein, 45 g carbohydrates, 4 g fiber, 4 g total fat, 1 g saturated fat, 4 mg cholesterol, 28 mg sodium

# LEMONY BLUEBERRY CHEESECAKE BARS

Makes 24
**Prep Time:** 25 minutes
**Cook Time:** 1 hour
**Healing Foods:** wheat, eggs, cheese, blueberries
**Ailments It Heals:** chronic fatigue syndrome, hyperthyroidism, osteoporosis, varicose veins

## CRUST
1½  cups whole wheat pastry flour
¼  tsp baking powder
¼  tsp baking soda
¼  tsp salt
2  Tbsp unsalted butter, softened
2  Tbsp canola oil
½  cup sugar
1  large egg, lightly beaten
1  tsp vanilla extract

## FILLING
12  oz (375 g) reduced-fat cream cheese (Neufchâtel)
½  cup sugar
1  Tbsp cornstarch
2  large eggs, lightly beaten
4  tsp freshly grated lemon zest
1½  tsp vanilla extract
3  cups fresh or frozen and partially thawed blueberries

1. Preheat oven to 350°F (180°C). Coat a 13 x 9-in (33 x 23 cm) baking dish with cooking spray.

2. To make the crust: In medium bowl, whisk flour, baking powder, baking soda, and salt. In mixing bowl, beat butter, oil, and sugar with electric mixer until smooth. Add egg and vanilla and beat until smooth. Add dry ingredients and mix with rubber spatula just until dry ingredients are moistened. Transfer dough to prepared baking dish. Use a piece of plastic wrap to press it into an even layer.

3. Bake crust, uncovered, for 20 minutes, or until puffed and starting to brown around edges.

4. To make the filling: Blend cream cheese, sugar, and cornstarch in a bowl with an electric mixer or in a food processor, until smooth and creamy. Add eggs, lemon zest, and vanilla. Beat or process until smooth. Spread blueberries over crust. Pour cream cheese batter over blueberries, spreading evenly.

5. Bake for 35 to 40 minutes, or until filling has set. Let cool completely in pan on wire rack. Cut into 24 bars with a sharp knife coated with cooking spray. Bars will keep, covered, in refrigerator for up to 4 days or in freezer for up to 1 month.

**Per serving:** 140 calories, 3 g protein, 17 g carbohydrates, 1 g fiber, 6 g total fat, 3 g saturated fat, 40 mg cholesterol, 105 mg sodium

# PUMPKIN MAPLE CHEESECAKE

**Serves 16**
**Prep Time:** 15 minutes
**Cook Time:** 1 hour 10 minutes plus cooling
**Healing Foods:** cheese, pumpkins, eggs
**Ailments It Heals:** arthritis, cystic fibrosis, Parkinson's disease

1 cup graham cracker crumbs
3 Tbsp vegetable oil
24 oz (750 g) ⅓-less-fat cream cheese, softened
½ cup firmly packed light brown sugar
15 oz (750 g) solid-pack pumpkin puree
½ cup maple syrup
3 large eggs
2 Tbsp cornstarch
2 tsp pumpkin pie spice
1 tsp vanilla extract
½ tsp salt

**1.** Preheat oven to 350°F (180°C). Lightly coat 9-in (23 cm) springform cake pan with cooking spray.

**2.** In small bowl, stir together cracker crumbs and oil. Press mixture over bottom and ½ in (1 cm) up side of pan. Bake for 10 minutes, or until crust just begins to color.

**3.** In large bowl, beat cream cheese and brown sugar until well blended. Beat in pumpkin, maple syrup, eggs, cornstarch, pie spice, vanilla, and salt until smooth. Pour filling into crust.

**4.** Bake for 55 to 60 minutes, or until center is just set. Transfer pan to wire rack. Let cool completely. Cover and refrigerate at least 4 hours before serving.

**Per serving:** 236 calories, 6 g protein, 22 g carbohydrates, 1 g fiber, 14 g total fat, 7 g saturated fat, 72 mg cholesterol, 291 mg sodium

# ANGEL FOOD CAKE WITH STRAWBERRIES

**Serves 12**
**Prep Time:** 20 minutes
**Cook Time:** 50 minutes plus cooling
**Healing Foods:** strawberries, oranges, eggs, flour
**Ailments It Heals:** cholesterol (high), irritable bowel syndrome, obesity

20 oz (600 g) frozen strawberries, thawed
½ cup orange juice
12 large egg whites, at room temperature
1¼ tsp cream of tartar
½ tsp salt
1¼ cups sugar
3 Tbsp grated lemon zest
1 tsp vanilla extract
1 cup flour

**1.** In large bowl, combine strawberries and orange juice. Refrigerate.

**2.** Preheat oven to 325°F (160°C). In large bowl, beat egg whites, cream of tartar, and salt with electric mixer until foamy. Gradually beat in sugar,

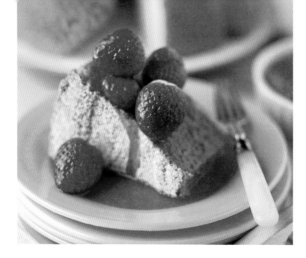

2 Tbsp at a time, until thick, soft peaks form. Beat in lemon zest and vanilla.

**3.** Gently fold flour into mixture, ¼ cup at a time, until incorporated. Spoon into ungreased 10-in (25 cm) angel food or tube pan (3 L). Bake for 50 minutes, or until top springs back when lightly pressed.

**4.** Invert cake pan to cool. If pan does not have legs, hang pan over neck of bottle. Cool cake completely. Run metal spatula around edges and center of pan, then invert onto cake platter. Serve with strawberries and their juice.

**Per serving:** 159 calories, 5 g protein, 35 g carbohydrates, 1 g fiber, 0 g total fat, 0 g saturated fat, 0 mg cholesterol, 153 mg sodium

# CARROT CAKE WITH CREAM CHEESE GLAZE

**Serves 12**
**Prep Time:** 10 minutes
**Cook Time:** 35 minutes plus cooling
**Healing Foods:** apples, eggs, wheat, carrots, nuts, milk
**Ailments It Heals:** iron overload, memory loss, stroke

½ cup applesauce
⅔ cup granulated sugar
2 large eggs
2 Tbsp canola oil
1 tsp vanilla extract
1¼ cups whole wheat pastry flour
1 tsp baking soda
1 tsp ground cinnamon
½ tsp salt
1½ cups shredded carrots (3 large)
½ cup chopped walnuts
1 oz (30 g) low-fat cream cheese
2 Tbsp low-fat milk
2 to 3 Tbsp confectioners' sugar

**1.** Preheat oven to 350°F (180°C). Coat 9-in (23 cm) round cake pan with cooking spray. In small bowl, whisk together applesauce, granulated sugar, eggs, oil, and vanilla.

**2.** In large bowl, whisk together flour, baking soda, cinnamon, and salt. Make a well in center, add applesauce mixture, and stir just until blended. Stir in carrots and walnuts. Pour batter into pan.

**3.** Bake for 35 minutes, or until a wooden pick inserted in center comes out clean. Transfer to a rack and let cool for 10 minutes, then remove from pan and let cool for 1 hour.

**4.** Meanwhile, in small bowl, whisk together cream cheese and milk until well combined. Add 2 Tbsp confectioners' sugar and whisk until smooth, adding more sugar if glaze is too thin. Place cake on serving plate and drizzle with glaze.

**Per serving:** 160 calories, 3 g protein, 23 g carbohydrates, 2 g fiber, 6 g total fat, 1 g saturated fat, 37 mg cholesterol, 236 mg sodium

# CHOCOLATE BANANA SOUFFLÉS

**Serves 8**
**Prep Time:** 25 minutes
**Cook Time:** 20 minutes
**Healing Foods:** bananas, chocolate, eggs
**Ailments It Heals:** Alzheimer's disease, blood pressure, diverticulitis, muscle cramps

- 4 large, very ripe bananas, peeled and cut into 2-in (5 cm) chunks
- ¼ cup water
- ¾ cup plus 2 Tbsp turbinado sugar
- 4 oz (125 g) bittersweet chocolate, cut into ¼-in (0.5 cm) pieces
- ⅛ tsp ground cinnamon
- 6 large egg whites

Pinch of salt

**1.** In a food processor or blender, add the bananas and puree. Measure 2 cups puree and set aside. Discard any extra puree.

**2.** In medium saucepan, combine water and ½ cup sugar. Bring to a boil over low heat, stirring occasionally. When mixture boils, stop stirring and continue cooking for 2 minutes, or until syrup thickens. Stir in banana puree. Remove from heat and stir in chocolate and cinnamon. Let stand a minute to melt chocolate, then whisk until smooth. Pour mixture into heatproof bowl and cool to room temperature, stirring occasionally.

**3.** Set rack in middle of oven and preheat to 400°F (200°C). Coat eight individual 4-oz (120 mL) ramekins with cooking spray, then coat the sprayed surface with 2 Tbsp sugar. Set aside on baking sheet.

**4.** In bowl of an electric mixer, combine egg whites and salt. Whip until egg whites just begin to hold a shape. Increase speed to medium high and whip in remaining ¼ cup sugar in a slow stream, until mixture holds a soft, glossy peak when whisk is lifted.

**5.** Gently fold banana puree into egg whites, working quickly to prevent egg whites from deflating. Divide soufflé batter evenly among ramekins, filling each to within ¼-in (0.5 cm) of the top. Bake for 12 to 15 minutes, or until well-risen.

**6.** Immediately remove baking sheet from oven. Use oven mitts to transfer ramekins to dessert plates and serve immediately.

**Per serving:** 229 calories, 4 g protein, 45 g carbohydrates, 3 g fiber, 6 g total fat, 3 g saturated fat, 0 mg cholesterol, 42 mg sodium

# CREAMY CITRUS AND VANILLA RICE PUDDING

**Serves 4**
**Prep Time:** 10 minutes
**Cook Time:** 32 minutes plus cooling
**Healing Foods:** rice, cinnamon, eggs
**Ailments It Heals:** anemia, celiac disease, jaundice, lactose intolerance

- 4 cups rice milk
- 3 strips (3 x ½ in or 7.5 x 1 cm each) orange zest
- 3 strips (3 x ½ in or 7.5 x 1 cm each) lime zest
- 1 cinnamon stick, split lengthwise
- ½ tsp salt
- ½ cup basmati, jasmine, or texmati rice
- ¼ cup sugar
- 2 large egg yolks
- ½ tsp vanilla extract

**1.** In large saucepan, stir together rice milk, orange and lime zests, cinnamon, and salt. Add rice and bring to a simmer over medium-low heat. Cover and cook for 15 minutes, stirring occasionally.

**2.** Meanwhile, in a medium bowl, whisk together sugar and egg yolks.

**3.** Uncover rice and cook, stirring frequently, for 15 minutes, or until rice is very tender. Whisk some of hot rice mixture into egg mixture to warm it, then whisk egg mixture into saucepan. Cook, stirring constantly, for 2 minutes, or until pudding is slightly thickened.

**4.** Transfer pudding to bowl and stir in vanilla. When cool, remove orange zest, lime zest, and cinnamon stick. Cool to room temperature, then cover and refrigerate until serving time.

**Per serving:** 279 calories, 5 g protein, 56 g carbohydrates, 0 g fiber, 5 g total fat, 1 g saturated fat, 106 mg cholesterol, 394 mg sodium

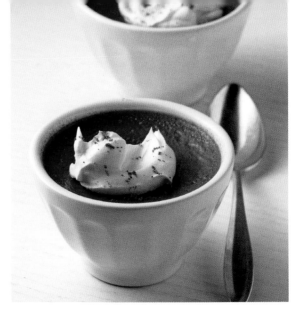

# PUMPKIN CUSTARDS

Serves 6
**Prep Time:** 20 minutes
**Cook Time:** 55 minutes plus cooling
**Healing Foods:** eggs, pumpkins, cinnamon, soy
**Ailments It Heals:** hyperthyroidism, Parkinson's disease, sore throat

|   |   |
|---|---|
| 2 | large eggs |
| 2 | large egg whites |
| ⅔ | cup sugar |
| ¾ | cup canned unseasoned pumpkin puree |
| 1½ | tsp ground cinnamon |
| ½ | tsp ground nutmeg |
| ¼ | tsp salt |
| ½ | tsp vanilla extract |
| 1½ | cups vanilla soymilk |
| 3 | Tbsp whipped cream or low-calorie whipped topping |

**1.** Preheat oven to 325°F (160°C). Line roasting pan with folded kitchen towel (this prevents the custard cups from sliding around). Put a kettle of water on to boil for water bath.

**2.** In large bowl, whisk eggs, egg whites, and sugar until smooth. Add pumpkin, cinnamon, nutmeg, salt, and vanilla. Whisk until blended. Gently whisk in the soymilk.

**3.** Divide mixture among six ¾-cup (175 mL) custard cups. Skim foam from surface of custards. Set custard cups on towel in roasting pan. Pour enough boiling water into pan to come halfway up sides of custard cups. Place roasting pan in oven and bake, uncovered, for 50 to 55 minutes, or until custards are set. Transfer custard cups to a rack and let cool. Then cover and refrigerate for 1 hour, or until chilled.

**4.** Just before serving, top each custard with a dollop of whipped cream (or whipped topping).

**Per serving:** 166 calories, 5 g protein, 28 g carbohydrates, 1 g fiber, 4 g total fat, 1 g saturated fat, 75 mg cholesterol, 165 mg sodium

# MELON BERRY COMPOTE WITH GREEN TEA AND LIME

Serves 6
**Prep Time:** 10 minutes plus steeping
**Healing Foods:** tea, limes, cantaloupe, blueberries
**Ailments It Heals:** bulimia, cancer, colds and flu, eye problems, varicose veins

2   green tea bags
⅔   cup boiling water
2   Tbsp sugar
1   tsp grated lime zest
2   Tbsp lime juice
½   cantaloupe, cut into 1½-in (3.5 cm) cubes (3 cups)
2   cups blueberries, rinsed and dried

**1.** Place tea bags in boiling water and let steep for 3 to 4 minutes. Remove tea bags. Add sugar to tea and stir until dissolved. Stir in lime zest and lime juice. Let cool to room temperature.

**2.** Combine cantaloupe and blueberries in large bowl. Pour green tea mixture over fruit and toss to coat well. The compote will keep, covered, in refrigerator for up to 2 days.

**Per serving:** 72 calories, 1 g protein, 18 g carbohydrates, 2 g fiber, 0 g total fat, 0 g saturated fat, 0 mg cholesterol, 13 mg sodium

# ORANGE AND POMEGRANATE COMPOTE

Serves 4
**Prep Time:** 15 minutes
**Healing Foods:** oranges, pomegranates
**Ailments It Heals:** cholesterol (high), infertility, urinary tract infections

2   Tbsp orange liqueur, such as Grand Marnier or Cointreau, or orange juice
1   Tbsp sugar
3   medium-large navel oranges
½   pomegranate

**1.** In medium bowl, stir orange liqueur (or orange juice) and sugar together. Peel oranges, removing white pith with paring knife. Quarter oranges and slice. Add orange segments to bowl and toss to coat.

**2.** Scoop seeds from pomegranate half into small bowl, discarding membrane. Sprinkle pomegranate seeds over oranges. The compote will keep, covered, in refrigerator for up to 2 days.

**Per serving:** 94 calories, 2 g protein, 23 g carbohydrates, 3 g fiber, 0 g total fat, 0 g saturated fat, 0 mg cholesterol, 1 mg sodium

# GUAVAS AND PLUMS WITH VANILLA SYRUP

Serves 4
**Prep Time:** 5 minutes
**Cook Time:** 5 minutes
**Healing Foods:** plums, guava, nuts
**Ailments It Heals:** cancer, constipation, obesity

14.5 oz (410 mL) can plums
14.5 oz (410 mL) can guava halves
1 tsp vanilla extract
⅓ cup chopped pistachio nuts

**1.** Drain plums, pouring syrup into large saucepan. Drain syrup from guava halves into same pan. Boil syrup on high for 4 to 5 minutes, or until reduced by about half.

**2.** Meanwhile, pit the plums if necessary and divide them among four bowls. Add guava halves.

**3.** Stir vanilla into syrup and spoon evenly over fruit. Sprinkle with pistachio nuts and serve.

**Per serving:** 201 calories, 3 g protein, 39 g carbohydrates, 7 g fiber, 5 g fat, 1 g saturated fat, 0 mg cholesterol, 22 mg sodium

# FRESH FIGS WITH RASPBERRIES AND ROSE CREAM

Serves 4
**Prep Time:** 15 minutes
**Healing Foods:** figs, raspberries
**Ailments It Heals:** constipation, diabetes, hemorrhoids

3½ oz (100 g) crème fraîche, or sour cream mixed with a little confectioners' sugar
2 tsp raspberry jam
Finely grated zest of 1 lime
1 to 2 Tbsp rosewater, or to taste
8 small ripe juicy figs
4 large fresh fig leaves (optional)
7 oz (210 g) fresh raspberries
Fresh mint leaves

**1.** Place crème fraîche in a bowl and beat in raspberry jam and lime zest until jam is well distributed. Add rosewater and stir to mix. Transfer rose cream to a serving bowl.

**2.** Cut each fig vertically into quarters without cutting all the way through, so they remain whole. Arrange fig leaves, if using, on four plates and place 2 figs on each plate.

**3.** Spoon a dollop of rose cream into center of each fig. Serve remaining cream separately. Scatter raspberries over plates, garnish with mint leaves, and serve.

**Per serving:** 162 calories, 2 g protein, 20 g carbohydrates, 5 g fiber, 10 g total fat, 6 g saturated fat, 34 mg cholesterol, 13 mg sodium

# FRUIT PARFAIT WITH GINGER TEA CREAM

Serves 4
**Prep Time:** 10 minutes
**Cook Time:** 5 minutes plus cooling
**Healing Foods:** milk, tea, berries
**Ailments It Heals:** arthritis, motion sickness, respiratory disorders

- 2 cups skim milk
- 1 envelope unflavored gelatin
- 2 ginger herbal tea bags
- 3 Tbsp sugar
- ⅛ tsp salt
- 4 cups mixed fruit such as cantaloupe cubes, sliced strawberries, and blueberries

**1.** Place 1 cup milk in small bowl. Sprinkle gelatin over cold milk. Set aside for 5 minutes, or until gelatin softens. Meanwhile, in large saucepan, bring the remaining 1 cup milk to a boil.

**2.** Add tea bags, sugar, salt, and softened gelatin mixture to boiling milk, stirring with each addition. Remove from heat and stir for 1 minute to dissolve gelatin and sugar. Set aside for 3 minutes to allow tea to steep.

**3.** Let mixture cool to room temperature, then refrigerate for 1 to 1½ hours, or until it begins to set. Spoon ¼ cup of tea cream into each of four large wine goblets or dessert cups. Top with fruit and remaining tea cream. Refrigerate at least 1 to 2 hours longer, until tea cream is set and chilled.

**Per serving:** 144 calories, 7 g protein, 30 g carbohydrates, 3 g fiber, 1 g total fat, 0 g saturated fat, 2 mg cholesterol, 146 mg sodium

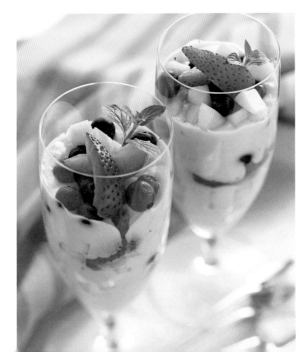

# GRILLED FRUIT EN BROCHETTE

Serves 8
**Prep Time:** 30 minutes
**Cook Time:** 8 minutes
**Healing Foods:** figs, pineapples, pears, peaches, bananas, raspberries
**Ailments It Heals:** blood pressure, cholesterol (high), hemorrhoids

### Coulis

- 2 cups fresh raspberries
- 1½ tsp grated orange zest
- ½ cup orange juice
- 1 Tbsp sugar

### Brochettes

- 4 fresh figs, or 4 dried figs, soaked and drained
- ½ large fresh pineapple (1 lb or 500 g)
- 2 large pears, ripe but firm (1 lb or 500 g)
- 2 large peaches, ripe but firm (1 lb or 500 g)
- 2 large bananas, ripe but firm
- ⅓ cup fresh lemon juice
- 1 Tbsp sugar
Fresh raspberries

1. Soak eight bamboo skewers, 10 to 12 in (25 to 30 cm) long, in cold water for 20 minutes.

2. To make coulis: In blender or food processor, puree raspberries, orange zest and juice, and sugar. Strain mixture to remove seeds, if you wish, but it's not necessary. Set aside.

3. Preheat grill or broiler.

4. To make brochettes: Cut figs lengthwise into 4 equal pieces (about 2 cups). Peel, core, and cut pineapple into bite-size chunks (3 cups). Core (do not peel) pears and cut into 1½-in (3.5 cm) cubes. Pit (do not peel) peaches and cut into 1½-in (3.5 cm) cubes. Peel bananas and cut crosswise into 1½-in (3.5 cm) pieces. Thread fruit onto soaked skewers, alternating them to make a colorful arrangement. Mix lemon juice and sugar in measuring cup. Baste brochettes with half of mixture.

5. Grill or broil brochettes for 4 minutes. Turn, baste with remaining lemon juice mixture, and grill or broil for 3 to 4 minutes, or until light golden brown.

6. For each serving, spread about ¼ cup coulis on a plate and arrange a fruit brochette on top. Garnish with raspberries, if you wish. Serve hot.

**Per serving:** 184 calories, 2 g protein, 47 g carbohydrates, 8 g fiber, 1 g total fat, 0 g saturated fat, 0 mg cholesterol, 6 mg sodium

# THREE-BERRY FOOL

**Serves 4**
**Prep Time:** 20 minutes plus standing
**Cook Time:** 7 minutes
**Healing Foods:** yogurt, raspberries, strawberries, blueberries
**Ailments It Heals:** arthritis, blood pressure, flatulence, herpes

1   qt (1 L) low-fat plain yogurt
2   cups frozen unsweetened raspberries, thawed
2   cups frozen unsweetened strawberries, thawed
½   cup sugar
1½  tsp vanilla extract
3   tsp cornstarch blended with 2 Tbsp water
2   cups frozen unsweetened blueberries
2   Tbsp orange juice
¼   tsp ground black pepper
¼   tsp allspice
1   Tbsp fresh lemon juice

1. Spoon yogurt into fine-mesh strainer or coffee filter set over bowl to catch drips. Let yogurt stand for 4 hours at room temperature.

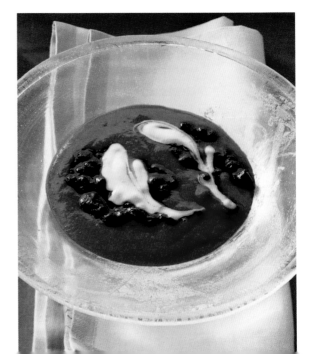

2. In food processor, combine raspberries, strawberries, ¼ cup sugar, and ½ tsp vanilla. Puree, then transfer to small saucepan and bring to a boil over medium heat. Stir in half of cornstarch mixture and bring to a boil. Cook, stirring constantly for 1 minute, until lightly thickened. Cool to room temperature, transfer to bowl, cover, and refrigerate.

3. In small saucepan, combine blueberries, orange juice, pepper, allspice, and 2 Tbsp sugar. Bring to a simmer over low heat. Cook, stirring frequently, for 5 minutes, or until blueberries are tender. Stir in remaining cornstarch mixture and bring to a boil. Cook, stirring constantly, for 1 minute, or until thickened. Transfer to bowl and stir in lemon juice. Cover and refrigerate.

4. In medium bowl, combine drained yogurt and remaining 2 Tbsp sugar and 1 tsp vanilla.

5. To serve, spoon raspberry-strawberry mixture into four bowls. Spoon blueberry mixture into the center and top with yogurt. Gently swirl mixture to lightly marble yogurt with fruit puree.

**Per serving:** 350 calories, 14 g protein, 68 g carbohydrates, 6 g fiber, 4 g total fat, 2 g saturated fat, 15 mg cholesterol, 172 mg sodium

# TROPICAL FRUIT SALAD

**Serves 6**
**Prep Time:** 20 minutes
**Healing Foods:** yogurt, grapefuit, kiwis, banana, melons, ginger
**Ailments It Heals:** circulatory disorders, menstrual problems, prostate problems

1  cup low-fat vanilla yogurt
1  tsp grated lime zest
2  red grapefruits

2  kiwis, peeled and cut into thin slices
2  bananas, sliced
1  small cantaloupe or large papaya, seeded and cut into chunks
2  Tbsp crystallized ginger

1. In small bowl, combine yogurt and lime zest.

2. Over large bowl, cut grapefruits into sections, then place in bowl. Squeeze membranes over bowl to release juice. Add kiwis, bananas, cantaloupe, and ginger. Toss to blend.

3. To serve, divide fruit among six bowls. Top each with 1½ Tbsp yogurt mixture.

**Per serving:** 154 calories, 3 g protein, 36 g carbohydrates, 4 g fiber, 1 g total fat, 0 g saturated fat, 3 mg cholesterol, 34 mg sodium

# KIWI-PASSION FRUIT SALAD

**Serves 4**
**Prep Time:** 15 minutes
**Healing Foods:** papayas, mangoes, kiwi, passion fruit
**Ailments It Heals:** acne, colds and flu, multiple sclerosis, stroke

1  large papaya
1  large mango
2  kiwi
½  cup (125 mL) orange juice
2  Tbsp lime juice
2  passion fruit

1. Peel and halve papaya and scoop out seeds. Slice fruit crosswise and arrange slices in two rows on serving platter, or cut into chunks and put into large serving bowl.

2. Peel mango, remove the pit, and cut lengthwise into wedges. Arrange wedges in a row between papaya slices. Or cut into chunks and add to serving bowl.

3. Peel kiwi and cut lengthwise into wedges or chunks. Scatter them over mango and papaya.

4. Mix orange juice with lime juice. Halve the passion fruit and scoop out seeds and pulp into juice mixture. Spoon over salad and serve immediately.

**Per serving:** 183 calories, 2 g protein, 45 g carbohydrates, 7 g fiber, 1 g total fat, 0 g saturated fat, 0 mg cholesterol, 20 mg sodium

2. Add strawberries, pear, and cucumber to bowl. Set aside 4 star-fruit slices for decoration. Dice remaining slices and add to bowl.

3. Drizzle Grand Marnier over fruit, sprinkle with mint, and toss gently to mix well. Cover with plastic wrap and refrigerate for 20 minutes.

4. Pile fruit mixture into shells and decorate with reserved star fruit.

**Per serving:** 107 calories, 1 g protein, 20 g carbohydrates, 3 g fiber, 1 g total fat, 0 g saturated fat, 0 mg cholesterol, 8 mg sodium

# MINTY MELON CUPS

Serves 6
**Prep Time:** 25 minutes plus chilling
**Healing Foods:** cantaloupe, honeydew, strawberries, pears, mint
**Ailments It Heals:** celiac disease, diverticulitis, rosacea

1  small cantaloupe (about 1 lb or 500 g)
1  small honeydew melon (about 1 lb or 500 g)
1  pint ripe strawberries, hulled and sliced (1½ cups)
1  large pear, cut into ½-in (1 cm) pieces
½  small cucumber, diced (½ cup)
2  star fruits, sliced ¼ in (0.5 cm) thick
6  Tbsp Grand Marnier or brandy
2  Tbsp shredded fresh mint
Fresh mint sprigs

1. Cut both melons in half crosswise and scoop out seeds from center. Using melon baller or small spoon, scoop out balls of melon into large bowl. With a tablespoon, scoop out any remaining melon into the bowl, leaving smooth shells.

# FRESH FRUIT SOUP

Serves 4
**Prep Time:** 30 minutes plus chilling
**Healing Foods:** peppers, chile, guava, kiwi
**Ailments It Heals:** acne, colds and flu, gout, jet lag

2  cups pineapple juice
2  cups orange juice
½  cucumber, diced
¼  red onion, finely chopped
1  small red bell pepper, seeded and chopped
½  red chile pepper, seeded and chopped
Juice of 1 lime
½  tsp sugar
1  guava, peeled and diced
1  kiwi, diced
1  Tbsp chopped fresh mint
2  Tbsp chopped fresh cilantro
Fresh mint sprigs (optional)

1. In large bowl, mix together pineapple and orange juices. Add cucumber, onion, bell pepper, chile pepper, lime juice, and sugar and stir well to mix. Cover and chill for 1 hour so flavors can develop.

2. Remove from refrigerator and stir in guava, kiwi, chopped mint, and cilantro.

3. Ladle soup into bowls and garnish with mint sprigs, if using, and serve at once.

**Per serving:** 171 calories, 2 g protein, 41 g carbohydrates, 3 g fiber, 1 g fat, 0 g saturated fat, 0 mg cholesterol, 8 mg sodium

# MIXED BERRY AND STONE FRUIT SOUP

Serves 8
**Prep Time:** 20 minutes
**Cook Time:** 0 minutes
**Healing Foods:** nectarines, plums, blueberries, blackberries, yogurt
**Ailments It Heals:** flatulence, stroke, varicose veins

¼ cup orange juice
1 Tbsp lemon juice
3 Tbsp sugar
2 medium nectarines, pitted and cut into 1 x ½-in (2.5 x 1 cm) pieces (1 ½ cups)
3 medium plums, pitted and cut into 1 x ½-in (2.5 x 1 cm) pieces (1 ½ cups)
1 cup fresh blueberries, rinsed
1 cup fresh blackberries, rinsed
2 Tbsp frozen orange juice concentrate
2 ice cubes, crushed
½ cup nonfat vanilla yogurt
Mint sprigs for garnish

1. In large bowl, combine orange juice, lemon juice, and sugar. Stir to dissolve sugar. Gently stir in nectarines, plums, blueberries, and blackberries. Transfer ¾ cup of fruit and juices to blender. Add

orange juice concentrate and ice cubes to blender and blend until smooth. Scrape puree into bowl containing remaining fruit. Stir gently to combine.

2. To serve, ladle soup into dessert bowls and garnish each serving with a dollop of yogurt and mint sprig.

**Per serving:** 88 calories, 2 g protein, 21 g carbohydrates, 2 g fiber, 0 g total fat, 0 g saturated fat, 0 mg cholesterol, 10 mg sodium

**DRINKS**

# CARROT-ORANGE JUICE

Serves 2
**Prep Time:** 5 minutes
**Healing Foods:** carrots, oranges, ginger
**Ailments It Heals:** colds and flu, fever, gout, varicose veins

1 ½ cups fresh or bottled carrot juice, chilled
⅔ cup fresh-squeezed orange juice (3 oranges)
½-in-thick (1 cm) slice peeled fresh ginger

1. In medium bowl, mix carrot juice and orange juice. Crush ginger in garlic press to fill ½ tsp. Stir crushed ginger into juice mixture and serve. (If making ahead, stir before serving.)

**Per serving:** 75 calories, 2 g protein, 17 g carbohydrates, 0 g fiber, 0 g total fat, 0 g saturated fat, 0 mg cholesterol, 93 mg sodium

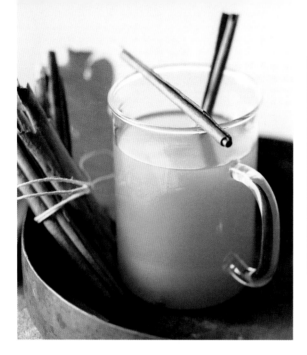

## SPICY VEGETABLE COCKTAIL

**Serves 4**
**Prep Time:** 8 minutes
**Healing Foods:** tomatoes, onions, parsley
**Ailments It Heals:** colds and flu, muscle cramps, respiratory disorders

3 cups tomato juice
¼ cup coarsely chopped, seeded green bell pepper
1 scallion, trimmed to 4 in (10 cm), thinly sliced
1 Tbsp coarsely chopped parsley
1 Tbsp horseradish sauce
1 tsp Worcestershire sauce
½ tsp sugar
½ tsp Tabasco, or to taste
Celery stalks and lemon slices, for garnish (optional)

**1.** In blender, combine tomato juice, pepper, scallion, parsley, horseradish sauce, Worcestershire sauce, sugar, and Tabasco. Process for 2 to 3 minutes, or until smooth.

**2.** Serve over ice. Garnish with celery and lemon, if using.

**Per serving:** 55 calories, 2 g protein, 10 g carbohydrates, 1 g fiber, 1 g total fat, 0 g saturated fat, 1 mg cholesterol, 686 mg sodium

## WARM PINEAPPLE-GINGER PUNCH

**Serves 4**
**Prep Time:** 5 minutes
**Cook Time:** 10 minutes
**Healing Foods:** pineapples, ginger, cloves
**Ailments It Heals:** arthritis, flatulence, motion sickness, sore throat

4 cups pineapple juice
1 cup sliced fresh ginger, unpeeled
1 Tbsp honey
1 cinnamon stick, split lengthwise
8 whole cloves
¼ tsp ground black pepper

**1.** In medium saucepan, combine pineapple juice, ginger, honey, cinnamon, cloves, and pepper. Bring to a boil. Reduce to a simmer and cook for 10 minutes. Strain and serve warm.

**Per serving:** 152 calories, 1 g protein, 38 g carbohydrates, 0 g fiber, 0 g total fat, 0 g saturated fat, 0 mg cholesterol, 4 mg sodium

# CHAI

Serves 2
**Prep Time:** 2 minutes
**Cook Time:** 5 minutes plus steeping
**Healing Foods:** ginger, tea, milk
**Ailments It Heals:** diabetes, fever, lupus, multiple sclerosis, osteoporosis

1½   cups water
¼   tsp ground cinnamon
¼   tsp ground cloves
¼   tsp ground ginger
⅔   cup low-fat milk or vanilla soymilk
3   black tea bags
2   tsp honey, or to taste

**1.** In small saucepan, combine water, cinnamon, cloves, and ginger. Bring to a simmer. Reduce heat to low, cover, and simmer for 5 minutes. Add milk (or soymilk) and heat until steaming but not boiling. Remove from heat.

**2.** Add tea bags, cover, and let steep for 3 to 4 minutes. Pour into 2 mugs and sweeten with honey to taste.

**Per serving:** 63 calories, 3 g protein, 11 g carbohydrates, 0 g fiber, 1 g total fat, 1 g saturated fat, 3 mg cholesterol, 49 mg sodium

# ELECTROLYTE DRINK

Serves 1
**Prep Time:** 5 minutes
**Healing Foods:** apples, lemons
**Ailments It Heals:** diarrhea, fever, urinary tract infections

1   cup apple juice
2   cups water
½ to 1 tsp salt
Juice from 1 lemon or 1 lime

In a pitcher, combine apple juice, water, salt, and lemon or lime juice. Store in refrigerator.

**Per serving:** 127 calories, 0 g protein, 34 g carbohydrates, 0 g fiber, 0 g total fat, 0 g saturated fat, 0 mg cholesterol, 1,174 mg sodium

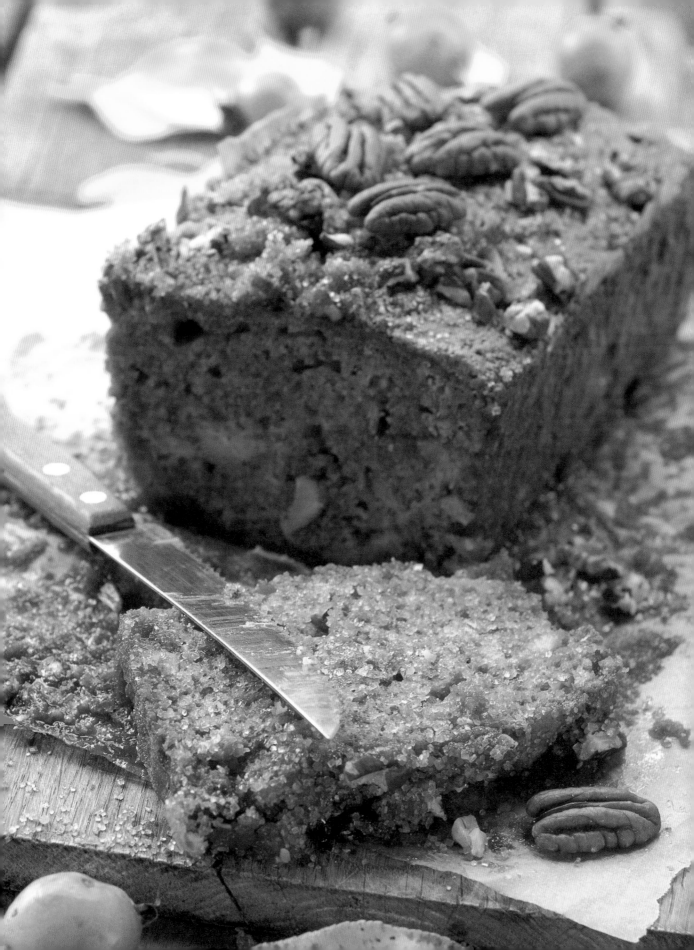

# AILMENTS

## Daily Meal Plans to Heal What Ails You

Now that you know food can be powerful medicine, it's time to take advantage of its healing powers. No food or diet is likely to cure an ailment, but eating the right foods and avoiding the wrong ones can go a long way toward improving your wellbeing. Healing foods provide nutrients your body needs to ease symptoms, fight disease, and repair itself.

To get started, check out an ailment that you or someone you know has been affected by. You can also be proactive by reviewing the diet advice for conditions you may be predisposed to develop because of a family history or other risk factors you may have. For instance, if you have a family history of diabetes, you may want to familiarize yourself with low glycemic and fiber-rich foods that help keep your blood sugar levels stable

Each entry begins with aquick lists, so you can see at a glance which foods may cause additional symptoms or worsen an ailment and which foods may improve or prevent it. These aren't compre-

hensive lists, but just highlight the best and worst foods to eat if you suffer from that condition. And because ailments often affect different people in different ways, we also highlight foods that you may consider limiting. If you suffer from migraines, for example, you may want to avoid aged cheeses, processed meats, red wine, or certain fruits and vegetables if they trigger your headaches.

At the heart of each entry is a sample one-day meal plan that shows you how to minimize harmful foods and maximize the healing ones. You'll also get a list of recipes to try (in the order they appear in Part 2) that feature one or more of the foods that heal. And to help you eat that way every day, we provide general diet advice for each condition.

Changing your diet is just one part of getting better, but its impact goes way beyond helping to heal a specific ailment. Some positive side effects include more energy, a stronger immune system, and a longer, healthier life.

# ACNE

## FOODS THAT HARM

Dairy products

High-glycemic foods, such as soft
drinks, white flour, and refined
sugars

## FOODS THAT HEAL

Broccoli

Cabbage

Oranges

Berries

Kiwi

Melons

Peppers

Spinach and other dark leafy greens

Fish

Poultry

Whole grains

Lentils

Avocados

Potatoes

Bananas

Oysters

Flaxseed

## FOODS TO LIMIT

Iodized salt

## HOW TO EAT

Limiting dairy and increasing your intake
of vitamins and minerals will keep your
skin looking its best. Here's a meal plan
that does exactly that while providing
alternate sources of calcium. Eat this way
regularly to prevent outbreaks and heal
them quickly when they happen.

**Enjoy a wide variety of fruits and vegetables,** including a mix of colors to get all
the skin-clearing vitamins such as beta-
carotene and C.

**Drink lots of water** and eat high-water
content fruits and veggies such as watermelon, strawberries, tomatoes, and zucchini. Staying hydrated keeps your skin
glowing.

**Get your vitamin B6 and zinc.** Found
in meat, fish (especially oysters), poultry,
whole grains, beans, lentils, avocados,
nuts, potatoes, bananas, and leafy greens,
this vitamin and mineral may reduce acne
by helping to regulate hormones impli-
cated in the development of acne lesions.

**Load up on healthy fat.** Omega-3 fatty
acids can help ward off the inflammation
of acne. Flaxseed and fish are rich in these
healthy fats.

## SAMPLE MEAL PLAN

**Breakfast:** ¾ cup of whole grain cereal
with ½ cup of soymilk; ½ sliced banana

**Lunch:** *Chicken Salad with Citrus* (page
161); 1 whole wheat pita pocket, sliced in
quarters

**Snack:** ¼ cup of bean dip with 6 whole
grain crackers

**Dinner:** 3 oz of grilled fish; ½ cup of
cooked brown rice; at least ½ cup of
chopped, steamed kale; *Avocado, Jicama,
and Orange Salad* (page 174)

**Dessert:** 2 cups of cubed cantaloupe

## OTHER RECIPES TO TRY

- Grilled Salmon Salad
- Spinach Salad with Chickpeas
- Orange Beef with Broccoli and Jicama
- Brown Rice with Cabbage and
  Chickpeas

# ADHD (ATTENTION DEFICIT/HY-PERACTIVITY DISORDER)

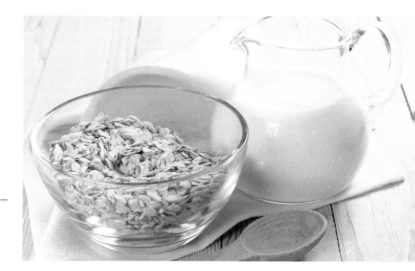

## FOODS THAT HARM

Some children with ADHD may be
sensitive to foods containing
salicylates, including:
Processed foods
Foods containing dyes,
  particularly red or orange dyes
Dried fruits

## FOODS THAT HEAL

Salicylate-free foods, such as:
Bananas
Pears
Lentils
Whole grain breads and cereals
Fish
Lean meat and poultry
Milk and cheese
Eggs

## FOODS TO LIMIT

Sugary foods, such as cookies and
  soft drinks

## HOW TO EAT

A diet filled with more complex carbs and
protein instead of sugary carbs may promote
better concentration and help you relax.

**Nix simple carbs** such as candy, honey,
sugar, fruit drinks, soft drinks, and foods
sweetened with corn syrup.

**Eat complex carbs,** especially later in
the day.

**Get more protein** like beans, eggs, low-
fat cheese, fish, and lean meat.

## SAMPLE MEAL PLAN

**Breakfast:** 1 cup of oatmeal prepared
with ½ cup of whole milk; 1 banana

**Lunch:** *Macaroni and Cheese with Spinach* (page 215); 1 cup of vegetable soup

**Snack:** 1 pear; 1 oz of low-fat cheese

**Dinner:** *Greek-Lamb Kebabs* (page 186);
baked potato topped with 1 Tbsp reduced-
fat sour cream, chopped chives, and ½ cup
of steamed vegetables

**Snack:** ½ peanut butter sandwich made
with 1 slice of whole grain bread

## OTHER RECIPES TO TRY

- Summer Greens Scramble
- Beef-Fillet Salad with Mustard
  Vinaigrette
- Sloppy Joes
- Zucchini-Carrot Crustless Quiche
  Squares
- Savory Lamb Stew with Sweet
  Potatoes

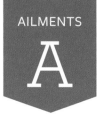
# AGE-RELATED MACULAR DEGENERA-TION

*See* Eye Problems, page 305

# AIDS AND HIV INFECTION

*See also* Diarrhea, page 303

### FOODS THAT HARM

Shellfish, hamburgers, sushi, homemade mayonnaise, and other undercooked food

### FOODS THAT HEAL

Fish

Lean meats

Poultry without skin

Legumes

Cooked fruits and vegetables

Quinoa

Barley

Buckwheat

Olive oil

Walnuts

Flaxseed

### FOODS TO LIMIT

Sugary foods, such as cookies and soft drinks

Raw fruits and vegetables

Red meat, butter, and other foods with saturated fats

### HOW TO EAT

Good nutrition can prevent or delay weight loss and other complications associated with the disease.

**Avoid empty calories**—foods like cookies and soft drinks provide calories but little to no nutrition.

**Aim for 5 to 6 servings** of vegetables and fruits per day.

**Choose whole grain carbohydrates** at least 50 percent of the time.

**Keep protein in check.** To avoid overtaxing your kidneys, limit protein to 0.4 to 0.5 g per pound of body weight. That's 60 to 75 g if you weigh 150 lbs (68 kg).

**Practice food safety.** Wash hands before handling food, during its preparation, and after. Keep hot foods hot and cold foods cold. Avoid contact between raw and cooked foods. Eggs should be boiled for at least 7 minutes; meat and fish should be well cooked, with an internal temperature of 160° to 165°F (71° to 74°C).

**Cook ahead.** To make healthy eating easier on days when you're not feeling well, prepare dishes when you feel good and freeze them.

### SAMPLE MEAL PLAN

**Breakfast:** *Hot Cereal with Apples and Dates* (page 121) topped with 1 tsp of ground flaxseeds

**Lunch:** 3 oz of baked skinless chicken breast; *Barley and Beet Salad* (page 168); 1 cup of chopped, steamed greens

**Snack:** small container of low-fat yogurt with ½ cup of fruit canned in its own juice

**Dinner:** *Flank Steak Roll with Carrots and Red Peppers* (page 181); small baked potato topped with 1 Tbsp of reduced-fat sour cream; 1 slice of whole grain bread

**Dessert:** 1 orange

## OTHER RECIPES TO TRY

- Cod and Vegetable Stew
- Three-Bean Chili
- Asian Grilled Tuna Burgers
- Spinach-Stuffed Meat Loaf
- Tuscan Veal Chops
- Springtime Quinoa
- Roasted Root Vegetables

# ALCOHOLISM

### FOODS THAT HARM

Alcohol in any form

### FOODS THAT HEAL

Legumes

Whole grain or fortified and
enriched grain products

Lean meat and poultry

Nuts

Mushrooms

Broccoli

Cabbage

Dairy products

Spinach

Kale

## HOW TO EAT

Alcoholism can lead to malnutrition, not only because chronic drinkers tend to have poor diets, but also because alcohol alters the digestion and metabolism of most nutrients. To prevent problems, eat a wide variety of nutrient-packed foods and don't skip meals.

**Add calcium.** Dairy foods and dark leafy greens are good sources of this bone-strengthening mineral. Many alcoholics are at higher risk of bone fractures and osteoporosis.

**Speak to a nutritionist.** A nutritionist can help you customize your diet to address underlying problems such as obesity or liver damage.

### SAMPLE MEAL PLAN

**Breakfast:** *Mushroom and Bell Pepper Frittata* (page 123); 1 slice of whole grain toast with 1 tsp of trans fat free soft spread; 1 cup of calcium-fortified orange juice

**Lunch:** *Pasta Primavera* (page 216), 2 cups of mixed green salad tossed with 2 Tbsp of low-fat dressing and 1 Tbsp of walnuts; 1 whole grain roll

**Snack:** 1 banana

**Dinner:** *Pork Chops and Cabbage* (page 188); ½ cup of cooked brown rice; ½ cup of steamed broccoli florets

**Dessert:** milkshake or protein smoothie, any flavor

## OTHER RECIPES TO TRY

- One-Egg Omelet with Chopped Broccoli, Tomatoes, and Cheddar
- Grilled Salmon with Sautéed Greens
- Roasted Pork with Pomegranate Sauce
- Baked Pasta with Garlic and Greens
- Orange-Walnut Broccoli

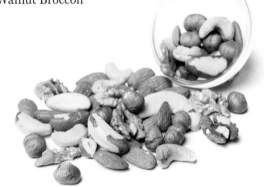

# ALLERGIES, FOOD

## FOODS THAT HARM

Almost any food can provoke an allergic reaction. Eight foods that account for 90% of allergic reactions are:

Milk and milk products

Eggs (especially egg whites)

Soy and soy products

Wheat and wheat products

Peanuts

Tree nuts

Fish

Shellfish

## HOW TO EAT

**Keep a food diary.** Record the foods you eat each day and when you eat them. (Don't forget to include snacks and beverages!) Record any allergy symptoms you experience, as well as the time the symptoms begin. Share your food diary with your doctor to help determine which foods may be triggering your symptoms.

**Read labels carefully.** Once you identify what you're allergic to, learn to read labels to avoid exposure.

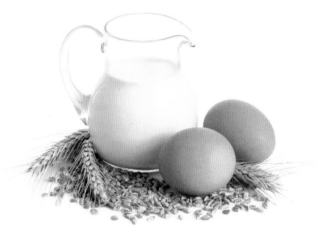

# ALLERGIES, SEASONAL

*See* Hay Fever, page 312

# ALZHEIMER'S DISEASE

## FOODS THAT HARM

Alcohol

## FOODS THAT HEAL

Olive oil

Tomatoes

Green beans

Zucchini

Cauliflower

Brussels sprouts

Eggplant

Peppers

Salmon

Mackerel

## FOODS TO LIMIT

Red meat, butter, and other foods with saturated fats

Sugary foods, such as cookies and soft drinks

## HOW TO EAT

There is evidence that some foods and nutrients are powerful allies in the battle against Alzheimer's. Here's how to protect against Alzheimer's and dementia or slow their effects if you have the disease.

**Adopt a Mediterranean eating style** that includes olive oil, tomatoes, fish, poultry, cruciferous vegetables, fruits, and leafy green vegetables, and less amounts of foods with saturated fat, such as butter and red meat.

**Eat fatty fish at least three times a week.** Good sources also include trout, sardines, herring, anchovies, halibut, bluefish, ocean perch, bass, and red snapper.

**Toss aluminum cookware.** Although a link between aluminum and Alzheimer's hasn't been proven, some scientists argue that increased concentration in the Alzheimer's brain worsens the condition. As a precaution, avoid using aluminum cookware because the metal can leach into food. Other sources: some antacids and drinking water in areas where aluminum compounds are used in city water treatment.

## SAMPLE MEAL PLAN

**Breakfast:** 1 cup of oatmeal or cream of wheat prepared with skim milk; at least ½ cup of fresh fruit

**Lunch:** *Penne with Fresh Tomato Sauce and Grilled Eggplant* (page 218); at least ½ cup of steamed green string beans; 1 whole grain roll

**Snack:** 1 cup of cubed cantaloupe or honeydew with ¼ cup of low-fat cottage cheese

**Dinner:** *Salmon and Asparagus Farfalle with Walnut-Feta Sauce* (page 201); 1 cup of mixed green salad tossed with grated carrots, drizzled with 2 Tbsp low-fat dressing

**Dessert:** *Sesame-Fig Bars* (page 251)

## OTHER RECIPES TO TRY

- Mediterranean Salad with Edamame
- Grilled Salmon with Sautéed Greens
- Roasted Mackerel with Cherry Tomatoes and Potatoes
- Roasted Tomatoes with Garlic and Herbs
- Trout with Lemon-Mushroom Stuffing
- Baked Pasta with Garlic and Greens
- Cauliflower and Spinach Casserole

# ANEMIA

### FOODS THAT HEAL

**Organ meats**

**Beef**

**Poultry**

**Fish**

**Egg yolks**

**Soy products (except soy sauce)**

**Green leafy vegetables**

**Iron-enriched breads and cereals**

**Citrus fruits**

**Broccoli**

**Red peppers**

### FOODS TO LIMIT

**Spinach**

**Rhubarb**

**Swiss chard**

**Chocolate**

**Bran**

**Nuts**

**Tea**

## HOW TO EAT

The most common type of anemia in North America is due to iron deficiency. Here are some general guidelines to boost iron levels to prevent or treat this type of anemia. Never take iron supplements without consulting your doctor.

**Consume as much iron from foods as possible.** The best sources are animal products—meat, fish, poultry, and egg yolks.

**If you're a vegetarian, eat more vitamin C–rich foods.** This vitamin enhances the body's absorption of iron from plant sources,

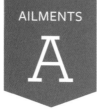

such as green leafy vegetables, dried fruits, soy and other legumes, nuts, seeds, and iron-enriched breads and cereals.

**Avoid drinking tea during meals.** Tea contains natural compounds called tannins that inhibit iron absorption.

**Watch for foods with oxalates,** such as spinach, rhubarb, Swiss chard, and chocolate, and phytates, such as nuts and bran cereal. Both interfere with your body's ability to absorb and use iron.

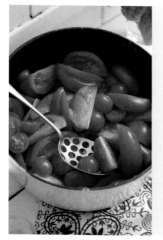

### QUICK TIP:
### Cook with iron pots

Tomatoes and other acidic foods prepared in iron pots add large amounts of iron to food. Four ounces (120 mL) of tomato sauce heated in a regular pot provides 0.7 mg of iron; cooking it in an iron pot adds 5 mg. Ironware may discolor food, but the taste is unaffected.

### SAMPLE MEAL PLAN

**Breakfast:** 2 scrambled eggs; 1 cup of Raisin Bran with ½ cup of skim milk; 1 orange

**Lunch:** *Chicken Salad with Citrus* (page 161) and 1 enriched soft breadstick; for vegetarians, a bowl of lentil soup, 1 enriched roll topped with 2 tsp of prepared red pepper pesto, and 1 cup of chopped steamed collards

**Snack:** ¼ cup of trail mix

**Dinner:** *Orange Beef with Broccoli and Jicama* (page 184), 1 cup of cooked brown rice, and a whole grain roll; for vegetarians, a bowl of chili, 1 cup of cooked brown rice, 1 cup of steamed kale, and 1 enriched roll

**Dessert:** *Chewy Date-Walnut Bars* (page 253)

### OTHER RECIPES TO TRY

- Fish Tacos
- Zucchini-Carrot Crustless Quiche Squares
- Buckwheat Noodles with Tofu and Green Vegetables
- Pot Roast with Root Vegetables
- Calf's Liver with Rigatoni
- Orange Beets
- Creamy Citrus and Vanilla Rice Pudding

# ANOREXIA NERVOSA

### FOODS THAT HEAL

Eggs
Milk and other dairy foods
Meat, fish, and poultry
Whole grains

### FOODS TO LIMIT

Low-calorie diet foods and soft drinks
Foods that have a diuretic or laxative effect (includes foods with sorbitol and some herbal teas like senna leaf tea)

### HOW TO EAT

Here are steps to help achieve a stable weight. Consult with a dietitian to make sure all nutritional needs are met.

**Start with small portions,** then gradually increase food intake.

**Choose nutritious and easily digestible foods,** such as eggs, custards, soups, and milkshakes.

**Suck on a lemon drop before meals.**
Sour foods increase saliva flow, which can
stimulate appetite.

**Monitor food intake closely.** Relapses
are common, and close monitoring may be
necessary to ensure that the person with
anorexia is really eating. But avoid making
food a constant source of attention and
conflict.

### SAMPLE MEAL PLAN

**Mini Breakfast:** 1 small container of 2%
Greek yogurt, topped with 3 to 4 Tbsp of
granola

**A.M. Mini Meal:** 1 sliced apple with
1 piece of string cheese

**Mini Lunch:** *Buffalo Chicken Fingers*
(page 246) with your favorite steamed
vegetables and rice

**P.M. Mini Meal:** 8 whole wheat pita chips
with *Asian Peanut Dip* (page 249), or try a
bean dip, guacamole, or cheese nachos

**Mini Dinner:** 1 cup of soup, any kind; ½
sandwich—try a turkey or tuna fish sandwich on whole grain bread—or have a grilled
chicken or bean burger on a whole wheat
bun; ½ cup of steamed vegetables or a small
leafy green salad with your favorite dressing

**Dessert:** *Fruit Salad with Spiced Coconut*
(page 176)

### OTHER RECIPES TO TRY

- One-Egg Omelet with Chopped
  Broccoli, Tomatoes, and Cheddar
- Zucchini-Carrot Crustless Quiche
  Squares
- Asian Noodle Salad
- Rice Salad with Chicken and Grapes
- Turkey Bacon and Apricot Bites
- Vegetable-Stuffed Mushrooms

# ANXIETY

*See* Mood Disorders, page 333

# ARTHRITIS

### FOODS THAT HARM

Red meat, butter, egg yolks, and
   other foods with saturated fat
Processed foods that contain trans
   fats
Refined carbohydrates, such as
   sugar and white flour

### FOODS THAT HEAL

Salmon
Sardines
Trout
Anchovies
Citrus fruits
Kiwi
Pumpkin
Peppers
Sweet potatoes
Cabbage
Collard greens
Rhubarb
Spinach
Chia seeds
Walnuts
Pineapple
Beans
Soy products (except soy sauce)

### HOW TO EAT

While medications are different for os-
teoarthritis and rheumatoid arthritis, the
diet advice is similar. Both conditions benefit from reducing inflammation and pain
with these tips.

**Eat fish two to three times a week.** The
human body uses omega-3 fatty acids to

manufacture prostaglandins, chemicals that play a role in inflammation and pain.

**Pump up antioxidants.** Vitamins C and E and beta-carotene help to make collagen, reduce inflammation, and slow the progression of this disease. In addition to the foods above, berries and melons are also packed with these vitamins.

**Find more omega-3s.** If you're not a fish fan or if you want more variety, try flaxseed, chia seed, and walnuts.

**Enjoy more bromelain.** This enzyme in pineapple may help reduce swelling.

**Get more phytoestrogens.** Food sources include beans and soy.

### SAMPLE MEAL PLAN

**Breakfast:** ½ cup of low-fat cottage cheese mixed with fresh kiwi slices and 1 Tbsp of crushed walnuts; 1 slice of whole grain toast with 1 Tbsp of apple butter

**Lunch:** *Pineapple-Chipotle Chicken* (page 195); 1 small baked sweet potato; a side of coleslaw made with low-fat mayonnaise

**Snack:** 1 orange

**Dinner:** 3 oz of broiled salmon; *Pasta with Walnut Cream Sauce* (page 217); ½ cup of steamed broccoli

**Dessert:** *Pumpkin Maple Cheesecake* (page 261)

### OTHER RECIPES TO TRY

- Carrot Ginger Yogurt Muffins
- Spinach, Sweet Potato, and Shiitake Salad Sesame Greens and Bean Sprouts
- Grilled Salmon with Sautéed Greens
- Bok Choy, Tofu, and Mushroom Stir-Fry
- Pasta with Cabbage, Apples, and Leeks

# ASTHMA

### FOODS THAT HARM

Dried fruit

Beer

Wine

White grape juice

Instant soup mix

Instant mashed potatoes

Cheese

Soy sauce

Mushrooms

### FOODS THAT HEAL

Salmon

Mackerel

Sardines

Berries

Green leafy vegetables

### HOW TO EAT

Food allergies can cause asthma attacks, so it's important to identify these types of triggers. See Allergies, Food (page 280) for more information. In addition, these general guidelines will help lessen your chances of attacks or complications.

**Double up on fresh fruits and veggies.** Aim to have at least 2 servings at every meal and one with every snack to protect lung function and boost immunity. However, beware of potential trigger foods.

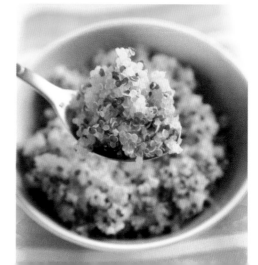

**Know your trigger foods and avoid them.** Common trigger foods are those that contain sulfites (such as dried fruits, white grape juice, instant soup mix, and instant potatoes), salicylates (such as dried fruits and some fresh fruits), molds (such as cheese and mushrooms), and those that are fermented (such as soy sauce, beer, and wine).

**Sip coffee or tea.** It may help squelch a mild attack because it relaxes bronchial muscles. Skip this tip if you are sensitive to salicylates or take a theophylline drug.

### SAMPLE MEAL PLAN

**Breakfast:** 1 cup of oatmeal with cinnamon, topped with ½ cup of skim milk; 1 cup of fresh fruit

**Lunch:** *Poached Salmon with Cucumber-Dill Sauce* (page 200); 1 cup of black bean soup; 1 small baked potato topped with 2 Tbsp of salsa and 1 cup of steamed vegetables

**Snack:** 1 banana

**Dinner:** 3 oz of baked chicken; 1 cup of a cooked whole grain such as brown rice, quinoa, or millet; at least ½ cup steamed green leafy vegetables and ½ cup steamed assorted other vegetables

**Dessert:** a bowl of fresh cherries

### OTHER RECIPES TO TRY

- Raspberry-Beet Smoothie
- Buckwheat Noodles with Tofu and Green Vegetables
- Grilled Salmon with Sautéed Greens
- Roasted Mackerel with Cherry Tomatoes and Potatoes

# ATHERO-SCLEROSIS

### FOODS THAT HARM

Processed foods that contain trans fats

### FOODS THAT HEAL

Olive oil
Almonds
Avocados
Oats
Lentils
Tofu
Salmon
Sardines
Apples
Pears
Citrus fruits

### FOODS TO LIMIT

Red meat, butter, and other foods with saturated fats
High-cholesterol foods, such as eggs, shrimp, and organ meats

### HOW TO EAT

Diet plays a critical role in both the development and treatment of atherosclerosis, or hardening of the arteries. Here are ways to delay or prevent the condition.

**Limit total fat intake to 10% to 30% of calories.**

**Cut down on saturated fat.** Some strategies include downsizing meat portions, substituting olive oil for butter or margarine, and eating low-fat dairy products.

**Eliminate trans fats,** which are found in packaged foods such as cookies and crackers and snack food such as chips.

**Limit dietary cholesterol to 300 mg a day**—about the amount in 1½ egg yolks.

**Go fish at least twice a week.** The omega-3 fatty acids in salmon, sardines, and other cold-water fish lower blood levels of triglycerides. They also reduce the tendency to form blood clots.

**Eat 5 to 10 g of soluble fiber per day.** Oat bran; oatmeal; lentils and legumes; pectin-containing fruits such as pears, apples, and citrus fruits; barley; guar gum; and psyllium all contain soluble fiber that lowers blood cholesterol—probably by interfering with the intestinal absorption of bile acids, which forces the liver to use circulating cholesterol to make more bile.

**Eat more soy.** Aim for 25 g of soy protein—about 1½ cups of edamame—per day.

### SAMPLE MEAL PLAN

**Breakfast:** 1 apple-oat bran muffin; 1 slice of honeydew and 3 large strawberries mixed with ½ cup of yogurt and topped with 1 Tbsp of toasted, sliced almonds

**Lunch:** *Buckwheat Noodles with Tofu and Green Vegetables* (page 171); 1 whole grain roll; orange.

**Snack:** 1 pear; a soy protein snack bar

**Dinner:** 3 oz of grilled salmon; *Mediterranean Salad with Edamame* (page 177); 1 large ear of grilled corn on the cob with 1 tsp of trans fat free soft spread

**Dessert:** *Chocolate Almond Biscotti* (page 257)

### OTHER RECIPES TO TRY

- Nutty Muesli
- Pear Rhubarb Muffins
- Lentil Soup with Canadian Bacon
- Grilled Salmon Salad
- Broiled Salmon with Avocado-Mango Salsa
- Chewy Oatmeal Raisin Cookies

**WARNING!**
**FOOD-DRUG INTERACTION**
If you are taking anticoagulant medication such as Coumadin, you should limit foods high in vitamin K because they can counteract the desired effect of the drug.

# BLEEDING PROBLEMS

**FOODS THAT HARM**
Alcohol

**FOODS THAT HEAL**
Green peas
Spinach
Broccoli
Liver
Lean meat
Legumes
Citrus fruits

### HOW TO EAT

Bleeding disorders can be inherited such as hemophilia, related to certain cancers such as leukemia, or caused by vitamin K deficiencies. Here are some general guidelines that may help no matter what the cause.

**Eat foods rich in vitamin K,** which is necessary for the blood to clot normally. Sources include green peas, broccoli, spinach, brussels sprouts, and organ meats.

**Eat more foods with vitamin C.** Vitamin C deficiency can cause bleeding gums.

**Up your iron intake.** Chronic blood loss can lead to anemia, a blood disorder that is characterized by inadequate levels of red blood cells.

### SAMPLE MEAL PLAN

**Breakfast:** 2 scrambled eggs; 2 slices of turkey bacon; 1 slice of whole grain toast with 1 tsp of jam; ½ cup of fresh grapefruit sections

**Lunch:** 3 oz of roasted turkey breast; *Brussels Sprouts with Caraway Seeds* (page 229); 1 small baked potato topped with 1 Tbsp reduced-fat sour cream

**Snack:** 1 tangerine; 1 oz of reduced-fat cheese; 4 low-sodium crackers

**Dinner:** 3 oz of baked chicken; *Springtime Quinoa* (page 220); ½ cup of lightly sautéed spinach and sliced carrots; 1 whole grain roll

**Dessert:** ½ cup of orange sherbet

## OTHER RECIPES TO TRY

- Beef and Blue Cheese Burgers
- Spinach-Stuffed Meat Loaf
- Calf's Liver with Rigatoni
- Sesame Greens and Bean Sprouts
- Orange-Walnut Broccoli

# BLOOD PRESSURE

## FOODS THAT HARM

Salty and processed foods, such as pickles

## FOODS THAT HEAL

Green leafy vegetables
Low-fat dairy products
Legumes
Bananas
Melons
Oranges
Dried fruit
Nuts and seeds
Whole wheat pasta
Carrots
Sweet potatoes

## FOODS TO LIMIT

Red meat, butter, and other foods with saturated fats
Alcohol
Caffeinated drinks

## HOW TO EAT

Following the DASH (Dietary Approaches to Stop Hypertension) diet, which is endorsed by numerous health organizations including the American Heart Association and the Mayo Clinic, will help lower blood pressure. Here is a synopsis of the DASH diet and accompanying strategies.

- Have 6 to 8 servings of grains daily.
- Eat 4 to 5 servings each of fruits and vegetables daily.
- Consume 2 to 3 servings of low-fat or nonfat dairy foods daily.
- Limit meats, poultry, and fish to 6 or fewer 1-oz servings daily.
- Eat 4 to 5 servings of nuts, seeds, or legumes per week.
- Limit fats to 2 to 3 servings daily.
- Limit sweets to 5 servings per week.

**Limit your salt intake.** A key component of what makes DASH effective is reducing sodium intake. The range of acceptable sodium intake per day is 1,500 to 2,300 mg. The best way to reduce sodium intake is to avoid adding salt and to avoid most processed foods, which are usually loaded with sodium. Check labels carefully—look for the term sodium to find hidden salt.

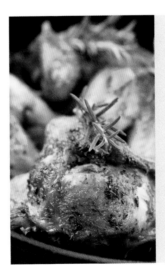

### QUICK TIP:
#### Flavor without salt

To limit your sodium intake but still add flavor to your food, use herbs and spices instead. For example use tarragon in roasted poultry dishes or add a dried bay leaf or two to your soups and stocks instead of your usual amount of salt. For more suggestions, see Herbs and Spices on page 61.

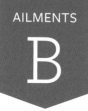
## SAMPLE MEAL PLAN

**Breakfast:** 1 cup of whole grain cereal with 1 cup of skim milk and 1 small sliced banana; 1 slice of whole grain cinnamon raisin bread with 1 tsp of trans fat-free soft spread

**Lunch:** 2 to 3 oz of baked chicken; *Rustic Grilled Vegetable and Rigatoni Salad* (page 172); 1 small baked sweet potato; 1 orange

**Snack:** 1 cup of fresh fruit salad—try grapes, cubed cantaloupe, and whole strawberries dipped in 1 cup of low-fat or fat-free yogurt

**Dinner:** 2 to 3 oz of lean meat, poultry, or fish; ½ cup of cooked brown rice; 1 cup of lightly sautéed carrots and collards; 1 whole grain roll

**Dessert:** *Grilled Fruit en Brochette* (page 267)

### OTHER RECIPES TO TRY

- Zucchini Frittata
- Strawberry-Yogurt Smoothie
- Endive, Apple, and Watercress Salad
- Rice-Stuffed Squash

# BRONCHITIS

*See* Respiratory Disorders, page 345

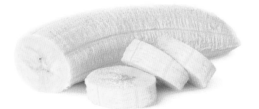

# BULIMIA

## FOODS THAT HARM

Trigger foods that are associated with binges

## FOODS THAT HEAL

Bananas

Berries

Apples

Pears

Whole grain cereals and breads

Lean meat

## HOW TO EAT

Like all eating disorders, bulimia can be difficult to treat and usually requires a team approach under the guidance of a dietitian or a physician. Here are some general guidelines.

**Eat more high-potassium foods** like bananas, cantaloupe, potatoes, and spinach.

**Emphasize foods high in protein** such as lean meats, salmon, chicken, fish, beans, low-fat dairy.

**Add fiber-filled foods** such as whole grain cereals and breads and fresh fruits and vegetables.

**Drink fluids regularly.** This will help to restore normal bowel function, which may have been affected by laxative use.

### SAMPLE MEAL PLAN

**Breakfast:** 1 cup of whole grain cereal with ½ cup of skim milk and ¼ cup of fresh berries

**Lunch:** chicken salad sandwich on 2 slices of whole grain bread with lettuce, tomato, and sprouts; small bunch of grapes

**Snack:** 1 pear; 1 oz of low-fat cheese

**Dinner:** 3 oz of grilled salmon; *Watermelon and Feta Salad* (page 180); 1 whole wheat pita bread

**Dessert:** 1 banana

## OTHER RECIPES TO TRY

- Multigrain Pancakes or Waffles
- Beef, Onion, and Pepper Fajitas
- Beef and Blue Cheese Burgers
- Cauliflower Salad with Cashews
- Pot Roast with Root Vegetables

# BURNS

## FOODS THAT HARM

Caffeinated drinks

Alcohol

## FOODS THAT HEAL

Lean meat

Poultry

Fish

Shellfish

Eggs

Legumes

Whole grains

Citrus fruit

Melons

Water

## HOW TO EAT

A well-balanced diet that provides extra calories will promote healing and tissue repair. Here are some additional suggestions.

**Up your zinc intake.** Good sources of this wound healer include seafood, meat, and poultry. You'll also get some from eggs, milk, beans, nuts, and whole grains.

**Choose vitamin C–rich fruits and vegetables.** Top sources include citrus fruits, melons, broccoli, and bell peppers, especially red ones.

**Stay hydrated.** Drink 4 to 6 cups of water a day, along with other noncaffeinated and nonalcoholic beverages.

## SAMPLE MEAL PLAN

**Breakfast:** 2 eggs poached, scrambled or sunny-side up; 2 slices of whole grain toast with 2 tsp of trans fat free soft spread; ½ cup fresh grapefruit sections

**Lunch:** *Curried Chicken Salad Sandwiches* (page 148); 12 baked crinkle-cut sweet potato fries; 1 orange; 1 protein shake

**Snack:** 1 thick slice of watermelon; a small handful of mixed nuts

**Dinner:** *Shrimp Seviche with Avocado and Pumpkin Seeds* (page 210); ½ cup of cooked brown rice; 1 cup of steamed broccoli; 1 whole grain roll with 1 tsp trans fat free soft spread

**Dessert:** 2 cups of cubed cantaloupe dipped in ½ cup of 2% Greek yogurt

## OTHER RECIPES TO TRY

- Cod and Vegetable Stew
- Three-Bean Chili
- Cantaloupe and Orange Soup
- Beef and Blue Cheese Burgers
- Crab Cakes with a Melon Relish
- Roasted Pork with Pomegranate Sauce
- Broiled Salmon with an Avocado-Mango Salsa
- Thai Roasted Shrimp

# CANCER

## FOODS THAT HARM

Foods that may contain pesticide residues and environmental pollutants

## FOODS THAT HEAL

Lean meat

Fish

Shellfish

Apples

Berries

Citrus fruit

Tomatoes

Onions and garlic

Green tea

Wheat bran and wheat germ

Brown rice

Brazil nuts

## FOODS TO LIMIT

Red meat, butter, and other foods with saturated fats

Alcohol

Foods that have been salt-cured, smoked, fermented, or charbroiled

## HOW TO EAT

The following guidelines will help protect you against cancer. If you're being treated for cancer, you can still follow the suggestions below, but you should consult a doctor or dietitian for a more personalized plan.

**Go overboard with fruits and vegetables.** Five servings a day is the minimum.

**Reduce fat intake.** Choose lean cuts of meat and trim away all visible fat. Eat vegetarian dishes several times a week. Adopt low-fat cooking methods such as baking and steaming, and limit use of added fats such as butter, margarine, mayonnaise, shortening, and oils.

**Fill up with fiber.** To hit the recommended 25 g a day for women and 38 g a day for men, eat plenty of beans, legumes, whole grain cereals and pasta, fruits, and vegetables.

**Limit processed meats** such as bacon, hot dogs, and luncheon meats.

## SAMPLE MEAL PLAN

**Breakfast:** 1 cup of whole grain cereal with ½ cup of skim milk, 2 tsp of wheat germ, and ½ cup of fresh berries; a cup of green tea

**Lunch:** *Salmon Cake Sandwiches* (page 152; 1 cup of tomato soup; 1 orange

**Snack:** 1 apple; 8 brazil nuts

**Dinner:** *Three-Bean Chili* (page 141); 1 cup of mixed green salad with grated carrots, sliced cucumbers, and 2 Tbsp low-fat dressing; 1 whole grain roll

**Dessert:** *Melon Berry Compote with Green Tea and Lime* (page 265)

## OTHER RECIPES TO TRY

- Beef, Onion, and Pepper Fajitas
- Couscous-Stuffed Peppers
- Beef Filet Salad with Mustard
- Warm Kasha and Seafood Salad
- Endive, Apple, and Watercress Salad

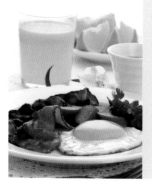

### QUICK TIP:
### Have oranges with bacon

Can't pass up the bacon when you go out for brunch? You can mitigate some of negative effects of eating processed meat by including good sources of vitamins C and E with your meal.

- Spinach Stuffed Meat Loaf
- Creamy Citrus and Vanilla Rice Pudding

# CANKER SORES

*See* Dental Problems, page 300

# CARDIOVASCULAR DISEASE

## FOODS THAT HARM

Salty foods, such as pickles

## FOODS THAT HEAL

Citrus fruits

Green leafy vegetables

Salmon

Trout

Tofu

Oats

Apples

Pears

Olive oil

Whole grain breads and cereals

Flaxseed

Nuts

## FOODS TO LIMIT

Red meat, butter, and other foods with saturated fats

Processed foods with trans fats

High-cholesterol foods, such as eggs, shrimp, and organ meats

## HOW TO EAT

Diet plays a significant role in preventing cardiovascular disease, and it can minimize problems if you already have heart disease. Here are the guidelines for a heart-healthy diet.

**Consume 2 or 3 servings of fish high in omega-3 fats a week.** Salmon, sardines, herring, trout, and other fatty cold-water fish are good sources. Plant sources of omega-3s include canola, soybean, and flaxseed oil, ground flaxseed, and nuts.

**Include 5 to 10 g of soluble fiber a day.** Oat bran, oats, psyllium, flax, lentils, legumes, apples, pears, grapes, and other fruits are high in soluble fiber.

**Swap out white bread and low-fiber cereals for whole wheat bread and whole grain cereals.** Look for products that list whole grain or whole wheat as one of their first ingredients and contain 3 g or more of fiber per serving.

**Use healthy oils,** such as olive and canola.

**Eat more soy.** It contains plant compounds called isoflavones that appear to benefit the heart by lowering cholesterol levels.

**Eat a small handful of nuts daily.** They're rich sources of fiber, vitamin E, essential fatty acids, and minerals—all linked to heart health.

**Try going meatless one day a week.** A combination of legumes and whole grains is a prudent, low-fat meat alternative.

**Limit alcohol intake.** A glass of red wine or beer may be "heart-healthy," but excessive amounts of alcohol over time may lead to increased blood pressure, obesity, or other health problems.

## SAMPLE MEAL PLAN

**Breakfast:** 1 cup of whole grain, high fiber cereal with ½ cup of soymilk and 2 tsp of ground flaxseeds; a couple sections of orange

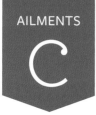
**Lunch:** *Open-Faced Grilled Vegetable Sandwich* (page 154); cup of lentil soup; 1 apple

**Snack:** small handful of nuts; 1 large pear

**Dinner:** *Broiled Salmon with Avocado-Mango Salsa* (page 199); ½ cup of cooked brown basmati rice; 2 cups of mixed salad greens with 2 tbsp of olive oil and vinegar dressing; 1 slice of whole wheat bread

**Dessert:** 1 cup of grapes or 5-oz glass of red wine

### OTHER RECIPES TO TRY

- Pear Rhubarb Muffins
- Berry-Flaxseed Smoothie
- Cantaloupe and Orange Soup
- Whole Wheat Noodles with Peanut Sauce and Chicken No-Bake Flax-seed-Nut Bars
- Grilled Salmon with Sautéed Greens
- Cider-Baked Acorn Squash with Apple Stuffing
- Spiced Almonds

# CARPAL TUNNEL SYNDROME

*See* Arthritis, page 283

# CATARACTS

*See* Eye Problems, page 305

# CELIAC DISEASE

## FOODS THAT HARM

Foods made with wheat, rye, barley, oats, bulgur, spelt, or triticale

Foods using wheat products as a thickening agent or coating, such as meat loaf and certain soups and sauces

Beverages containing gluten, such as beer

Many commercial salad dressings, except pure mayonnaise

## FOODS THAT HEAL

Skim milk

Eggs

Fish

Meat and poultry

Fresh fruits and vegetables

Legumes

Potatoes

Rice

Quinoa

## HOW TO EAT

These recommendations can help make living with celiac disease a little easier.

**Be a gluten sleuth.** Read all labels. Gluten is used in some surprising places—candy, ice creams, supplements, medications, sausages bound with bread crumbs, and foods coated with batter.

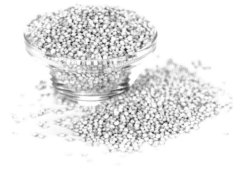

**Don't deprive yourself.** Try gluten-free items such as rice pasta and baked goods made with corn, rice, potato, or soy flours.

**Prepare most foods at home** to ensure a healthy diet without risking exposure to gluten.

## SAMPLE MEAL PLAN

**Breakfast:** *Spinach and Goat Cheese Omelet* (page 122); 1 slice of gluten-free bread, toasted, with 1 tsp of trans fat free soft spread; 1 cup of your favorite fresh fruit

**Lunch:** 3 oz of grilled chicken breast; *Quinoa with Chiles and Cilantro* (page 200); at least ½ cup steamed sliced carrots with 1 tsp trans fat free soft spread

**Snack:** 1 apple; 1 oz of low-fat cheddar cheese

**Dinner:** 3 oz of grilled tilapia; 1 medium baked potato with 1 Tbsp of reduced-fat sour cream; ½ cup of succotash; 1 gluten-free roll

**Dessert:** 1 frozen fruit sorbet bar

## OTHER RECIPES TO TRY

- Summer Greens Scramble
- Three-Bean Chili
- Tuscan Bean Soup
- Pork Chops and Cabbage
- Springtime Quinoa
- Rice Salad with Chicken and Grapes
- Minty Melon Cups

# CHOLESTEROL, HIGH

## FOODS THAT HARM

- Heavily marbled red meat
- Pizza
- Hard margarines
- Store-bought baked goods
- Fast foods and junk foods
- Full-fat dairy products
- Fried foods

## FOODS THAT HEAL

- Sterol-fortified orange juice
- Oats and oat bran
- Kidney beans
- Apples
- Pears
- Fish
- Extra-virgin olive oil

## FOODS TO LIMIT

- Salt and salty foods

## HOW TO EAT

Diet plays a key role in keeping cholesterol levels in the healthy range or lowering them if they are high. Here's how.

**Choose lean meats.** Trim all visible fat before cooking. Remove poultry skin before (or at least after) cooking.

**Get 2 g of sterols a day.** Find them in labeled buttery spreads, orange juice, and yogurt drinks.

**Eat 5 to 10 g of soluble fiber a day.** Good sources include kidney beans, apples, pears, and prunes.

**Moderate alcohol** to one (for women) or two (for men) drinks a day.

**Add omega-3s** from fish, soybeans, and nuts.

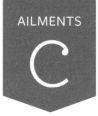

**SAMPLE MEAL PLAN**

**Breakfast:** *Pear Rhubarb Muffins* (page 128); 1 small container of low-fat yogurt; 8 oz of sterol-fortified orange juice

**Lunch:** *Tuna and Cannellini Salad with Lemon* (page 165); 2 whole wheat bread sticks; 1 sliced apple

**Snack:** 3 pitted prunes; small handful of nuts

**Dinner:** grilled chicken sandwich on a whole grain roll; 1 cup of vegetable-pasta salad; 1 ear of corn on the cob with 1 Tbsp of a sterol-containing spread

**Dessert:** 8-oz of sterol-fortified orange juice

**OTHER RECIPES TO TRY**

- Fish Tacos
- Grilled Salmon Salad
- Poached Salmon with Cucumber-Dill Sauce
- Cod with Gremolata Crust
- Scallops Florentine
- Toasted Oat-Raisin Bread
- Chewy Oatmeal Raisin Cookies
- Grilled Fruit en Brochette

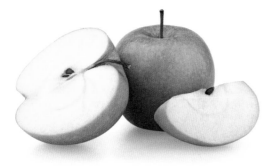

# CHRONIC FATIGUE SYNDROME

**FOODS THAT HARM**

Alcohol

**FOODS THAT HEAL**

Complex carbohydrates, such as whole grain cereals and breads
Green leafy vegetables
Fish
Nuts
Oysters
Eggs
Melons
Kiwi
Sunflower seeds
Salty foods (only for those with low blood pressure)

**FOODS TO LIMIT**

Caffeinated drinks

**HOW TO EAT**

Although there is no known cure, certain nutrients may help prevent or manage chronic fatigue syndrome.

**Eliminate food allergies.** Work with a registered dietitian to examine your diet and discover potential food allergies.

**Eat more immune-boosting zinc and vitamin C.** Foods rich in zinc include seafood (especially oysters), meat, poultry, eggs, milk, beans, nuts, and whole grains. Good sources of vitamin C include citrus fruits, berries, melons, kiwi, broccoli, and cauliflower.

**Consume more essential fatty acids** from fish, nuts, seeds, flaxseed and flaxseed oil, canola oil, wheat germ, and leafy green vegetables.

**QUICK TIP: Add a shake of salt**

If low blood pressure is part of your diagnosis, you may benefit from an increase in your sodium intake. Pickles, capers, anchovies, potato chips, and other salty foods can help.

**Get more magnesium.** Good sources include legumes, nuts, sunflower seeds, green vegetables, avocados, and amaranth.

## SAMPLE MEAL PLAN

**Breakfast:** 1 cup of whole grain amaranth flakes (dry cereal) with 1 cup of skim milk, ¼ cup of fresh berries, and 2 tsp of ground flaxseed

**Lunch:** *Crab and Avocado Salad* (page 167); 1 oz of sweet potato chips

**Snack:** 1 hard-cooked egg; a small handful of roasted sunflower seeds

**Dinner:** *Thai Roasted Shrimp* (page 211) served over ½ cup of cooked brown rice and 1 cup of lightly steamed watercress

**Dessert:** a couple slices of kiwi and cubed cantaloupe stirred into ½ cup of 2% Greek yogurt

## OTHER RECIPES TO TRY

- Fish Tacos
- Watermelon and Feta Salad
- Grilled Salmon with Sautéed Greens
- Cod with Gremolata Crust
- Shrimp Seviche with Avocado and Pumpkin Seeds
- Sesame Greens and Bean Sprouts
- Whole Wheat Flaxseed Bread
- Oysters with Tomato Salsa

# CIRCULATORY DISORDERS

(Including aneurysms, intermittent claudication, phlebitis, and Raynaud's disease)

*See also* Atherosclerosis, page 285; Blood Pressure, page 287

## FOODS THAT HEAL

**Citrus fruits**
**Onions**
**Garlic**
**Salmon**
**Sardines**

## FOODS TO LIMIT

**Fried foods**
**Salty foods, such as pickles**

## HOW TO EAT

There are no specific dietary treatments for circulatory disorders. However, these suggestions may help prevent or manage some conditions.

**Adopt a low-fat, low-salt diet.** Aim for less than 30% of calories from fat and under 2,000 mg of sodium.

**Add more fish.** Eat at least 2 servings a week of fatty fish or other sources of omega-3 fatty acids.

**Get your vitamin E.** Good sources include sunflower seeds, almonds, wheat germ, and sunflower and safflower oils.

## SAMPLE MEAL PLAN

**Breakfast:** *Tropical Fruit Salad* (page 269); 1 multigrain bagel, toasted, with 2 Tbsp of trans fat free soft spread

**Lunch:** 6 oz-serving of vegetable lasagna; 1 cup of mixed green salad with grated carrots, sliced cucumbers, and 2 Tbsp of low-fat dressing

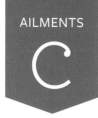
**Snack:** 1 oz of almonds or roasted sunflower seeds, unsalted

**Dinner:** 3 oz of baked salmon; *Roasted Tomatoes with Garlic and Herbs* (page 000); 3 baked red-skinned potatoes; ½ cup of steamed broccoli florets

**Dessert:** 2 tangerines

### OTHER RECIPES TO TRY

- Turkey, Spinach and Rice in Roasted Garlic Broth
- Grilled Salmon Salad
- Broiled Salmon with Avocado-Mango Salsa
- Grilled Salmon with Sautéed Greens
- Orange Beets

# CIRRHOSIS

### FOODS THAT HARM

Salty foods, such as pickles

Alcohol

### FOODS THAT HEAL

Berries

Papayas

Bell peppers

Fortified and enriched cereals and breads

Soy products (except soy sauce)

Peas

Legumes

Fish

Water

### FOODS TO LIMIT

Fatty foods

### HOW TO EAT

A healthy, low-sodium diet can help to slow the progression of the disease. Here are more diet suggestions that can help.

**Eat small, frequent meals** or snacks to combat appetite loss.

**Up your protein.** People with cirrhosis need more protein—a recommended 0.54 g per pound (1.2 g per kg) of body weight. Include vegetable proteins like soy, peas, and legumes.

**Have healthy fats.** Moderate amounts of mono- and polyunsaturated fats (oily fish, olive oil, safflower oil) provide needed calories without overburdening the liver.

### SAMPLE MEAL PLAN

**Mini Breakfast:** 2 slices of french toast made with enriched low-sodium bread and drizzled with 2 Tbsp of syrup

**A.M. Mini Meal:** ½ cup of cottage cheese mixed with ¼ cup of berries or sliced papaya

**Mini Lunch:** *Couscous-Stuffed Peppers* (page 158); 1 slice of enriched low-sodium bread

**P.M. Mini Meal:** 1 cup of low-sodium bean soup; 4 low-sodium crackers

**Mini Dinner:** 2 oz of baked skinless chicken breast; 2 small roasted red potatoes; at least ½ cup of cooked peas and carrots

**Dessert:** 1 cup of fresh strawberries dipped in ½ cup of soy yogurt

### OTHER RECIPES TO TRY

- Multigrain Pancakes or Waffles
- Jamaican Jerked Chicken Salad
- Papaya and Avocado Salad

- Whole Wheat Noodles with Peanut Sauce and Chicken
- Carrot-Flecked Corn Bread

# COLD SORES

*See* Herpes, page 315

# COLDS AND FLU

## FOODS THAT HEAL

Citrus fruits
Berries
Brussels sprouts
Chicken soup and other broths
Yogurt
Wheat germ and wheat bran

### HOW TO EAT

You won't cure a cold or flu by eating certain foods, but there are some nutrients to focus on that may protect you from getting sick—or if you do, they may ease symptoms and speed your recovery.

**Get your vitamin C.** Besides citrus, other good sources are peppers, kiwi, broccoli, brussels sprouts, cantaloupe, and tomato juice.

**Drink lots of fluids.** A minimum of eight to 10 glasses of fluids, such as water, tea, and broth, are recommended daily.

**Abstain from alcohol** to keep your immune system on its toes.

**Spice up your meals** with capsaicin, hot peppers, chiles, garlic, and turmeric.

**Eat foods rich in zinc.** You'll find this immune booster in seafood (especially oysters), red meat and poultry, yogurt and other dairy products, wheat germ, wheat bran, and whole grains.

### SAMPLE MEAL PLAN

**Breakfast:** 1 poached egg; 1 slice of whole wheat toast; *Carrot-Orange Juice* (page 000); if you're still hungry, add ½ cup of yogurt with berries and 1 tsp of wheat germ

**Lunch:** *Quick Chicken Noodle Soup* (page 136); 6 whole wheat crackers; if you feel hungry, try ½ roasted turkey sandwich on whole wheat bread and a little cranberry relish

**Snack:** fruit juice, vegetable juice, a banana, applesauce, tea, toast, peanut butter crackers, an orange, or pudding (optional if you are hungry)

**Dinner:** As you start to feel better and your appetite picks up, add more variety to your meal plan such as 2 oz of baked fish or chicken, ½ cup of soft cooked whole grains, and ½ cup of cooked vegetables

**Dessert:** a cup of herbal tea

### OTHER RECIPES TO TRY

- Blueberry and Cranberry Granola
- Berry Salad with Passion Fruit
- Wheat Germ Smoothie
- Chicken-Kale Soup with Roasted Pepper Puree
- Cantaloupe and Orange Soup
- Chicken Salad with Citrus
- Fruity Brussels Sprouts

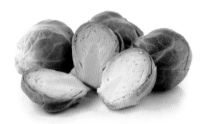

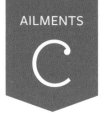

# CONSTIPATION

## FOODS THAT HEAL

Bran cereals

Beans

Legumes

Berries

Water

## HOW TO EAT

Your diet can contribute to constipation, or it can relieve it. Here are suggestions for what to eat to get and keep things moving.

**Get 25 to 38 g of fiber daily.** To do that, eat more whole grain products, legumes, fruits, and vegetables. See the Sample Meal Plan below, which reflects a fiber intake that's within this goal. Gradually increase fiber intake until you reach this goal.

**Down the H$_2$O.** Aim for 8 glasses of nonalcoholic fluids every day.

**Avoid alcohol.** It can cause dehydration and prevents the body from properly absorbing nutrients.

**Drink hot liquids.** Try herbal tea, a glass of hot water with lemon, or coffee in the morning.

## SAMPLE MEAL PLAN

**Breakfast:** ½ cup of hot oat bran cereal prepared with skim milk; 1 tangerine

**Lunch:** *Black Bean and Sweet Potato Burritos* (page 211)

**Snack:** 1 container low-fat vanilla yogurt with ¼ cup of berries

**Dinner:** 3 oz of grilled halibut; *Tuscan Bean Soup* (page 141); ½ cup of cooked brown rice; at least ½ cup of steamed vegetables (or if you prefer, have 1 cup of mixed green salad and 2 Tbsp of low-fat dressing)

**Dessert:** 1 frozen fruit sorbet bar

## OTHER RECIPES TO TRY

- Hot Cereal with Apples and Dates
- Blueberry-Oatmeal Muffins
- Lentil Soup with Canadian Bacon
- Three-Bean Chili
- Lentil and Rice Paella with Clams
- Artichokes with Lentils and Lima Beans
- Edamame Hummus with Pita Crisps

# CROHN'S DISEASE

*See* Inflammatory Bowel Disease, page 320

# CYSTIC FIBROSIS

## FOODS THAT HEAL

Meat

Poultry

Eggs

Milk and yogurt

Pasta

Cookies

Cakes

Salty foods

Juices

## HOW TO EAT

While there isn't a special diet to treat cystic fibrosis, eating certain foods can have an effect on managing the disease. Here are some general guidelines, but it's also important to consult with a dietitian.

**Eat larger portions** and lots of snacks.

**Eat more protein.** Along with sources listed at left, enrich whole milk by adding 1 cup of dried milk per quart or liter.

**Combine sugary foods with protein,** such as peanut butter and jelly, milk-shakes, or trail mix.

**Consume more sodium,** especially during hot weather or exercise.

**Stay hydrated.** In addition to high-calorie juices and nectars, sip water to help prevent constipation.

## SAMPLE MEAL PLAN

**Breakfast:** *Huevos Rancheros* (page 124); a glass of whole milk, or coffee or tea with half-and half

**Snack:** cheese and crackers or peanut butter crackers; 1 cup of fruit juice

**Lunch:** *Shrimp and Vegetable Stir-Fry* (page 209); a bowl of cream soup such as cream of broccoli, cream of potato soup, or New England clam chowder; 1 roll with 2 tsp of butter

**Snack:** a milkshake: blend ½ cup of whole milk, ½ cup of half and half, 2 cups of vanilla ice cream, 2 Tbsp of malt powder, and an envelope of instant breakfast powder (any flavor)

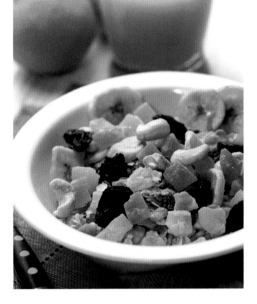

**Dinner:** 3 to 4 oz of baked salmon or 2 pieces of fried chicken; *Baked Rice with Wild Mushrooms and Cheese* (page 221); steamed broccoli with ¼ cup of cheese sauce

**Dessert:** strawberry shortcake topped with fresh strawberries and lots of whipped cream

**Snack:** *Walnut Shortbread* (page 254); ½ cup of pudding

## OTHER RECIPES TO TRY

- Hot Cereal with Apples and Dates
- Zucchini-Carrot Crustless Quiche Squares
- Shrimp Seviche with Avocado and Pumpkin Seeds
- Thai Roasted Shrimp
- Macaroni and Cheese with Spinach
- Pasta with Walnut Cream Sauce
- Fried Rice with Tofu and Vegetables
- Buffalo Chicken Fingers

## QUICK TIP:
### Bump up the calories

Add shredded cheese or butter to soups, sauces, casseroles, vegetables, mashed potatoes, rice, noodles or meat loaf. For heartier entrées, bread meat, poultry, and fish before frying or broiling it.

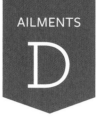

# D DENTAL PROBLEMS

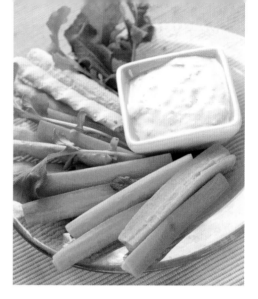

### FOODS THAT HARM

Starchy snacks and sugary foods, such as sweetened cereals and cookies

Acidic drinks sipped over prolonged periods of time, such as wine or unsweetened fruit juice

### FOODS THAT HEAL

Low-fat dairy products

Aged cheeses

Fortified soy beverages

Eggs

Legumes

Carrots

Sweet potatoes

Broccoli

Oranges

Dark leafy green vegetables, especially spinach

Apples

Celery

Yogurt

Rice

### FOODS TO LIMIT

Dried fruit and other sticky foods

### HOW TO EAT

Calcium is important for your teeth and gums, so a diet high in calcium is essential. Here are more eating tips for your teeth.

**Finish a meal with aged cheese.** It helps prevent cavities. Other postmeal teeth protectors are fresh fruit such as apples, carrots, and celery.

**Chew gum with xylitol.** It helps counter harmful bacteria if you chew it for at least 5 minutes right after a meal.

### SAMPLE MEAL PLAN

**Breakfast:** 1 sunny-side up egg; 1 slice of whole grain toast; ½ cup of fresh fruit

**Lunch:** cheese sandwich made with 2 slices of whole grain bread, 2 oz of low-fat colby cheese, sliced tomato, lettuce, mustard, and 1 Tbsp of your favorite spread; a cup of bean soup; 1 orange

**Snack:** ½ cup of raw vegetables dipped in ¼ cup of low-fat dressing—try a mix of baby carrots, celery sticks, and broccoli florets.

**Dinner:** *Savory Lamb Stew with Sweet Potatoes* (page 133); at least ½ cup of cooked spinach; 1 whole grain roll

**Dessert:** ½ cup vanilla yogurt with ¼ cup chopped apples

### OTHER RECIPES TO TRY

- Carrot Soup with Dill
- Broccoli Salad with Almonds and Dried Cranberries
- Spinach, Sweet Potato, and Shiitake Salad
- Calf's Liver with Rigatoni
- Carrot and Parsnip Puree

# DEPRESSION

## FOODS THAT HARM

Aged cheeses and other foods and drinks that contain tyramine, if you are taking MAO inhibitors

## FOODS THAT HEAL

Turkey

Almonds and other nuts

Pumpkin seeds and other seeds

Watercress and other green leafy vegetables

Lentils and other beans

Whole grains

Corn

Asparagus

Peas

## FOODS TO LIMIT

Sugary foods, such as cookies and soft drinks

## HOW TO EAT

The right foods can help to stabilize your mood. For example, carbohydrates can have a calming, relaxing effect. Here's how to eat to beat depression.

**Combine tryptophan with carbs.** This serotonin booster is found in turkey, almonds, and pumpkin seeds. Eating them with carbs like beans and whole grains helps to convert the tryptophan into serotonin.

**Get your B vitamins.** In addition to the healing foods listed above, good sources are meat, fish, poultry, potatoes, orange juice, and fortified soy and rice beverages.

**Add omega-3 fats.** Seek sources such as salmon, trout, mackerel, and flaxseed.

**Eat a small piece of dark chocolate occasionally.** The naturally occurring substance in chocolate called phenylethylamine (PEA) has been found to elevate endorphin levels and act as a natural antidepressant. Just don't go overboard.

## SAMPLE MEAL PLAN

**Breakfast:** ½ cup of fruit and nut whole grain cereal with 1 cup of skim milk; 2 Tbsp of roasted pumpkin seeds

**Lunch:** 3 oz of baked salmon; *Endive, Apple, and Watercress Salad* (page 177); ½ cup cooked basmati or wild rice blend

**Snack:** bowl of lentil, split pea, or low-fat cream of asparagus soup; 1 crusty whole grain roll; 1 orange

**Dinner:** 3 oz of roasted turkey breast; baked sweet potato; ½ cup of corn; 1 cup of steamed collards or kale

**Dessert:** small piece of dark chocolate

## OTHER RECIPES TO TRY

- Three-Bean Chili
- Pork, Pear, and Potato Salad
- Bulgur with Spring Vegetables
- Brown Rice with Cabbage and Chickpeas
- Spiced Cauliflower with Peas
- Edamame Hummus with Pita Crisps

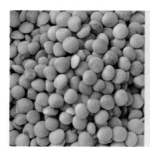

**QUICK TIP: Eat more beans**

They're a rich source of carbohydrates, which have been associated with relaxation. Beans also help convert tryptophan into serotonin, a feel-good hormone.

## WARNING! FOOD-DRUG INTERACTION

If you are taking an antidepressant in the class called monoamine oxidase (MAO) inhibitors, such as phenelzine (Nardil) and tranylcypromine (Parnate), your blood pressure could rise dangerously when you eat foods rich in the amino acid tyramine. Tyramines are found in protein-rich foods that have been aged, dried, fermented, pickled, or bacterially treated—such as aged cheeses, tofu or soy, and alcohol.

# DIABETES

### FOODS THAT HARM

- Red meat, butter, and other foods with saturated fats
- Processed foods that contain trans fats

### FOODS THAT HEAL

- Whole grain breads, cereals, and pasta
- Oats
- Barley
- Peas
- Low-fat dairy products
- Avocados
- Apples
- Pears
- Oranges
- Chicken breast
- Mushrooms

### FOODS TO LIMIT

- High glycemic foods such as potatoes, soft drinks, white flour, and refined sugars

### HOW TO EAT

Diet is the cornerstone of diabetes management, and it can help you avoid developing diabetes in the first place. Here are some guidelines.

**Balance, balance, balance.** Meals and snacks should provide a mixture of carbohydrates, fats, and proteins.

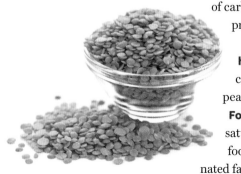

**Seek fiber-rich carbohydrates** like barley, oat cereals, oatmeal, beans, peas, and lentils.

**Follow a low-fat diet.** Limit saturated fats from animal foods and avoid hydrogenated fats in packaged foods.

Monounsaturated and polyunsaturated fats—vegetable oils, nuts, fish, and avocados—are good in moderation.

**Eat foods low on the glycemic index (GI).** This index (see page 354) is a measure of how quickly foods are broken down into glucose. The faster a food is digested and absorbed into the bloodstream, the higher its GI. High-GI foods cause a rapid rise in blood sugar, which can be dangerous, especially for people with diabetes. People who have diets with lot of high-GI foods have higher rates of obesity, diabetes, heart disease, and cancer.

**Get enough chromium,** found in foods such as wheat bran, whole grains, chicken breast, mushrooms, and blackstrap molasses. Aim for 50 to 200 mg a day.

**Drink coffee.** Studies suggest that the caffeinated variety may reduce your risk of developing type 2 diabetes.

**Keep carbs steady throughout the day.** In order to avoid swings in blood sugar levels, don't go more than 3 or 4 hours without eating something.

### SAMPLE MEAL PLAN

**Breakfast:** *Individual Breakfast Tortilla* (page 125); ½ cup of low-fat cottage cheese with ¼ cup of fresh red or black raspberries

**Snack:** 1 plum; a small handful of nuts

**Lunch:** *Whole Wheat Noodles with Peanut Sauce and Chicken* (page 196); ½ cup of cooked carrots and peas

**Snack:** ½ whole wheat pita with 2 Tbsp hummus or guacamole dip

**Dinner:** *Spinach-Stuffed Meat Loaf* (page 183); a cup of barley-mushroom soup; 3 roasted new potatoes; 1 cup of mixed green salad with 2 Tbsp low-fat dressing

**Evening snack:** 1 apple, sliced with 2 tsp of peanut butter

## OTHER RECIPES TO TRY

- Blueberry Oatmeal Muffins
- Barley and Beet Salad
- Wheat Berry Salad with Dried Apricots
- Buckwheat Noodles with Tofu and Green Vegetables
- White Beans Stewed with Swiss Chard
- Vegetable-Stuffed Mushrooms

# DIARRHEA

## FOODS THAT HEAL

Water
Herbal teas
Ginger ale
Broth
Bananas
Rice
Applesauce
Toast
Salted crackers
Chicken soup

## FOODS TO LIMIT

Dairy products
Apple juice
Prunes
Sugarless chewing gum

## HOW TO EAT

When diarrhea starts up, stop eating solid food and focus on rehydrating. Sip warm or tepid drinks. Drink half a cup of fluid—water, mineral water, herbal teas, clear broths, or ginger ale—every 15 minutes. As you start to feel better, you can reintroduce solid foods by following the tips below.

Repeat a meal plan like the one below for 1 or 2 days. Once symptoms start to taper off more completely, try additional foods such as gelatin, cooked oatmeal, cream of wheat, cooked eggs, plain cooked pasta, or skinless baked potatoes. If symptoms last longer than 1 or 2 days, consult your doctor. Note that this diet is designed for adults and children over age 3. Please consult your doctor for recommendations for infants.

**Slowly introduce low-fiber foods.** When you feel like eating (but preferably not within the first 24 hours), try crackers, toast, rice, bananas, cooked carrots, boiled potatoes, applesauce, or chicken. See the meal plan below for suggestions.

**Keep food as bland as possible.** It's easier on the GI system.

**Choose flat soda,** if you're drinking clear carbonated beverages such as ginger ale or 7Up. If you have diabetes, opt for diet soda.

## SAMPLE MEAL PLAN

**Breakfast:** banana; cream of rice cereal; applesauce; toast; broth or tea

**Lunch:** a bowl of chicken soup; soft cooked grains; soft noodles; cooked carrots; lightly buttered toast or saltines

**Dinner:** a bowl of chicken noodle or rice soup; boiled potatoes; soft cooked grains; soft cooked vegetables; stewed chicken; applesauce; banana; tea or ginger ale

## OTHER RECIPES TO TRY

- Basic Chicken Stock
- Electrolyte Drink

# DIVERTICU-LITIS

## FOODS THAT HEAL

Berries

Bananas

Figs

Bran

Brown rice

Black beans

Split peas

Artichokes

Water

Broth

## HOW TO EAT

Diets lacking in dietary fiber can lead to the formation of diverticula, small pouches in the intestinal wall. This condition is called diverticulosis. When the diverticula become inflamed or infected, you have diverticulitis. A bout of acute diverticulitis can be extremely painful. In severe and acute cases, your doctor may need to hospitalize you and your diet may be temporarily modified to a liquid diet until the inflammation has subsided. When you resume eating after an acute bout of diverticulitis, your doctor may temporarily prescribe lower fiber before advancing you to a higher fiber diet. To prevent or delay diverticulosis or diverticulitis, eat a high-fiber diet such as the one below.

**Eat more vegetables and whole grains.** Raw fruits and vegetables, especially with the skin on, are particularly good.

**Drink fluids.** At least eight glasses a day of water, tea, or other clear liquids will help prevent constipation while you add fiber.

## SAMPLE MEAL PLAN

**Breakfast:** 1 cup of cooked oat bran cereal prepared with skim milk; ½ cup of blueberries or sliced strawberries

**Lunch:** chicken salad wrap made with a whole wheat tortilla, lettuce, grated carrots, and tomato; 1 cup of black bean soup

**Snack:** ½ cup of low-fat yogurt; 1 banana

**Dinner:** 3 oz of baked fish, *Baked Rice with Wild Mushrooms and Cheese* (page 221); 1 cup vegetable medley with steamed broccoli, cauliflower, and carrots

**Dessert:** 3 dried figs

## OTHER RECIPES TO TRY

- Hot Cereal with Apples and Dates
- Blueberry-Oatmeal Muffins
- Three-Bean Chili
- Black Bean and Sweet Potato Burritos
- Brown Rice with Cabbage and Chickpeas
- Rice Salad with Chicken and Grapes
- Chewy Oatmeal Raisin Cookies

# ECZEMA

## FOODS THAT HARM

Milk, eggs, nuts, or any other foods that trigger or worsen eczema

## FOODS THAT HEAL

Apricots

Carrots

Mangoes

Bananas

Squash

Green leafy vegetables

Legumes

Salmon

Flaxseed

Canola oil

Brown rice

Wheat germ

## HOW TO EAT

The trick is to avoid foods that may trigger eczema and to fill up on those that may help alleviate it. Here are some guidelines.

**Test for allergies.** Common culprits include eggs, dairy products, seafood, walnuts, and pecans.

**Consume more antioxidants.** Brightly colored fruits and vegetables like apricots, squash, mangoes, carrots, pumpkin, and sweet potatoes may prevent breakouts by countering the formation of free radicals.

**Eat foods rich in essential fatty acids (EFAs),** such as vegetable oils, fatty fish, and flaxseed to decrease swelling.

**Get lots of vitamin B6 to protect against sensitivity rashes.** Good sources include lean meat, fish, poultry, legumes, brown rice, wheat germ, avocado, banana, potato, and leafy green vegetables.

**Drink 3 cups of oolong tea.** Polyphenols in the tea suppress allergic responses.

## SAMPLE MEAL PLAN

**Breakfast:** 1 cup of whole grain cereal with 1 cup of soy or almond milk and 2 Tbsp of toasted wheat germ; 1 banana; a cup of oolong tea

**Lunch:** *Fruit Salad with Spiced Coconut* (page 176); 1 whole wheat soft bread stick; a cup of oolong tea

**Snack:** 1 oz of carrot chips; 3 pieces of dried mango

**Dinner:** *Grilled Salmon with Sautéed Greens* (page 200); ½ cup of cooked brown rice; ½ of a baked acorn squash

**Dessert:** a cup of oolong tea

## OTHER RECIPES TO TRY

- Ginger Butternut Squash Soup
- Grilled Salmon Salad
- Lentil and Rice Paella with Clams
- Rice-Stuffed Squash
- Sesame Greens and Bean Sprouts

# EMPHYSEMA

*See* Respiratory Disorders, page 345

# EYE PROBLEMS

## FOODS THAT HARM

Red meat, butter, and other foods with saturated fats

## FOODS THAT HEAL

Carrots

Corn

Red bell peppers

Dark leafy greens like kale or collard greens

Fish

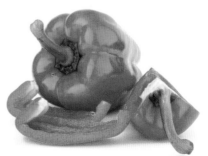

## HOW TO EAT

You can protect yourself against age-related eye problems such as cataracts and macular degeneration, which can both lead to blindness, by following these tips.

**Start your day with fruit.** Add a vision-saving burst of antioxidants to your morning meal with a glass of orange or tomato juice, grapefruit, kiwi, strawberries, or cantaloupe.

**Eat a variety of veggies.** While carrots are good for your eyes and you should eat them, dark leafy greens, corn, and red peppers actually have more peeper-protecting antioxidants.

**Maintain a healthy weight.** Excess pounds may increase your risk for cataracts.

**Eat fish at least twice a week.** Studies show that it can protect against macular degeneration.

**Cut back on saturated fats.** These artery-clogging fats may contribute to problems by blocking arteries in the retina.

## SAMPLE MEAL PLAN

**Breakfast:** 1 cup of whole grain cereal with ½ cup of skim milk and ½ cup of sliced strawberries; 1 cup of orange juice

**Lunch:** *Grilled Eggplant Sandwiches with Red-Pepper-Walnut Sauce* (page 156)

**Snack:** ½ cup of roasted red bell pepper, carrots, and 4 olives dipped in ¼ cup of hummus

**Dinner:** 3 oz of baked salmon with 2 Tbsp of fruit chutney; *Spinach Salad with Chickpeas* (page 173); 1 piece of corn bread

**Dessert:** 2 cups of cubed cantaloupe

## OTHER RECIPES TO TRY

- Chicken-Kale Soup with Roasted Pepper Puree
- Tuna and Carrot Sandwiches on Rye
- Grilled Salmon with Sautéed Greens
- Mackerel Tandoori Style
- Snapper and Snaps in a Packet
- White Beans Stewed with Swiss Chard

# FEVER

## FOODS THAT HEAL

Water
Fruit juice
Chicken broth or soup
Herbal teas
Bananas
Rice
Applesauce
Toast
Eggs
Rice cereals

## HOW TO EAT

A fever is one of the body's natural ways of fighting disease and should not be suppressed unless very high or accompanied by other symptoms. The following tips will help you feel better while you have a fever.

**Don't starve.** The old adage "Feed a cold, starve a fever" has no medical basis. If anything, you need more calories than normal because your metabolic rate rises when you have a fever.

**Load up on liquids.** Sip often on water, fruit juice, herbal teas, broth, soup, or even frozen fruit juice bars.

**Try the BRAT diet.** Eat bananas, rice, applesauce, and toast for fever-related diarrhea. Also good: chicken or beef broth, chicken-rice soup, rice cereals, and boiled or poached eggs. See Diarrhea, page 303.

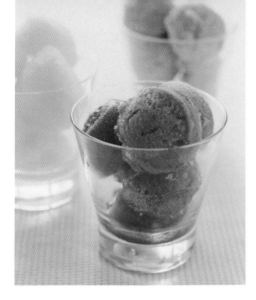

## SAMPLE MEAL PLAN

**Breakfast:** 1 slice of toast with 1 tsp trans fat free soft spread; 1 scrambled egg; 1 piece of fruit; a cup of fruit juice or tea

**Lunch:** 1 cup of soup or broth; 1 cup of spaghetti with plain marinara sauce; 1 slice of bread; a cup of fruit juice or tea

**Snack:** ½ cup of cottage cheese with ¼ cup of sliced fruit

**Dinner:** 2 oz cooked lean beef or poultry; 1 cup of chicken rice soup; ½ cup of mashed potatoes; ½ cup of cooked carrots and greens

**Dessert:** frozen fruit sorbet bar or ½ cup of sherbet

## OTHER RECIPES TO TRY

- One-Egg Omelets with Chopped Broccoli, Tomatoes, and Cheddar
- Basic Chicken Stock
- Quick Chicken Noodle Soup
- Vegetable Stock
- Miso Soup with Tofu
- Cantaloupe and Orange Soup
- Carrot-Orange Juice
- Chai

# FIBROIDS

### FOODS THAT HARM
Beer

### FOODS THAT HEAL
Dairy products
Broccoli
Spinach
Swiss chard
Brussels sprouts
Oranges

### FOODS TO LIMIT
Breads, pasta, and other foods made with white flour

## HOW TO EAT

Hormones are likely to play a role in the development of fibroids, and your diet can affect hormone levels. Here's how to eat to reduce your risk and minimize the impact of fibroids if you have them.

**Cut carbs,** especially refined white flour ones. The blood sugar spikes they cause over time may affect hormone levels that can fuel the development of fibroids.

**Get milk** and other dairy products to lower your risk of fibroids.

**Gobble oranges.** In one study, they protected women. However, OJ didn't have the same effect.

**Graze on green veggies.** Eating more than a serving a day may slash your risk by up to 50%.

**Watch calories.** Being overweight increases your risk of fibroids.

## SAMPLE MEAL PLAN

**Breakfast:** 1 whole grain English muffin, toasted, with 2 tsp of fruit spread; ½ cup of low-fat cottage cheese mixed with a couple of mandarin oranges

**Lunch:** a cup of low-fat cream of broccoli soup; 3 oz of roasted chicken or turkey; 1 baked potato topped with 1 Tbsp reduced-fat sour cream; 1 cup of cooked spinach

**Snack:** apple slices; 1 piece of string cheese

**Dinner:** 3 oz of roasted pork loin; *Fruity Brussels Sprouts* (page 228); ½ cup of baked squash (acorn, butternut, or buttercup); 1 whole grain roll

**Dessert:** ½ cup 2% Greek yogurt

### OTHER RECIPES TO TRY

- Endive, Apple, and Watercress Salad
- Sesame Greens and Bean Sprouts
- Orange-Walnut Broccoli
- Brussels Sprouts with Caraway Seeds
- Cauliflower and Spinach Casserole
- White Beans Stewed with Swiss Chard
- Carrot-Orange Juice

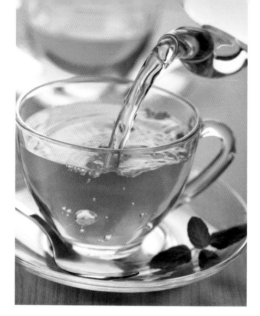

# FLATULENCE

### FOODS THAT HARM

Carbonated drinks

Chewing gum

Bran

Milk, for those who are lactose
  intolerant

### FOODS THAT HEAL

Peppermint, chamomile, fennel,
  or ginger tea

Yogurt

Anise

Rosemary

Bay leaf

Kombu seaweed

### FOODS TO LIMIT

Kidney beans and other dried beans

Brussels sprouts

Onions

Corn

Asparagus

Sorbitol

### HOW TO EAT

Unfortunately, flatulence can be an unpleasant side effect of eating a healthier, high-fiber diet. Passing gas also seems to worsen with age. Here are some dietary changes that may help:

**Gulp less air when eating.** Eating smaller portions, chewing food thoroughly, and not gulping liquids can help minimize episodes.

**Drink herbal tea after meals.** It helps improve digestion.

**Try yogurt with live cultures.** It may help cut gas production.

**Soak dried beans first.** Aim for at least 4 hours (preferably 8 or more) to reduce the amount of gas they may produce.

**Spice up gas producers.** You may be able to reduce gas by adding anise, ginger, rosemary, bay leaves, and fennel seeds to cruciferous veggies like broccoli and cauliflower and other veggies that tend to cause

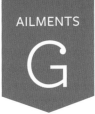
gas. Add kombu seaweed to cooking water (find it in Asian markets and natural food stores) for the same purpose.

**Stay away from artificial sweeteners,** such as sorbitol.

## SAMPLE MEAL PLAN

**Breakfast:** 2 pancakes with 2 tsp of maple syrup; ¼ cup of sliced fresh fruit; 1 slice of turkey bacon; a cup of peppermint tea

**Snack:** low-fat yogurt (choose a brand with live cultures, probiotics); ¼ cup of sliced fruit

**Lunch:** *Tuna and Cannellini Salad with Lemon* (page 165); 1 slice whole wheat crusty bread; an orange.

**Snack:** ½ cup of kefir

**Dinner:** beef stew (made with lean meat, potatoes, carrots, broth, and simple seasonings such as rosemary, thyme, and bay leaf); 1 whole grain roll; applesauce

**Dessert:** cup of chamomile, ginger, or fennel tea

## OTHER RECIPES TO TRY

- Strawberry-Yogurt Smoothie
- Three-Berry Fool
- Mixed Berry and Stone Fruit Soup

# FOOD POISONING

*See* Diarrhea, page 303

# GALLSTONES

### FOODS THAT HEAL

Tomatoes
Salmon
Brown rice
Whole wheat bread
Barley
Avocado
Olive oil
Walnuts
Flaxseeds

### FOODS TO LIMIT

Red meat, butter, and foods with saturated fat
Processed foods that contain trans fats
Sugary foods, such as cookies and soft drinks

## HOW TO EAT

Consistently following a low-fat diet can help prevent gallstones or minimize symptoms if you already have them. Here are more tips that can help.

**Always eat breakfast.** A substantial breakfast causes the gallbladder to empty itself and flush out any small stones and stagnant bile.

**Consume small, frequent meals.** They help to spur the gallbladder to empty stones and bile.

**Avoid extreme dieting.** Bile is more likely to form stones after fasting.

## SAMPLE MEAL PLAN

**Mini Breakfast:** 1 cup of bran flakes with ½ cup of skim milk, 2 tsp of flaxseeds, and ¼ cup of sliced peaches

**A.M. Mini Meal:** ½ whole wheat bagel with 1 tsp of trans fat free soft spread

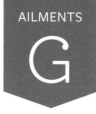
**Mini Lunch:** veggie burger on whole wheat bun with lettuce, tomato, avocado, and sprouts; *Brown Rice with Cabbage and Chickpeas* (page 222)

**P.M. Mini Meal:** 1 cup of barley-mushroom soup; 2 whole grain crackers

**Mini Dinner:** 3 oz of baked or grilled salmon; ½ cup of cooked brown rice or barley; a small mixed green salad with sliced cucumbers, tomatoes, grated carrots, and 2 Tbsp of low-fat dressing

**Dessert:** ½ cup of fresh fruit salad topped with 6 walnuts

### OTHER RECIPES TO TRY

- Barley and Beet Salad
- Papaya and Avocado Salad
- Broiled Salmon with Avocado-Mango Salsa Whole Wheat Flaxseed Bread
- Grilled Salmon with Sautéed Greens
- Salmon and Asparagus Farfalle with Walnut-Feta Sauce
- Rice-Stuffed Squash
- Roasted Tomatoes with Garlic and Herbs

# GASTRITIS

*See* Indigestion and Heartburn, page 318

# GASTROEN-TERITIS

*See* Diarrhea, page 303

# GASTRO-ESOPHAGEAL REFLUX (GERD)

*See* Indigestion and Heartburn, page 318

# GOUT

### FOODS THAT HARM

Organ meats

Game meats

Anchovies

Sardines

Herring

### FOODS THAT HEAL

Water

Fruit juice

Herbal teas

Vegetable broth

Soy products

### FOODS TO LIMIT

Cauliflower

Asparagus

Dried beans and peas

Oats

Whole grain cereals

Wheat germ and wheat bran

Mushrooms

Poultry

Alcohol

### HOW TO EAT

Gout is a type of arthritis that is caused by an inherited defect in the kidney's ability to excrete uric acid. You can reduce your production of uric acid and enhance the beneficial effect of drug treatment with these dietary guidelines.

**Limit meat, fish, and poultry to 4 to 6 oz (125 to 175 g) a day.** Animal proteins are high in purines that promote the overproduction of uric acid.

**Get your protein from plants,** such as soy.

**Chug at least 2 qt (2 L) of liquids daily.** It helps to dilute urine.

**Pass on alcohol.** It interferes with the elimination of uric acid.

**Avoid low-carb diets.** They encourage the formation of ketones, metabolic by-products that hamper the body's ability to excrete uric acid.

**Don't skip meals or fast.** Both, along with rapid weight loss, can raise blood levels of uric acid.

## SAMPLE MEAL PLAN

**Breakfast:** 1 cup of cornflakes with ½ cup of soymilk and ¼ cup sliced strawberries; a cup of fruit juice such as apple, cranberry, orange, or black cherry

**Lunch:** *Miso Soup with Tofu* (page 140); 1 slice of sourdough bread; 8 oz of water

**Snack:** 4 whole grain crackers with 2 tsp of soy nut butter; ½ cup of fruit juice

**Dinner:** 3 oz of cheese lasagna; 2 cups of mixed green salad and chopped fresh vegetables drizzled with 2 Tbsp of low-fat dressing; 1 small dinner roll; 8 oz of water

**Dessert:** ½ cup of fruited gelatin or ½ cup of Italian ice

## OTHER RECIPES TO TRY

- Vegetable Stock
- Cantaloupe and Orange Soup
- Romaine Lettuce with Chunky Tomato Vinaigrette
- Carrot-Orange Juice

# HALITOSIS

**FOODS THAT HARM**
- Garlic
- Onions

**FOODS THAT HEAL**
- Water
- Red bell pepper
- Broccoli
- Fennel seeds
- Chewing gum with xylitol

## HOW TO EAT

Your food choices have a big impact on your breath. Here's how to keep it fresh.

**Drink plenty of water.** Have a glass at the end of every meal or snack.

**Make gum your aperitif.** Sugar-free gum sweetened with xylitol helps cleanse the breath and curbs bacteria growth. Chew for at least 5 minutes for best results.

**Reach for raw veggies.** They help remove food particles stuck between teeth. And those rich in vitamin C, like broccoli and red bell peppers, create an unfriendly environment for bacteria.

**Chew a few fennel seeds** after mealtime to freshen your breath.

## SAMPLE MEAL PLAN

**Breakfast:** 1 cup of low-fat yogurt mixed with ¼ cup of granola; ½ cup of sliced fresh fruit

**Lunch:** 3 oz of lean roasted pork; a baked sweet potato with 1 tsp of brown sugar; 2 cups of mixed green salad with chopped fresh vegetables and 2 Tbsp low-fat dressing

**Snack:** raw veggies such as carrots and red pepper strips dipped in low-fat dressing

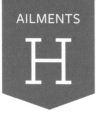
**Dinner:** 3 oz of roasted lean meat, fish, or poultry; *Broccoli Salad with Almonds and Dried Cranberries* (page 175); ½ cup of brown rice pilaf; 1 whole grain roll

**Dessert:** 1 cup of fresh fruit cocktail, canned in its own juice

## OTHER RECIPES TO TRY

- Mushroom and Bell Pepper Frittata
- Asian Grilled Tuna Burgers
- Asian Noodle Salad
- Orange-Walnut Broccoli
- Broccoli and Cauliflower with Cream Sauce
- Braised Carrot, Celery, and Fennel

# HAY FEVER

### FOODS THAT HARM

Artichokes

Chamomile tea

Endives

Escarole

Tarragon

Beer and wine

Sourdough bread

Blue cheese

Dried fruit

Mushrooms

Sausages

Sauerkraut

Soy sauce

Vinegar

Honey

### FOODS THAT HEAL

Salmon

Herring

Flaxseeds

## HOW TO EAT

The best strategy is to avoid foods that may trigger a flare-up.

**Get to know the family.** If ragweed triggers symptoms, so can foods in the sunflower plant family, such as artichokes, chamomile tea, chicory, dandelions, endives, escarole, Jerusalem artichokes, salsify, safflower (found in vegetable oils and margarines), sunflower seeds and oil, and tarragon.

**If you're allergic to mold, avoid fermented foods.** These include alcoholic beverages, beer, wine, and other drinks made by fermentation; breads made with lots of yeast or sourdough varieties; cheeses, especially blue cheese; dried fruits; mushrooms; processed meats or fish, including hot dogs, sausages, and smoked fish; sauerkraut and other fermented or pickled foods, including soy sauce; and vinegar and vinegary products, such as salad dressings, mayonnaise, ketchup, and pickles.

**Watch out for honey.** It may harbor bits of pollen.

**Make friends with fatty fish** and other foods high in omega-3s like flaxseed, soybean oil, and walnuts.

## SAMPLE MEAL PLAN

**Breakfast:** *Berry-Flaxseed Smoothie* (page 131); 2 toaster waffles drizzled with 2 Tbsp of reduced-calorie syrup (stay away from honey), or topped with ½ cup fresh fruit slices

**Lunch:** a cup of bean soup; a low-fat cheese sandwich

**Snack:** 1 small banana; 6 walnuts; ½ cup of plain vanilla yogurt

**Dinner:** 3 oz grilled salmon steak topped with fresh fruit relish; baked potato with

2 Tbsp reduced-fat sour cream; ½ cup of cooked vegetables

**Dessert:** ½ cup of vanilla pudding

**OTHER RECIPES TO TRY**

- Salmon and Fennel Lettuce Wraps
- Broiled Salmon with Avocado-Mango Salsa
- Salmon and Asparagus Farfalle with Walnut-Feta Sauce
- Walnut Shortbread

# HEARTBURN

*See* Indigestion and Heartburn, page 318

# HEMORRHOIDS

**FOODS THAT HEAL**

Water
Black beans
Lima beans
Barley
Bran flakes
Raspberries
Apples
Pears
Oats
Flaxseeds

**HOW TO EAT**

These guidelines can help prevent the formation of hemorrhoids or ease some of the pain and bleeding if you have them.

**Drink lots of water** or other caffeine-free beverages. It helps to soften stools.

**Fill up on fiber.** Try to include two high-fiber servings (3 or more grams) at every meal. Good options include whole grains, popcorn, baked potato with skin, nuts, beans, fruits, and vegetables. Women need 21 to 25 g daily; men, 30 to 38 g.

**Top with flax.** Sprinkle ground flaxseeds on top of cereal, smoothies, or yogurt for more fiber.

**SAMPLE MEAL PLAN**

**Breakfast:** 1 cup of bran flakes with ½ cup of skim milk and 1 tsp of ground flaxseeds; *Pear Rhubarb Muffins* (page 128); ½ cup of fruit juice with pulp

**Lunch:** *Three-Bean Salad with Manchego Cheese* (page 174); a cup of barley soup topped with chopped scallions

**Snack:** 1 apple

**Dinner:** 3 oz of baked fish or chicken; ½ cup of mashed potatoes; at least ½ cup of succotash; 1 cup of mixed green salad with grated carrots, croutons, and 2 Tbsp of low-fat dressing

**Dessert:** ½ cup of vanilla yogurt with ½ cup of fresh raspberries

**OTHER RECIPES TO TRY**

- Hot Cereal with Apples and Dates
- Tuscan Bean Soup
- Broccoli and Pearl Barley Salad
- Black Bean and Sweet Potato Burritos
- Whole Wheat Flaxseed Bread

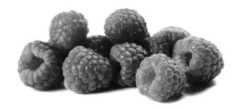

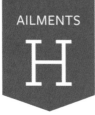
# HEPATITIS

**FOODS THAT HARM**

Alcohol

Raw shellfish

Sweets

**FOODS THAT HEAL**

Lean meat

Poultry

Fish

Eggs

Dairy

Legumes

Whole grains

**FOODS TO LIMIT**

Fried and fatty foods

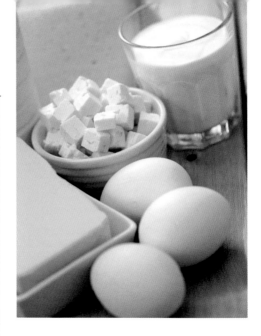

## HOW TO EAT

The following strategies can help ease symptoms of all forms of hepatitis such as appetite loss and nausea.

**Try to have breakfast.** Often, appetite decreases and nausea increases as the day progresses. Breakfast may be the best-tolerated meal.

**Graze throughout the day.** It can help encourage eating when you don't have much of an appetite.

**Get some protein at every meal.** Choose from animal and vegetable sources.

**Have a little fat.** It provides calories and adds flavor. Good sources are dairy products and eggs because they're easy to digest.

## SAMPLE MEAL PLAN

**Mini Breakfast:** 1 sunny-side up or scrambled egg; 1 slice of whole wheat toast with 1 tsp of jam; 1 banana

**A.M. Mini Meal:** ½ whole grain bagel with 2 tsp of peanut butter

**Mini Lunch:** *Pesto Chicken Spirals with Roasted Peppers* (page 246); a cup of low-sodium bean soup

**P.M. Mini Meal:** 4 oz enriched high-protein shake

**Mini Dinner:** *Cod with Gremolata Crust* (page 203); ½ cup of mashed potatoes; ½ cup of steamed broccoli, peas, or carrots; 1 small dinner roll

**Dessert:** ½ cup of frozen vanilla yogurt with 2 Tbsp of crushed peanuts and a maraschino cherry

## OTHER RECIPES TO TRY

- One-Egg Omelet with Chopped Broccoli, Tomatoes, and Cheddar
- Zucchini Frittata
- Strawberry-Yogurt Smoothie
- Cod and Vegetable Stew
- Beef, Onion, and Pepper Fajitas
- Asian Chicken Salad
- Braised Chicken with Winter Vegetables
- Turkey Bacon and Apricot Bites

# HERPES

## FOODS THAT HEAL

Lean meat

Fish

Yogurt

Milk

Whole grains

Fresh fruits and vegetables

## FOODS TO LIMIT

Alcohol

Caffeinated drinks

## HOW TO EAT

To help prevent recurrences, eat a well-balanced diet.

**Load up on lysine.** This amino acid, found in meat, fish, milk, and dairy products, may reduce the frequency of breakouts.

**Choose yogurt with live or "active" cultures.** *Lactobacillus acidophilus,* a healthy bacteria found in yogurts, may help prevent recurrences of cold sores.

## SAMPLE MEAL PLAN

**Breakfast:** 2 slices of whole grain toast with 2 tsp of trans fat free soft spread; ½ cup of low-fat cottage cheese with ½ cup sliced mangoes, peaches, or pineapple chunks

**Lunch:** *Beef in Lettuce Wraps* (page 143); an Asian-inspired noodle salad; ½ cup of vegetables, steamed, grilled, or baked

**Snack:** 1 cup of low-fat yogurt with ½ cup sliced fresh fruit

**Dinner:** *Roasted Pork with Pomegranate Sauce* (page 189); a medium baked sweet potato; ½ cup of steamed string bean

**Dessert:** 1 cup of kefir

## OTHER RECIPES TO TRY

- Fish Tacos
- Broccoli and Pearl Barley Salad
- Pot Roast with Root Vegetables
- Spinach-Stuffed Meat Loaf
- Orange Beef with Broccoli and Jicama
- Pork Chops and Cabbage

# HIATAL HERNIA

*See* Indigestion and Heartburn, page 318

# HIVES

## FOODS THAT HARM

Yellow food color no. 5 (tartrazine)

Shellfish

Nuts

Berries

Apricots

Grapes

Dried fruits

Tea

## FOODS THAT HEAL

Poultry

Seafood

Seeds

Fortified and enriched cereals and breads

## HOW TO EAT

Follow these tips to avoid an outbreak.

**Steer clear of trigger foods.** Some common ones are shellfish, nuts, and berries. Keep a food diary to identify ones that are problematic for you.

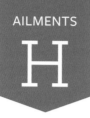

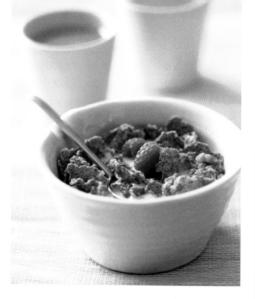

- Maple-Glazed Chicken with Root Vegetables
- Carrot-Flecked Corn Bread

# HYPER-THYROIDISM

**FOODS THAT HARM**
Caffeinated drinks

**FOODS THAT HEAL**
Dairy products
Soy products
Collard greens
Mustard greens

## HOW TO EAT

Dietary changes won't prevent or reverse this condition, but you can protect yourself with this advice.

**Get enough calcium and vitamin D** to keep your bones strong. An overactive thyroid may contribute to bone loss. Find D in salmon, tuna, mackerel, and fortified milk, soy beverages, and orange juice. Good calcium sources include milk, yogurt, cheese, broccoli, and kale.

### SAMPLE MEAL PLANS

**Breakfast:** 2 slices of whole grain toast with 2 Tbsp of jam; a glass of calcium-fortified orange juice

**Lunch:** grilled chicken sandwich made with 3 oz of boneless, skinless chicken breast, 2 Tbsp low-fat mayonnaise, lettuce, and tomato; 1 cup of steamed collards

**Snack:** 1 cup soy yogurt

**Seek out foods that are high in niacin,** such as chicken, tuna, beef, whole grains, and enriched cereals.

**Read food labels to avoid tartrazine.** This food additive (yellow food color no. 5) causes hives in some people.

### SAMPLE MEAL PLAN

**Breakfast:** 1 cup of fortified and enriched whole grain cereal with 1 cup of skim milk; 1 small banana

**Lunch:** *Turkey Cobb Salad Sandwiches* (page 150); 8 baked potato chips.

**Snack:** handful of roasted sunflower seeds; 1 pear

**Dinner:** *Scallops Florentine* (page 209); 1 medium baked potato with 2 Tbsp of reduced-fat sour cream; 1 cup mixed green salad with 2 Tbsp low-fat dressing.

**Dessert:** *Carrot Ginger Yogurt Muffins* (page 129)

### OTHER RECIPES TO TRY

- Papaya and Avocado Salad
- Watermelon and Feta Salad
- Braised Chicken Thighs with Winter Vegetables

**WARNING!**
**FOOD-DRUG INTERACTION**
If you're taking a synthetic thyroid hormone, limit dietary fiber. Certain foods (walnuts, soybean flour), supplements (iron, calcium), and medications (some antacids, ulcer medications, and cholesterol drugs) can also affect the effectiveness of the treatment. To avoid potential interactions, eat these foods or use these products several hours before or after you take your thyroid medication.

**Dinner:** *Pasta Primavera* (page 216); ½ cup of lightly steamed mustard greens

**Dessert:** 1 cup of frozen strawberry yogurt

## OTHER RECIPES TO TRY

- Spinach and Goat Cheese Omelet
- Zucchini-Carrot Crustless Quiche Squares
- Mediterranean Salad with Edamame
- Braised Mixed Greens with Dried Currants
- Lemony Blueberry Cheesecake Bars
- Pumpkin Custards

# HYPO-GLYCEMIA

## FOODS THAT HEAL

Apples
Lentils
Barley
Oats

## FOODS TO LIMIT

Alcohol
Sugary foods, such as candy

## HOW TO EAT

You may need to consult a dietitian or your physician to adjust your meals and snacks further, but here are some strategies to prevent drops in your blood sugar that can trigger a hypoglycemic episode.

**Think small, frequent meals.** Eating at regular intervals—about every 2 to 3 hours—helps to keep blood sugar levels more stable.

**Balance your meals.** Get an even mix of carbohydrates, fats, and proteins in every meal. This will help your body metabo-lize the foods slowly to allow for a steady release of energy. The meals below all have between 30 to 45 g of carbohydrates.

**Fill up on fiber.** Make sure you have a high-fiber food at every meal. In addition to those listed at left, other good sources include fruits, vegetables, and whole grains.

**Choose low glycemic load (GL) foods.** GL is a measurement of how readily foods are converted to blood glucose. See page 357 for foods.

**Choose sugar-free or no-added sugar beverages,** unless you are having a low-blood sugar episode.

## SAMPLE MEAL PLAN

**Mini Breakfast:** 1 soft cooked egg; 1 slice of whole grain toast with 1 tsp of trans fat free soft spread; ½ cup of citrus fruit

**A.M. Mini Meal:** *Blueberry-Oatmeal Muffins* (page 127)

**Mini -Lunch:** *Lentil Soup with Canadian Bacon* (page 134); ½ whole wheat pita; ½ cup steamed collards

**P.M. Mini Meal:** 4 whole grain crackers with 1 oz low fat cheese; ½ cup skim milk

**Mini Dinner:** 3 oz of baked boneless, skinless, chicken breast; ⅔ cup of cooked brown rice or risotto; ½ cup of diced carrots and peas

**Dessert:** 1 apple, sliced, with 2 tsp of peanut butter

## OTHER RECIPES TO TRY

- Broccoli and Pearl Barley Salad
- Herbed Chicken and Apple Burgers
- Lentil and Rice Paella with Clams
- No-Bake Flaxseed-Nut Bars

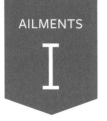

# HYPO-THYROIDISM

## FOODS THAT HARM
Walnuts
Soybean flour

## FOODS THAT HEAL
Carrots
Sweet potato
Papaya
Cantaloupe
Spinach
Turnip greens

## HOW TO EAT

These dietary strategies, along with medication, can help control hypothyroidism, a condition in which the thyroid gland isn't producing enough hormones.

**Eat more foods rich in beta-carotene.** You may need a higher intake because the hormone thyroxine, which is used to treat hypothyroidism, accelerates the conversion of beta-carotene to vitamin A in the body.

**Cook your broccoli.** Cabbage, broccoli, and other cruciferous vegetables contain substances called goitrogens, which block the effects of thyroid hormones. Cooking these foods inactivates the goitrogens.

## SAMPLE MEAL PLAN

**Breakfast:** ½ multigrain bagel with 1 oz of smoked salmon, red onions, and 1 Tbsp low-fat cream cheese; 1 cup of fruit salad made with fresh cantaloupe, mango, and strawberry slices

**Lunch:** *Carrot Soup with Dill* (page 138); 3 oz of grilled chicken; 1 cup of cooked cauliflower or broccoli florets

**Snack:** 1 oz of sweet potato chips; 1 apple

**Dinner:** 3 oz of broiled lean beef or roasted pork tenderloin; *Twice-Baked Stuffed Sweet Potatoes* (page 235); ½ cup of cooked spinach

**Dessert:** 1 cup sliced fruit—try papaya, mango, and kiwi drizzled with 1 tsp of honey.

## OTHER RECIPES TO TRY

- Cantaloupe and Orange Soup
- Papaya and Avocado Salad
- Braised Mixed Greens with Dried Currants

# IMPOTENCE

*See* Sex Drive, Diminished, page 347

# INDIGESTION AND HEARTBURN

## FOODS THAT HARM
Fatty foods

## FOODS THAT HEAL
Small meals at regular intervals

## FOODS TO LIMIT
Alcohol
Caffeinated drinks
Chocolate
Spicy foods
Peppermint
Tomatoes

Pickles
Vinegar
Citrus fruits

## HOW TO EAT

Follow this dietary advice to prevent or ease symptoms of occasional or chronic indigestion.

**Eat small, frequent meals.** They're easier to digest.

**Adopt a low-fat, balanced diet.** Fatty foods take longer to digest, staying in the stomach for more time and increasing the chance of heartburn or indigestion.

**Keep your distance from prime offenders,** such as acidic and spicy foods and drinks.

**Watch out for chocolate or peppermint.** They relax the diaphragmatic muscle, making it easier for stomach acid to flow up into the esophagus.

**Chew nonmint gum for dessert.** It stimulates saliva, which neutralizes acid in the esophagus.

**Close the kitchen 2 hours before bedtime.** You shouldn't eat anything within 2 hours of going to sleep.

### SAMPLE MEAL PLAN

**Mini Breakfast:** Spinach and mushroom omelet using ½ cup of fat-free liquid egg substitute; 1 slice of whole grain toast with 1 tsp of jam

**A.M. Mini Meal:** ½ cup low-fat yogurt; 1 small cookie

**Mini Lunch:** 2 oz of sliced turkey; *Rice-Stuffed Squash* (page 223); ½ cup of steamed green string beans, carrots, or broccoli

**P.M. Mini Meal:** Banana-Peanut Bread (page 243)

**Mini Dinner:** 2 oz of grilled or baked boneless, skinless chicken breast; 2 cups mixed green salad with 2 Tbsp low-fat dressing; *Carrot-Flecked Corn Bread* (page 243)

**Dessert:** ½ cup of fruited gelatin

### OTHER RECIPES TO TRY

- Yogurt Parfait
- Cauliflower Salad with Cashews
- Asparagus and Chicken Stir-Fry
- Braised Chicken with Winter Vegetables
- Snapper and Snaps in a Packet
- Cider-Baked Acorn Squash with Apple Stuffing

# INFERTILITY

## FOODS THAT HEAL

Enriched or fortified cereals
Brussels sprouts
Broccoli
Turnip greens
Yogurt
Legumes
Lean meat
Fish
Orange juice

## FOODS TO LIMIT

Caffeinated drinks (for women)
Alcohol

## HOW TO EAT

While nutrition is not a leading cause of infertility, it's important for both men and women to consume a healthful diet to enhance the chances of conceiving and delivering a healthy baby. The best way to do that is to eat a variety of foods from all food groups and follow these tips.

**Get more folate.** Women with a high intake are less likely to have children with neural tube defects such as spina bifida. Good sources include fortified breakfast cereals, leafy greens, legumes, and orange juice.

**Seek out zinc.** Inadequate intakes may lower male fertility. Good sources include oysters, lean roast beef, and peanuts.

**Go for B12.** Even in men who aren't deficient, vitamin B12—found in fortified breads and cereals, lean meat, poultry, and seafood—may improve sperm count and motility.

**Cut back on coffee.** Research has found that women who drink more than 3 cups of coffee a day reduce their chances of conceiving in any given month by 25%.

### SAMPLE MEAL PLAN

**Breakfast:** 1 cup of fortified whole grain cereal with ½ cup of skim milk; ½ cup low-fat fruit yogurt; ½ cup of orange juice

**Lunch:** *Grilled Oysters with Fennel and Spinach* (page 247); 6 whole grain crackers; at least 1 cup of steamed broccoli florets

**Snack:** ½ cup of yogurt with sliced fruit or berries

**Dinner:** 3 oz of cooked lean roast beef or pork; *Brussels Sprouts with Caraway Seeds* (page 229); ½ cup of mashed sweet potatoes; at least ½ cup of steamed turnip greens or kale

**Dessert:** ½ cup frozen vanilla yogurt with 2 Tbsp of chopped peanuts and a cherry on top

### OTHER RECIPES TO TRY

- Strawberry-Yogurt Smoothie
- Beef Fillet Salad with Mustard Vinaigrette
- Pork, Pear, and Potato Salad
- Calf's Liver with Rigatoni
- Whole Wheat Noodles with Peanut Sauce and Chicken
- Brown Rice with Cabbage and Chickpeas
- Orange-Walnut Broccoli
- Fruity Brussels Sprouts

# INFLAMMATORY BOWEL DISEASE

### FOODS THAT HARM

Fried foods, artificial sweeteners, or any other trigger foods

Alcohol

Caffeinated beverages

### FOODS THAT HEAL

Water

Bananas

Rice

Applesauce

Toast

White meat poultry

### FOODS TO LIMIT

Bran

Whole grains

Nuts

Dried fruits

## HOW TO EAT

While diet doesn't cause IBD and can't cure it, some foods may ease symptoms while others may trigger a flare-up. These are different for each person, so identify your trigger foods. Then stick to your safe foods and follow these tips.

**Eat five to six smaller meals.** This puts less strain on the intestinal tract.

**Drink up between meals.** It's important to stay hydrated, and drinking lots of fluids helps prevent kidney problems and gallstones. However, taking in liquids at the same time as food may sometimes cause diarrhea, so do your sipping in between meals.

**Focus on soluble fiber** found in oats, poached and peeled fruits, and cooked leafy green vegetables. Insoluble fiber (found in the Foods to Limit offerings at left) tends to be more irritating to the colon.

**Choose soft foods** like those in the meal plan below. They are easier to digest.

### SAMPLE MEAL PLAN

**Mini Breakfast:** 1 slice of toast with 1 Tbsp of apple butter; 1 banana

**A.M. Mini Meal:** ½ cup of cottage-cheese with ¼ cup of sliced peaches, fresh or canned

**Mini Lunch:** 2 oz of baked salmon; 1 cup of vegetable soup; ½ cup of cooked white rice (or brown rice if you tolerate it); ½ cup of sautéed greens such as spinach, bok choy, or cabbage

**P.M. Mini Meal:** 4 saltines with 2 tsp of nut butter

**Dinner:** 2 oz of poached chicken; ½ cup of cooked white rice (or brown rice if you tolerate it); ½ cup of cooked carrots

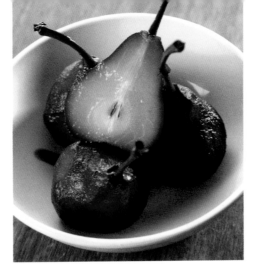

**Dessert:** 1 poached pear

### OTHER RECIPES TO TRY

- Zucchini Frittata
- Quick Chicken Noodle Soup
- Carrot Soup with Dill
- Braised Chicken with Winter Vegetables
- Grilled Salmon with Sautéed Greens
- Chewy Oatmeal Raisin Cookies

# INSOMNIA

### FOODS THAT HARM

Alcohol

Caffeinated drinks

### FOODS THAT HEAL

Milk and honey

Turkey sandwich

Banana

## HOW TO EAT

Your eating habits can certainly affect your sleeping habits. Here's some diet advice that can help you get a better night's sleep.

**Skip caffeine.** If you can't cut it out completely, at least avoid having any about 8 hours before bed.

**Combine foods for better sleep.** Milk and turkey contain sleep-inducing tryptophan, which works by increasing the amount of serotonin, a natural sedative, in the brain. But you need carbs—like honey or bread—to get tryptophan into your brain.

**Don't go to bed full.** Too much food can cause digestive discomfort that can keep you awake.

**Try rice for dinner.** In one study, eating a high-carb meal, in this case featuring jasmine rice, 4 hours before bed can halve the time it takes to fall asleep.

**Stop drinking fluids a couple of hours before bed.** It will reduce your chances of having to get up during the night.

### SAMPLE MEAL PLAN

**Breakfast:** 1 cup of whole grain cereal with ½ cup of skim milk; 1 sliced banana

**Lunch:** *Turkey Cobb Salad Sandwiches* (page 150); 1 oz of carrot chips

**Snack:** 4 honey mustard pretzels, or a serving of nugget-size pretzels

**Dinner:** *Rice Salad with Chicken and Grapes* (page 223) made with jasmine rice; a bowl of lentil soup; 1 piece of French bread

**Dessert:** a cup of warm skim milk with 1 tsp of honey

### OTHER RECIPES TO TRY

- Turkey, Spinach, and Rice in Roasted Garlic Broth
- Turkey Braciola Stuffed with Provolone and Spinach
- Thai Coconut Rice

# INTERSTITIAL CYSTITIS

### FOODS THAT HARM

Hot peppers

Coffee

Cranberry juice

Artificial sweeteners

### FOODS THAT HEAL

Water

Fresh fruits and vegetables

Dairy products

### FOODS TO LIMIT

Processed foods containing preservatives and other chemicals

### HOW TO EAT

Many foods are reported to worsen symptoms, but people react differently to different foods. Once you've identified your trigger foods, be especially careful not to eat them when you're starting a new drug therapy.

**Eliminate one at a time.** Rather than cutting suspected food triggers from your diet all at once, eliminate one at a time for several days and note if your symptoms improve. Foods that are common troublemakers are listed above.

**Consider going organic.** Buy fresh food as much as possible and organic food whenever you can.

**Sip water.** Keeping urine diluted may help. Speak with your doctor about how much you should drink.

### SAMPLE MEAL PLAN

**Breakfast:** *Carrot Ginger Yogurt Muffins* (page 129); ½ cup of low-fat cottage cheese with ¼ cup of fresh sliced fruit

**Lunch:** *Zucchini-Carrot Crustless Quiche Squares* (page 157); at least 1 cup of your favorite steamed vegetables

**Snack:** 1 pear

**Dinner:** *Pasta Primavera* (page 216); 2 cups of mixed salad greens with 2 Tbsp low-fat dressing; 1 slice of whole grain bread with 1 tsp trans fat free spread

**Dessert:** organic fresh fruit

## OTHER RECIPES TO TRY

- Cauliflower Salad with Cashews
- Papaya and Avocado Salad
- Baked Pasta with Garlic and Greens
- Macaroni and Cheese with Spinach
- Twice-Baked Stuffed Sweet Potatoes
- Cider-Baked Acorn Squash with Apple Stuffing

# IRON OVERLOAD

## FOODS THAT HARM

Alcohol (if there is liver damage)
Raw shellfish

## FOODS TO LIMIT

Iron-rich foods, such as lean red
meats and organ meats
Dark green leafy vegetables

## HOW TO EAT

Hemachromatosis is the most common form of iron overload disease and can be inherited or caused by anemia or alcoholism. Left untreated, it can cause irreversible damage and lead to serious conditions such as cancer, heart disease, and liver

disease. That's why it's important to see your doctor and work with a registered dietitian to develop a personal nutrition plan to meet your specific needs. Here are some general guidelines.

**Eat more low-iron foods.** Choose fresh fruit over dried; unfortified grain, cereal, or bread; chicken and fish instead of red meat; and veggies except for leafy greens.

**Avoid foods that increase iron absorption.** Vitamin C boosts absorption of iron, so it's best to eat foods high in vitamin C between meals or with foods that contain little iron.

# IRRITABLE BOWEL SYNDROME

## FOODS THAT HARM

Fatty and fried foods
Sugar alcohols, such as sorbitol,
lactitol, mannitol, and maltitol

## FOODS THAT HEAL

Water
Whole grain breads
and cereals
Berries
Lentils
Artichokes
Bananas

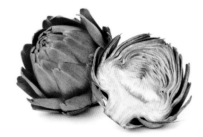

### HOW TO EAT

What you eat definitely affects your symptoms, although the effects of certain foods can vary from person to person. A food diary can help you to identify those foods that exacerbate or calm IBS for you. Here is some general advice.

**Eat several small meals** to reduce symptoms.

**Chew food thoroughly.** Poorly chewed food is harder to digest. Eating too fast also causes you to swallow more air that can result in irritating intestinal gas.

**Drink lots of water** to promote better digestion.

**Know which fiber you need.** Insoluble fiber, found in whole grain cereals and vegetables like peas and broccoli, helps to bulk up stools and ease elimination, relieving constipation. Foods high in soluble fiber, such as oats, barley, apples, and kidney beans, absorb water and are helpful for bouts of diarrhea.

### SAMPLE MEAL PLAN

**Mini Breakfast:** 1 cup of whole grain cereal with ½ cup of skim milk; *Blueberry-Oatmeal Muffins* (page 127)

**A.M. Mini Meal:** ½ cup of yogurt; 1 banana

**Mini Lunch:** 2 oz of baked chicken; ½ cup of mashed potatoes topped with chives or parsley; ½ cup of cooked wax beans

**P.M. Mini Meal:** *Warm Artichoke and Bean Dip* (page 251) with ½ whole wheat pita

**Mini Dinner:** 2 oz of broiled lean meat; 1 cup of lentil soup; ½ cup of cooked broccoli, or 2 cups of mixed green salad with 2 Tbsp of low-fat dressing; 1 slice of whole grain bread

**Dessert:** *Angel Food Cake with Strawberries* (page 261)

### OTHER RECIPES TO TRY

- Berry Salad with Passion Fruit
- Berry-Flaxseed Smoothie
- Lentil Soup with Canadian Bacon
- Cauliflower Salad with Cashews
- Artichokes with Lentils and Lima Beans
- Rhubarb-Blackberry Crumble

# JAUNDICE

### FOODS THAT HARM

Alcohol

### FOODS THAT HEAL

Lean meat

Poultry

Fish

Eggs

Dairy products

Quinoa

Lentils

### FOODS TO LIMIT

Fatty and fried foods

Sugary foods

### HOW TO EAT

Eating a nutritious, well-balanced diet can help to resolve some types of jaundice. Here are some guidelines.

**Be a grazer.** Several small meals throughout the day may be the best way to get a balanced diet since appetite tends to decrease and nausea is common.

**For hepatitis suffers, eat a diet high in protein.** Consume a healthy diet with sufficient protein daily, from both animal and vegetable sources. (See Hepatitis, page 314.)

**Opt for fats in dairy and eggs.** They're easier to digest than other fatty foods.

**Stay away from sweets.** They may squelch your appetite for more nutritious foods.

## SAMPLE MEAL PLAN

**Mini Breakfast:** an omelet made with broccoli and cheese; 1 slice of whole wheat toast; 1 small banana

**A.M. Mini Meal:** ½ cup of low-fat cottage cheese with ¼ cup sliced peaches (peeled or from a can, with no added sugar)

**Mini Lunch:** 3 oz of chicken salad stuffed into a small pita pocket; *Lentil Soup with Canadian Bacon* (page 134)

**P.M. Mini Meal:** 1 apple; 1 oz low-fat string cheese; 4 whole grain crackers

**Mini Dinner:** 3 oz of cooked lean roast beef, baked fish, or roasted chicken or turkey; *Springtime Quinoa* (page 220); ½ cup of lightly sautéed vegetables, or a small mixed green salad with 2 Tbsp of low-fat dressing

**Dessert:** ½ cup of *Creamy Citrus and Vanilla Rice Pudding* (page 263)

## OTHER RECIPES TO TRY

- Zucchini Frittata
- Quick Chicken Noodle Soup
- Sloppy Joes
- Fish Tacos
- Pineapple-Chipotle Chicken
- Cod with Gremolata Crust
- Pasta Primavera

# JET LAG

### FOODS THAT HEAL
Water
Cucumber
Celery
Watermelon
Grapes
Papaya

### FOODS TO LIMIT
Alcohol
Caffeinated beverages

## HOW TO EAT

To minimize jet lag, you'll need to change your eating habits 2 days before your flight if you're traveling within a country. If you're traveling farther, you'll need to follow this diet plan for about 4 days before takeoff.

**Feast and fast.** The scientifically tested anti–jet lag diet alternates feast days (high-protein breakfasts and lunches, high-carb dinners) with fast days (low-cal, low-carb meals) to trick your body to be right on time.

**Lose the booze.** Don't drink any alcohol the day before your flight, during the flight, and the day after the flight. The same goes for caffeine.

**Eat your water.** In addition to drinking lots of water, bring watery fruits and vegetables, such as those listed above, as snacks.

## SAMPLE MEAL PLAN
### DAY 1—FEAST
(2 to 4 days before you leave)

**Breakfast:** *One-Egg Omelet with Chopped Broccoli, Tomatoes, and Cheddar* (page 123); 2 oz of turkey bacon, smoked salmon, or lean meat; decaffeinated coffee or tea

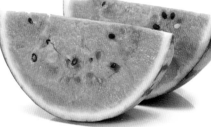

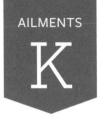

**Lunch:** 3 to 4 oz of baked, grilled, broiled, or roasted lean meat, chicken, turkey, or fish; 1 cup of bean soup, or 2 oz of low-fat cheese; decaffeinated coffee or tea

**Dinner:** *Baked Pasta with Garlic and Greens* (page 213); 1 whole grain roll; 1 slice of pie a la mode; decaffeinated coffee or tea

## DAY 2—FAST
(the day before you leave)

Eat lightly; choose small salads, broth or thin soups, fruit or fruit juice. Break your fast with a high-protein breakfast when you arrive at your destination the next day.

### OTHER RECIPES TO TRY

- Individual Breakfast Tortilla
- Curried Chicken Salad Sandwich
- Turkey Cobb Salad Sandwiches
- Japanese Sushi Rolls
- Potato Salad with Sun-Dried Tomatoes, Scallions, and Basil
- Watermelon and Feta Salad
- Macaroni and Cheese with Spinach
- Cherry Crisp

# KIDNEY DISEASE
(including kidney stones, nephritis, kidney failure)

### FOODS THAT HARM
Salty foods, such as pickles

### FOODS THAT HEAL
Water
Cranberry juice
Lemon juice

### FOODS TO LIMIT
Berries
Soybeans
Beet greens
Quinoa
Chocolate
Tea

### HOW TO EAT
Diet modifications will vary depending on the type and severity of the kidney disorder. It is best to seek the advice of a physician or registered dietitian who can help you with your diet as it relates to your disorder. Here are some general guidelines, including a meal plan that can help prevent and ease problems with kidney stones, one of the most common types of kidney problems.

**For kidney stones,** drink plenty of fluids throughout the day, include vegetarian sources of protein, and reduce oxalate-rich foods such as rhubarb, spinach, nuts, sweet potatoes, tea, soy, and chocolate (see meal plan below).

**For nephritis,** including cranberry juice daily in your diet may be helpful.

**For stages of kidney failure,** most people will need to limit sodium, protein, phosphorus-containing foods such as dairy products, and potassium-containing foods such as potatoes, citrus, and bananas. Fluids may or may not be restricted. If you are on dialysis, your diet may need to be modified further.

### SAMPLE MEAL PLAN

**Breakfast:** *Zucchini Frittata* (page 124); 2 slices of white toast with 2 Tbsp of apple-butter spread; 8 oz of juice or water

**Lunch:** chicken sandwich made with 3 oz of grilled chicken on a kaiser roll, stuffed with iceberg lettuce and drizzled with

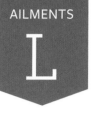
2 Tbsp of low-fat dressing; ½ cup steamed broccoli or peas; 1 cup of cantaloupe chunks; 8 oz of juice or water

**Snack:** 6 low-fat vanilla wafers; 8 oz of juice or water

**Dinner:** *Vegetable Pot Pie* (page 000); 1 whole grain roll; 8 oz of juice or water

**Dessert:** *Angel Food Cake with Strawberries* (page 213)

## OTHER RECIPES TO TRY

- Open-Faced Grilled Vegetable Sandwich
- Cod with a Gremolata Crust
- Savory Cranberry Chutney

# LACTOSE INTOLERANCE

## FOODS THAT HARM

Milk
Soft cheeses

## FOODS THAT HEAL

Lactose-free dairy products
Broccoli
Fortified and enriched breads
Fortified and enriched juices
Fortified soy beverages
Canned salmon (with bones)
Pinto beans
Rhubarb

## FOODS TO LIMIT

Yogurt
Hard cheeses

## HOW TO EAT

You can control symptoms of lactose intolerance by limiting dairy products in your diet. Here are some helpful strategies.

**Read labels carefully.** Look for ingredients like milk, milk solids, cream, whey, cheese flavors, curds, and nonfat milk powder. Such dairy products can be an ingredient or component of various food products such as cookies, breads, processed meats, hot dogs, some artificial sweeteners, and even some medications.

**Eat lactose-reduced or lactose-free products.** Most lactose-intolerant people can eat cultured dairy products, like yogurt. Others options are hard cheeses, like cheddar, edam, and gouda.

**Try adding milk to your diet slowly.** Start with a quarter-cup of milk and gradually increase the amount. Avoid drinking milk on an empty stomach.

**Get calcium from other sources, if you are very intolerant.** Good sources include sardines (with bones), black beans, kale, and almonds.

**Eat foods rich in vitamin D.** Since vitamin D is also needed for strong bones, eat eggs, salmon, and yogurt.

## SAMPLE MEAL PLAN

**Breakfast:** 2 pieces of French toast (made with almond or fortified rice milk) with 2 Tbsp reduced-calorie syrup; 2 slices of lean bacon or low-fat sausage links

**Lunch:** *Salmon and Fennel Lettuce Wraps* (page 152); 8 whole grain crackers; ½ cup of steamed carrots, cauliflower, and snow peas

**Snack:** 1 medium orange

**Dinner:** 3 oz of roasted turkey; *Broccoli and Pearl Barley Salad* (page 169); 1 cup of cooked spinach

**Dessert:** *Rhubarb-Blackberry Crumble* (page 259) made with soymilk

### OTHER RECIPES TO TRY

- Turkey, Spinach, and Rice in Roasted Garlic Broth
- Calf's Liver with Rigatoni
- Creamy Citrus and Vanilla Rice Pudding

# LUPUS

### FOODS THAT HARM

Alfalfa
Celery
Parsnips
Parsley
Lemons
Limes
Mushrooms
Smoked food
Grapefruit

### FOODS THAT HEAL

Broccoli
Cabbage
Cauliflower
Spinach
Milk
Fortified soy and rice beverages
Salmon
Mackerel
Herring
Nuts
Flaxseeds
Wheat germ

### FOODS TO LIMIT

Fatty, high-protein foods, especially animal products

**WARNING!**
**FOOD-DRUG INTERACTION**

Do not consume grapefruit or grapefruit juice if you are taking cyclosporine, a powerful immune system suppressor. They can dramatically increase the body's ability to absorb cyclosporine, leading to severe toxicity. If you are taking corticosteroids, cut back on salt. It will increase water retention and contribute to high blood pressure.

## HOW TO EAT

Lupus is an inflammatory disease so eating more foods that fight and reduce inflammation (fruits and veggies) and avoiding those that promote inflammation (animal products) is prudent. Here are more diet guidelines that may help.

**Go for variety.** Eating a colorful array of fruits, vegetables, and whole grains can also protect you from heart disease in addition to providing essential nutrients.

**Chomp on cruciferous veggies regularly.** Foods such as broccoli, cabbage, and cauliflower contain indoles that alter the metabolism of estrogen in a way that has a positive impact on lupus.

**Fish for omega-3s.** Their anti-inflammatory effects may relieve the joint pain, soreness, and stiffness associated with lupus.

**Eat foods rich in vitamin D.** Because most lupus patients must avoid exposure to the sun, they need to get this bone-strengthening vitamin from milk and fortified soy and rice beverages. Extra calcium is also beneficial.

**Avoid alfalfa in any form.** Even herbal supplements containing alfalfa worsen lupus symptoms. Other legumes may have a similar effect.

### SAMPLE MEAL PLAN

**Breakfast:** 1 cup of whole grain cereal with ½ cup skim milk or fortified soy or rice beverage, and 1 tsp of ground flaxseeds on top; ½ cup of fresh fruit

**Lunch:** 1 can of mackerel or sardines in olive oil (well-drained) on 8 whole grain low-sodium crackers; 1 cup of mixed green salad with chopped tomatoes, cucumbers, low-fat grated cheese, and 2 Tbsp of low-fat dressing

**Snack:** small handful of nuts

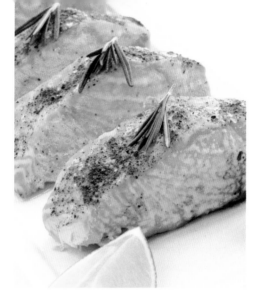

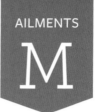

**Dinner:** 3 oz of baked salmon; *Cauliflower and Spinach Casserole* (page 231); 1 cup of cooked orzo with chopped fresh herbs

**Dessert:** *Wheat Germ Smoothie* (page 132)

## OTHER RECIPES TO TRY

- Berry-Flaxseed Smoothie
- Grilled Salmon with Sautéed Greens
- Pasta with Cabbage, Apple, and Leeks
- Spiced Almonds

# MEMORY LOSS

## FOODS THAT HEAL

Lean meat

Whole grains

Beans

Oranges

Cantaloupes

Eggs

Nuts and seeds

Spinach

Soybeans

## HOW TO EAT

A healthy diet can help to keep your brain sharp. Here are a few dietary changes that can make a difference.

**Make time for a good breakfast.** A Toronto study found that breakfast helped men and women ages 61 to 79 score better on memory tests. And when kids eat a morning meal, their exam scores improve.

**Get plenty of beta-carotene** and vitamin C found in sweet potatoes, butternut squash, carrots, red peppers, and broccoli.

**Add vitamin E.** Rich sources of this antioxidant include wheat germ, vegetable oils, and nuts.

**Get enough iron.** Lean meat, soybeans, and dark leafy greens like spinach are good sources.

**Drink some coffee.** A University of Arizona study showed that seniors who drank 12 oz (355 mL) of caffeinated coffee in the morning and afternoon maintained their memory better than the group of seniors who drank decaffeinated coffee.

**Limit alcohol.** In one study, adults who drank one to six alcoholic beverages a week were 54% less likely than abstainers to develop dementia over 6 years. However, 14 or more drinks weekly increased the risk of dementia by 22%.

## SAMPLE MEAL PLAN

**Breakfast:** 1 sunny-side up egg; 1 slice of whole grain toast; ½ cup low-fat fruit-flavored yogurt sprinkled with 2 tsp of wheat germ; ½ cup of orange juice

**Lunch:** grilled salmon burger on a whole wheat bun; *Lentil Soup with Canadian Bacon* (page 134); ½ cup of cooked spinach

**Snack:** *Sweet and Spicy Snack Mix* (page 252)

**Dinner:** *Flank Steak Roll with Carrots and Red Pepper* (page 181); 1 cup of cooked angel hair pasta sautéed in 2 tsp of olive oil and crushed garlic, and tossed with parmesan cheese to taste; 1 whole grain roll

**Dessert:** 2 cups of cubed cantaloupe

### OTHER RECIPES TO TRY

- Cantaloupe and Orange Soup
- Beef, Onion, and Pepper Fajitas
- Pork, Pear, and Potato Salad
- Buckwheat Noodles with Tofu and Green Vegetables
- Spinach Salad with Chickpeas
- Spinach-Stuffed Meatloaf

# MENOPAUSE

### FOODS THAT HEAL

Fortified and enriched cereals

Spinach

Tofu and other soy products

Nuts and seeds, especially flaxseeds

Vegetable oil

### FOODS TO LIMIT

Alcohol

Caffeinated drinks

Chocolate

Spicy foods

### HOW TO EAT

Enjoy a diet rich in whole grains, fruits, vegetables, and low-fat dairy products to help ease the symptoms of menopause and reduce your risk for chronic disease. Follow these additional strategies for even greater benefits.

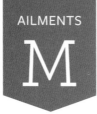

**Watch out for trigger foods.** Some foods can worsen symptoms like hot flashes, insomnia, and mood swings. Common culprits include coffee, tea, chocolate, colas, alcohol, and spicy foods.

**Include soy foods.** Studies have shown that they can help ease hot flashes.

**Try vitamin E.** For some women, vitamin E, found in many of the healing foods at left, helps tame hot flashes.

**Eat 1 to 2 Tbsp of ground flaxseed a day.** Grind the seeds and add to cereal, yogurt, or oatmeal.

### SAMPLE MEAL PLAN

**Breakfast:** spinach omelet; *Whole Wheat Flaxseed Bread* (page 242), toasted, with 2 tsp of jam; 1 cup of fresh orange or grapefruit sections

**Lunch:** 3 oz of baked or grilled salmon; *Mediterranean Salad with Edamame* (page 177); 1 medium baked potato with 1 tsp of trans fat free soft spread

**Snack:** *Cranberry-Peanut Cereal Bars* (page 254)

**Dinner:** *Fried Rice with Tofu and Vegetables* (page 222); a bowl of soup

**Dessert:** ½ cup of low-fat yogurt with sliced bananas and 1 Tbsp of ground flaxseeds

### OTHER RECIPES TO TRY

- Spinach and Goat Cheese Omelet
- Buckwheat Noodles with Tofu and Green Vegetables
- Spinach Salad with Chickpeas
- Bok Choy, Tofu, and Mushroom Stir-Fry
- Edamame Hummus with Pita Crisps

# MENSTRUAL PROBLEMS

## FOODS THAT HARM
Fatty and highly refined foods

## FOODS THAT HEAL
Apples

Pears

Whole grain and fortified and
enriched cereals

Lean meat

Green leafy vegetables

Sunflower seeds

Nuts

Lentils

Dairy products

Soy products

Figs

Salmon

Avocados

Potatoes

Raspberry leaf tea

Chamomile tea

## FOODS TO LIMIT
Alcohol

Salty foods

## HOW TO EAT

Follow these suggestions to prevent or ease some of the symptoms of premenstrual syndrome, the most common menstrual problem.

**Eat low glycemic foods.** Fiber-rich choices such as apples and pears keep blood sugar more stable to tame cravings. See the glycemic index chart on page 357.

**Get more calcium.** Low levels may contribute to mood swings, cramping, and bloating. Best sources include dairy products, fortified soy beverages, canned salmon or sardines, and leafy greens.

**Add more magnesium.** Munch on a handful of sunflower seeds, nuts, figs, and green vegetables to reduce your chances of PMS-induced headaches and depression.

**Boost vitamin B6.** Beef, pork, chicken, fish, whole grain cereals, bananas, avocados, and potatoes are good sources of this vitamin, which may reduce anxiety and depression.

**Indulge cravings carefully.** Too many sugary, empty calories may stimulate more cravings.

**Sip herbal teas for painful cramps.** Try raspberry leaf or chamomile tea.

**Load up on iron-rich foods, if you bleed a lot.** When eating red meat, legumes, fortified cereals, leafy green vegetables, and dried fruits include some vitamin C-rich foods like cantaloupe or kiwis to improve iron absorption.

## SAMPLE MEAL PLAN

**Breakfast:** 1 cup of whole grain cereal or a fruit and nut muesli, with 1 cup of skim or soy milk; 1 slice of cantaloupe

**Lunch:** *Crab and Avocado Salad* (page 167); 1 medium ear of corn on the cob with 1 tsp of trans fat free soft spread; 1 medium apple

**Snack:** 1 oz low-fat cheese; 1 medium pear; a small handful of unsalted nuts

**Dinner:** veggie burger on a whole wheat bun with lettuce, tomato, sprouts, 1 Tbsp of your favorite spread; a cup of lentil soup; 8 baked potato fries; ½ cup of steamed collard greens

**Dessert:** *Sesame-Fig Bars* (page 254); a cup of chamomile or raspberry leaf tea

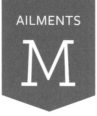
### OTHER RECIPES TO TRY

- Hot Cereal with Apples and Dates
- Raspberry-Beet Smoothie
- Pork, Pear, and Potato Salad
- Buckwheat Noodles with Tofu and Green Vegetables
- Mediterranean Salad with Edamame
- Papaya and Avocado Salad
- Potato Salad with Sun-Dried Tomatoes, Scallions, and Basil
- White Beans Stewed with Swiss Chard

# METABOLIC SYNDROME

*See* Diabetes, page 302

# MIGRAINES AND OTHER HEADACHES

### FOODS THAT HARM

Individual trigger foods, such as aged cheeses, processed meats, fermented foods, and more

### FOODS TO LIMIT

Caffeinated drinks

### HOW TO EAT

When it comes to migraines, the key dietary advice is to avoid foods that bring on the pain. Here's what you need to know, along with a meal plan featuring bland foods that are less likely to trigger a headache.

**Know and avoid common dietary triggers.** Keep a diary to learn what foods prompt symptoms, and then eliminate those foods. Common culprits in addition to those listed at left include pickles; legumes, especially dried beans, lentils, and soy products; nuts, seeds, and peanut butter; chocolate; organ meats and meats that are salted, dried, cured, smoked, or contain nitrites; sardines and anchovies; fruits, including avocados, bananas, citrus, figs, grapes, pineapples, raspberries, red plums, and raisins; red wine; artificial sweeteners; sulfites; and monosodium glutamate (MSG).

**Don't skip meals.** Eating regular meals will prevent hunger or low blood sugar, which can trigger a headache.

**Cut caffeine.** Drinking too much can contribute to the frequency of headaches. However, if you are completely off caffeine, you may be able to use it to fend off an attack because it constricts dilated blood vessels. At the first sign of an aura or pain, drink a cup of strong coffee or a cola, take two aspirin, and lie down in a dark, quiet room. The episode may pass within an hour or so.

### SAMPLE MEAL PLAN

**Breakfast:** 2 scrambled eggs with chopped vegetables; 1 slice of toast with 1 tsp trans fat free soft spread; ½ cup of sliced peaches

**Lunch:** Roast turkey sandwich on 2 slices of whole wheat bread with 2 oz of turkey breast, warmed, 2 strips of nitrite-free bacon, cooked, 1 Tbsp cranberry sauce, 1 slice tomato, 1 leaf lettuce, 1 Tbsp low-fat mayonnaise; *Ginger Butternut Squash Soup* (page 139)

**Snack:** 1 medium apple

**Dinner:** *Braised Chicken with Winter Vegetables* (page 191); 1 soft whole grain dinner roll

**Dessert:** 1 piece of angel food cake topped with sliced strawberries

## OTHER RECIPES TO TRY

- Cod and Vegetable Stew
- Bok Choy, Tofu, and Mushroom Stir-Fry
- Springtime Quinoa
- Roasted Root Vegetables
- Carrot-Flecked Corn Bread

# MOOD DISORDERS

## FOODS THAT HARM

Foods with additives, if allergic

## FOODS THAT HEAL

Turkey
Milk
Eggs
Pasta
Breads
Kale
Orange juice
Corn
Asparagus
Tuna
Salmon

## FOODS TO LIMIT

Caffeinated drinks
Alcohol
Sugary foods

## HOW TO EAT

Food can have an effect on the brain chemicals that control your mood. Here's how to ensure the effect is positive.

**Don't skip meals.** Eating small amounts of food frequently throughout the day can keep your energy level and mood more constant.

**Combine tryptophan and carbs.** This feel-good amino acid found in turkey, milk, and eggs works best when consumed with carbohydrates like bread.

**Fill your plate with veggies.** Leafy greens and other veggies listed at left are high in folate. Many depressed people are deficient in this mineral. Other good sources include lentils, peas, nuts, and seeds.

**Feast on fish.** Aim to eat fish three times a week or more.

## SAMPLE MEAL PLAN

**Breakfast:** *Asparagus, Egg, and Ham Sandwiches* (page 121); 1 cup of sliced fresh fruit, or ½ cup of orange juice

**Lunch:** *Tossed Tuna Salad Niçoise* (page 165); 1 whole grain roll

**Snack:** small handful of nuts or seeds; 1 banana

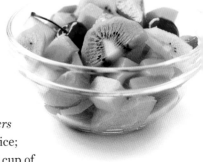

**Dinner:** *Indian-Style Turkey Burgers* (page 150); ½ cup cooked basmati rice; 1 medium ear of corn on the cob; ½ cup of steamed greens such as collards or kale

**Dessert:** 1 cup of milk with 1 tsp of honey

## OTHER RECIPES TO TRY

- Summer Greens Scramble
- Chicken-Kale Soup with Roasted Pepper Puree
- Cantaloupe and Orange Soup

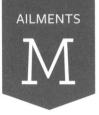

- Turkey Cobb Salad Sandwiches
- Herbed Turkey Meatballs and Fusilli
- Braised Mixed Greens with Dried Currants
- Jerk Turkey Breast with Ginger Barbecue Sauce
- Carrot-Flecked Corn Bread

# MOTION SICKNESS

### FOODS THAT HEAL

Ginger
Saltines or other dry crackers
Ginger ale
Water

### FOODS TO LIMIT

Alcohol
Fatty and fried foods
Salty foods, such as pickles
Dairy products
Caffeinated drinks

## HOW TO EAT

Try these suggestions to avoid feeling queasy. If you get sick and aren't up to making the recipes at right, or if they sound unappetizing, opt for simple, bland foods until you're feeling better.

**Nix feasting.** Keep meals light during the 24 hours before your trip. And avoid salty foods and dairy products. (See meal plan at right for suggestions.)

**Season pretravel meals with ginger.** Add 1 Tbsp of chopped ginger to fish, eggs, chicken, or turkey dishes.

**Hydrate ahead of time.** Down at least 8 glasses of water, ginger ale, or iced tea 24 hours before you travel.

**Sip while en route.** Ginger ale and ginger tea are good choices.

**Munch on dry crackers** if your stomach gets queasy.

### SAMPLE MEAL PLAN

**Breakfast:** toasted English muffin with 2 tsp apple butter or jam; a cup of peppermint or ginger tea

**Lunch:** *Chicken Breasts with Peaches and Ginger* (page 193); ½ cup of cooked rice

**Snack:** a cup of vegetable soup garnished with a smidge of grated gingerroot; a couple of unsalted crackers or saltines

**Dinner:** 1 lean turkey or chicken burger on a soft kaiser roll with 1 Tbsp of low-fat mayonnaise, lettuce, and a sliced tomato; a plain baked sweet potato

**Dessert:** *Warm Pineapple-Ginger Punch* (page 272)

### OTHER RECIPES TO TRY

- Indian-Style Turkey Burgers
- Asparagus and Chicken Stir-Fry
- Pineapple-Chipotle Chicken
- Jerk Turkey Breast with Ginger Barbecue Sauce
- Fruit Parfait with Ginger Tea Cream

### QUICK TIP: Snack on Protein

Before you hop in the car or board a plane, train, or boat, have a protein bar or drink. According to research from Penn State University, travellers who ate protein pre-travel fared better than those who filled up on carbohydrates.

# MULTIPLE SCLEROSIS

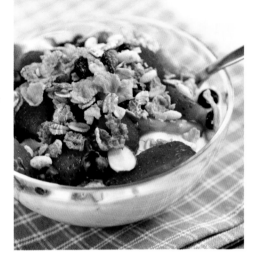

## FOODS THAT HEAL

Prune juice

Berries

Whole grain breads and cereals

Split peas

Artichoke

Nuts

Papaya

Milk

Fish

Cranberry juice

Water

## FOODS TO LIMIT

Alcohol

Spicy foods

## HOW TO EAT

Diet can help minimize MS symptoms such as fatigue, constipation, urinary tract infections, and problems with chewing and swallowing.

**Think low fat, high fiber.** Eating this way will provide energy and nutrients to maintain and repair tissues, fight infections, and reduce your risk of constipation. (See the meal plan below.)

**Eat foods rich in antioxidants** to counter free radical damage that may promote the progression of MS. Good sources of beta-carotene, vitamins C and E, and selenium include oranges, carrots, vegetable oils, nuts, seeds, and seafood, along with the healing foods above.

**Get plenty of vitamin D** from milk or fortified soy and rice beverages. It may help slow progression of the disease and will keep your bones strong.

**Increase fluid intake,** but avoid caffeine. Prune juice and cranberry juice are good choices, and help prevent constipation and urinary tract infections, respectively.

**Eat small, frequent meals** and don't skip breakfast.

**Choose soft textures** if you have difficulties with chewing or swallowing. For example, substitute shakes, yogurt, fruit and vegetable purees, puddings, and thick soups for firm or dry dishes.

### SAMPLE MEAL PLAN

**Mini Breakfast:** 1 serving of a high-fiber, whole grain cold cereal with 1 cup of skim milk and ¼ cup of fresh berries

**A.M. Mini Snack:** a tangerine; a small handful of nuts

**Mini Lunch:** 1 cup of split pea soup; ½ a grilled cheese sandwich

**P.M. Mini Meal:** a small high fiber-muffin; ½ cup of cranberry or prune juice

**Mini Dinner:** 3 oz of grilled fish; *Fruity Butternut Squash Casserole with Papaya* (page 239); ½ cup of steamed collards or kale

**Dessert:** 1 cup of strawberries dipped in ¼ cup of yogurt.

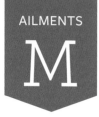
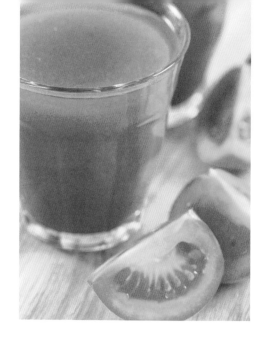

## OTHER RECIPES TO TRY

- Berry-Flaxseed Smoothie
- Papaya and Avocado Salad
- Whole Wheat Noodles with Peanut Sauce and Chicken
- Artichokes with Lentils and Lima Beans
- Carrot and Parsnip Puree
- Carrot-Flecked Cornbread
- Warm Artichoke and Bean Dip

# MUSCLE CRAMPS

### FOODS THAT HEAL

Bananas

Tomato juice

Milk

Water

Oranges

Melons

### FOODS TO LIMIT

Caffeinated drinks

### HOW TO EAT

You can ward off cramps or lessen their severity by following these guidelines.

**Guzzle H2O throughout the day.** Drink an extra 16 oz for every hour of exercise to help flush cramp-causing waste products from muscles.

**Eat lots of high-potassium foods.** A daily serving of one of the foods listed above can help banish cramps and prevent recurrences.

**Avoid caffeine.** It decreases circulation, which may contribute to cramps.

### SAMPLE MEAL PLAN

**Breakfast:** *Multi-Grain Pancakes or Waffles* (page 130) with 2 Tbsp of reduced-calorie syrup; 1 medium piece of fresh fruit such as an orange or a banana; 1 cup of milk

**Lunch:** roasted turkey sandwich (without the skin) on whole wheat bread with 1 Tbsp low-fat mayonnaise, lettuce, tomato, honey mustard, and a slice swiss cheese; 1 cup of tomato juice or V-8

**Snack:** 2 cups of cubed cantaloupe, honeydew, or watermelon

**Dinner:** 3 oz of grilled or baked chicken; 2 small ears of corn on the cob; 1 cup of steamed broccoli drizzled with 2 tsp melted trans fat free soft spread

**Dessert:** *Banana-Peanut Bread* (page 243); 1 cup of milk

### OTHER RECIPES TO TRY

- Cantaloupe and Orange Soup
- Avocado, Jicama, and Orange Salad
- Cauliflower Salad with Cashews
- Chocolate Banana Soufflés

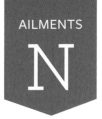

# NAIL PROBLEMS

## FOODS THAT HEAL

- Lean meat
- Poultry
- Fish, especially salmon and mackerel
- Citrus fruits
- Dried apricots
- Dark green leafy vegetables
- Fortified and enriched cereals and breads
- Legumes
- Peas
- Flaxseed oil

## HOW TO EAT

While most nail problems aren't related to your diet, nutritional deficiencies can impact your nails. Here are a few guidelines to keep your nails healthy.

**Get enough protein.** It's essential so your body can make keratin, a strong protein that's a major component of nails, hair, and skin.

**Add iron-rich foods.** Iron-deficiency anemia can prevent adequate nutrients from getting to your nails. For maximum absorption, consume iron-rich foods along with foods high in vitamin C.

**Consume more folate.** Some types of anemia that affect the nails are caused by a deficiency of folate, an essential B vitamin found in foods listed above.

**Bump up essential fatty acids.** Try 1 Tbsp of flaxseed oil a day (use it for salad dressing), or sprinkle ground flaxseeds on your cereal or smoothie.

## SAMPLE MEAL PLAN

**Breakfast:** 2 scrambled eggs; 1 slice of enriched bread, toasted, with 1 tsp of trans fat free soft spread; ½ grapefruit

**Lunch:** grilled salmon burger on an enriched or whole wheat bun; ½ cup of steamed green peas; 1 tangerine

**Snack:** 3 to 5 dried apricots; a small handful of nuts

**Dinner:** *Whole Wheat Pasta with Sausage and Greens* (page 190); ½ cup of steamed cauliflower; 1 whole grain roll

**Dessert:** fruit smoothie with 1 Tbsp of flaxseed oil

## OTHER RECIPES TO TRY

- Chicken-Kale Soup with Roasted Pepper Puree
- Celeriac and Spinach Soup
- Three-Bean Chili
- Beef, Onion, and Pepper Fajitas
- Wheat Berry Salad with Dried Apricots
- Asparagus and Chicken Stir-Fry
- Broiled Salmon with Avocado-Mango Salsa
- Snapper and Snaps in a Packet

### QUICK TIP: Try biotin

Some research suggests that this B vitamin can help make nails firmer and harder. Good sources include Swiss chard, carrots, eggs, milk, strawberries, raspberries, halibut, onions, cucumbers, cauliflower, walnuts, and almonds.

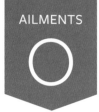

# NEURALGIA

**FOODS THAT HARM**

Alcohol

**FOODS THAT HEAL**

Lean meat

Poultry

Fish

Spinach

Potatoes

Nuts and seeds

Wheat germ

Vegetable oils

## HOW TO EAT

Deficiencies in certain vitamins can contribute to neuralgia. Here's how to eat to protect yourself.

**Maintain vitamin B12 levels.** Lean meat and poultry are some options.

**Keep up vitamin B6.** If you take hydralazine (a powerful antihypertensive medication) or isoniazid (used to treat tuberculosis), you need extra vitamin B6. In addition to the foods above, good sources are bananas, avocado, and bran.

**Pump up vitamin E.** Try fortified and enriched cereals and eggs along with foods listed above.

## SAMPLE MEAL PLAN

**Breakfast:** 1 cup of whole grain cereal with 1 cup of skim milk, ½ sliced banana, 1 Tbsp of wheat germ, 1 Tbsp of almonds, and 1 Tbsp of sunflower seeds

**Lunch:** 1 slice of spinach quiche; a small baked potato topped with 1 Tbsp of reduced-fat sour cream; a small bunch of grapes

**Snack:** fruit and nut bar

**Dinner:** *Pork, Pear, and Potato Salad* (page 159); 1 soft whole grain bread stick

**Snack:** 2 cups of popcorn tossed with 1 Tbsp of vegetable oil and salt, to taste

## OTHER RECIPES TO TRY

- Wheat Germ Smoothie
- Savory Lamb Stew with Sweet Potatoes
- Beef and Blue Cheese Burgers
- Jerk Turkey Breast with Ginger Barbeque Sauce
- Cauliflower and Spinach Casserole
- Multigrain Seeded Loaf

# OBESITY

**FOODS THAT HEAL**

Chickpeas

Carrots

Zucchini

Broccoli

Fish

Chicken

Beans

Skim milk and other dairy products

Whole wheat pasta

**FOODS TO LIMIT**

Alcohol

Sugary desserts

Salty processed snack foods

## HOW TO EAT

Here are some guidelines to help you drop pounds.

**Limit calories.** A reasonable approach is 1,500 a day for women and 2,000 for men.

**Watch empty calories.** No foods should be totally forbidden, but limit the ones that don't provide any nutrition, such as those noted at left.

**Eat in the AM.** Research shows that breakfast eaters weigh less than those who skip this meal.

**Fill up on fiber.** High-fiber foods—such as fruits and vegetables—have few calories, little fat, and lots of bulk to keep you satisfied longer.

**Add protein to every meal and snack.** Fish, chicken, or beans are good sources.

**Get enough low-fat dairy.** Being deficient can make you hungrier.

**Grab a handful of healthy nuts.** They'll fill you up.

## SAMPLE MEAL PLAN

**Breakfast:** 1 cup of high-fiber cereal with ½ cup of skim milk topped with ½ cup of your favorite fresh fruit; 1 slice of whole grain toast with 1 tsp of trans fat free soft spread

**Lunch:** *Tuscan Bean Soup* (page 141); 2 cups of mixed green salad with chopped fresh vegetables, 3 oz chicken or turkey (without the skin), and 2 Tbsp of reduced-fat dressing; 1 whole grain roll

**Snack:** 1 cup 2% Greek yogurt

**Dinner:** 1 cup of bean soup; *Grilled Salmon Salad* (page 164); ½ cup of cooked brown rice

**Dessert:** 1 slice of angel food cake with sliced fresh strawberries

## OTHER RECIPES TO TRY

- Cod and Vegetable Stew
- Fish Tacos
- Asian Chicken Salad
- Broccoli and Pearl Barley Salad
- Spinach Salad with Chickpeas
- Brown Rice with Cabbage and Chickpeas
- Flank Steak Roll with Carrots and Red Pepper

# OSTEO-ARTHRITIS

*See* Arthritis, page 283

# OSTEOPOROSIS

## FOODS THAT HARM

Salty foods

High levels of protein

## FOODS THAT HEAL

Skim milk and other dairy foods

Tofu

Romaine lettuce

Cabbage

Kale

Fortified soy or rice beverages

Flaxseed

Eggs

Citrus fruit

Melons

Berries

## FOODS TO LIMIT

Caffeinated drinks

Spinach

## HOW TO EAT

While calcium is needed for strong bones, it can't get the job done all by itself. Here are other essential nutrients to help you ward off osteoporosis.

**Go overboard with calcium.** In addition to the above foods, other good sources are canned fish eaten with the bones, nuts, dried beans, peas, and dark green leafy vegetables. The darker the greens, the more calcium they contain. An exception is spinach, which inhibits calcium absorption.

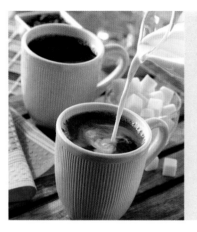

**QUICK TIP: Add milk to your coffee**

Caffeine can cause calcium to be excreted, so your best bet is to avoid caffeinated drinks as much as possible. If you really can't do without your morning joe, though, moderate your consumption to under 400 mg per day (or less, if you already have osteoporosis), make sure you meet your daily calcium requirement, and add at least 3 Tbsp skim milk, fortified soy milk, or almond milk to your coffee or tea.

**Don't forget calcium's BFF.** The body needs vitamin D to absorb calcium. You can get it from milk, fortified soy or rice beverages, egg yolks, and fatty fish like mackerel.

**Slip in some tofu.** Isoflavones found in soy products may help conserve bone mass.

**Add flaxseed.** Compounds called lignans may help keep your bones strong.

**Don't forget C.** This vitamin helps to form the connective tissue that holds bones together, and studies have linked higher intakes of C to higher bone density.

### SAMPLE MEAL PLAN

**Breakfast:** 1 cup of fortified whole grain cereal with 1 cup of skim milk; ¼ cup of sliced fresh strawberries; 1 tsp of flaxseeds

**Lunch:** *Romaine Lettuce with Chunky Tomato Vinaigrette* (page 179); a slice of vegetable quiche

**Snack:** 2 cups of honeydew or cantaloupe; 1 cup calcium-fortified soy or rice beverage

**Dinner:** *Pasta with Cabbage, Apples, and Leeks* (page 217); 1 whole grain roll

**Dessert:** *Lemony Blueberry Cheesecake Bars* (page 260); 1 cup of skim milk

### OTHER RECIPES TO TRY

- Summer Greens Scramble
- Yogurt Parfait
- Berry-Flaxseed Smoothie
- Cantaloupe and Orange Soup
- Buckwheat Noodles with Tofu and Green Vegetables
- Pork Chops and Cabbage
- Fried Rice with Tofu and Vegetables
- Whole Wheat Flaxseed Bread

# PARKINSON'S DISEASE

### FOODS THAT HEAL

Broccoli
Spinach
Whole grain cereals and breads
Soft or pureed foods

### FOODS TO LIMIT

High-protein foods, if taking medications such as levodopa

### HOW TO EAT

Diet can help ease some of the symptoms of Parkinson's disease.

**Put easy-to-chew foods on the menu.** If you have trouble chewing or swallowing, eat more cooked cereals or well-moistened dry cereals, poached or scrambled eggs, soups, mashed vegetables, rice, soft-cooked pasta, tender chicken or turkey, well-cooked boneless fish, pureed fruits, custard, yogurt, and juices.

**Don't forget vitamin K.** Get it from green vegetables such as broccoli and spinach to keep up your energy level.

**Make dining easier.** Take small bites, chew thoroughly, and swallow everything before taking another bite. Sip a liquid between bites to help wash food down.

**Try smaller but more frequent meals,** if eating is tiring.

## SAMPLE MEAL PLAN

**Mini Breakfast:** ½ cup of cooked oatmeal or cream of rice made with ½ cup of skim milk; 1 bran muffin with 1 tsp of trans fat free soft spread

**A.M. Mini Snack:** 1 cup of vegetable soup; 4 crackers

**Mini Lunch:** 1 cup of spinach lasagna; ½ cup of steamed broccoli; 1 soft roll

**P.M. Mini Snack:** ½ cup of sliced soft fruit, applesauce, or stewed fruit

**Mini Dinner:** *Spinach-Stuffed Meat Loaf* (page 183); *Carrot and Parsnip Puree* (page 230); 1 slice of soft bread

**Dessert:** ½ cup of gelatin with whipped cream

## OTHER RECIPES TO TRY

- Quick Chicken Noodle Soup
- Broccoli Potato Soup
- Sloppy Joes
- Herbed Chicken and Apple Burgers

- Herbed Turkey Meatballs and Fusilli
- Farfalle with Winter Squash Sauce
- Macaroni and Cheese with Spinach
- Cauliflower and Spinach Casserole

# PEPTIC ULCERS

### FOODS THAT HARM

Coffee, including decaffeinated, and other sources of caffeine

Alcohol

Peppermint

Tomatoes

Black pepper

Chile peppers

Garlic

Cloves

### FOODS THAT HEAL

Lean meat

Poultry

Fortified and enriched breads and cereals

Dried fruits

Legumes

Yogurt

### FOODS TO LIMIT

Fatty foods

Milk

Citrus juice

### HOW TO EAT

You can reduce the pain of peptic ulcers and possibly avoid them in the future with these eating strategies.

**Avoid trigger foods.** Common culprits are listed on page 341.

**Close the kitchen after dinner.** Late-evening eating can stimulate acid secretion during sleep.

**WARNING!**
**FOOD-DRUG INTERACTION**
If you're taking levodopa, some physicians advise having it 20 to 30 minutes before meals to be most effective. If this provokes nausea, it can be taken with a carbohydrate snack, such as crackers or bread. Protein delays the absorption of levodopa, so avoid high-protein diets while on this medication. Some doctors suggest eating the day's protein in the evening, when it's less likely to create problems.

**Reduce fat and dairy.** See the meal plan below for how to achieve this without missing out on key nutrients like calcium.

**Turn down the spice.** Some, like those listed on page 341, stimulate stomach acid. Citrus juices may also cause discomfort.

**Spoon some yogurt.** The kind with live lactobacilli and bifidobacteria may help reduce symptoms.

**Up your iron,** if you have iron-deficiency anemia due to bleeding ulcers.

**Sip aloe vera juice.** This home remedy recommends ½ cup three times a day.

### SAMPLE MEAL PLAN

**Breakfast:** omelet with fresh chopped vegetables; 2 slices of turkey bacon; a glass of calcium-fortified soy or rice beverage

**Lunch:** *Ham and Celeriac Pitas* (page 147); a bowl of bean or vegetable soup; 6 whole grain crackers; a small box of raisins

**Snack:** 1 cup of yogurt with ¼ cup of sliced papaya or mango stirred in.

**Dinner:** *Asparagus and Chicken Stir-Fry* (page 190); 1 dinner roll

---

**QUICK TIP: Check out licorice**

One home remedy for peptic ulcers that seems to work well is a form of licorice called deglycyrrhizinated licorice (DGL). DGL is sold in wafer form at health food stores. Follow the dosage instructions on the package. Don't use regular licorice, though, especially if you have high blood pressure, as it can raise blood pressure if eaten in large enough amounts.

---

**OTHER RECIPES TO TRY**

- Yogurt Parfait
- Lamb Burgers with Fruit Relish
- Rice Salad with Chicken and Grapes
- Beef, Scallion, and Asparagus Roll-Ups

# PMS

*See* Menstrual Problems, page 331

---

# PNEUMONIA

*See* Respiratory Disorders, page 345

---

# PCOS (POLY-CYSTIC OVARY DISEASE)

---

**FOODS THAT HARM**

High-glycemic foods such as white bread and refined cereals

**FOODS THAT HEAL**

Apples
Pears
Berries
Beans
Peas
Whole grains

**FOODS TO LIMIT**

Alcohol

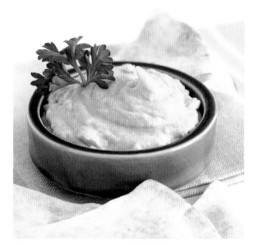

**Dinner:** veggie burger on a whole grain roll; 1 cup of bean soup; 1 cup of steamed vegetables

**Dessert:** 2 cups of berries

## OTHER RECIPES TO TRY

- Berry Salad with Passion Fruit
- Pear Rhubarb Muffins
- Raspberry-Beet Smoothie
- Tuscan Bean Soup
- Herbed Chicken and Apple Burgers
- Springtime Quinoa
- Beef, Scallion, and Asparagus Roll-Ups

# PROSTATE PROBLEMS

### FOODS THAT HEAL

Tomatoes and tomato products

Red grapefruit

Watermelon

Brazil nuts

Salmon

Trout

Arctic char

Wheat bran and wheat germ

Oats

Brown rice

Soy products (except soy sauce)

Broccoli

Cauliflower

Cabbage

Whole grains

Water

### FOODS TO LIMIT

Fatty foods, especially animal products

Caffeinated drinks

## HOW TO EAT

Dietary advice is similar to what doctors recommend for people with type 2 diabetes, but women with PCOS may have a more difficult time losing weight because of hormone imbalances.

**Be vigilant about portions.** Downsize all of your plates to make portion control and weight loss easier. Losing just 5% of your weight can improve symptoms.

**Increase fiber intake.** Aim for at least 5 g of fiber per meal or snack to satisfy an increased appetite, which can be a symptom of PCOS.

**Choose low-glycemic foods,** which can help improve insulin resistance, a problem for PCOS sufferers. See page 357.

## SAMPLE MEAL PLAN

**Breakfast:** *Hot Cereal with Apples and Dates* (page 121); 1 cup of fresh fruit

**Lunch:** pita sandwich made with 1 whole wheat pita bread, 3 oz of cooked chicken breast or roasted turkey (without the skin), ½ cup veggies (shredded lettuce, grated carrots, sliced cucumbers, and sprouts), and 2 Tbsp of low-fat dressing; 1 medium pear

**Snack:** ¼ cup of hummus with 6 whole grain high-fiber crackers

### HOW TO EAT

A low-fat diet that limits animal proteins is healthy for many reasons, including better prostate health. Here are more ways a man can prevent problems.

**Mix in foods with lycopene.** Red fruits and veggies like tomatoes and watermelon tend to be the best sources. Lycopene is fat soluble and absorbed best when eaten with a little fat, such as turkey meatballs, grated cheese, or olive oil.

**Go nuts.** They tend to be a good source of both selenium and vitamin E, nutrients that may protect against cancer. Other good sources are listed on page 343.

**Seek out soy.** It may help prevent prostate enlargement and protect against cancer.

**Eat more fish and use vegetable oils high in omega-3 fats.** They seem to reduce cancer risk.

**Dish out plenty of veggies,** especially the cruciferous kind like broccoli.

### SAMPLE MEAL PLAN

**Breakfast:** 1 cup of whole grain cereal with ½ cup of soymilk; 1 slice of whole wheat toast with trans fat free soft spread; 1 cup of red grapefruit juice

**Lunch:** *Penne with Fresh Tomato Sauce and Grilled Eggplant* (page 218); 1 cup of mixed green salad with 2 Tbsp of reduced-fat dressing; 1 whole wheat roll

**Snack:** a protein shake made with soy protein; brazil nuts

**Dinner:** *Roasted Mackerel with Cherry Tomatoes and Potatoes* (page 204); 1 cup of chopped greens such as collards, kale, or broccoli rabe (steam or sauté with a little vegetable oil); 1 whole grain roll

**Dessert:** watermelon slices or red grapefruit

### OTHER RECIPES TO TRY

- Wheat Germ Smoothie
- Potato Salad with Sun-Dried Tomatoes, Scallions, and Basil
- Watermelon and Feta Salad
- Monkfish and Mussel Kebabs
- Trout with Lemon-Mushroom Stuffing
- Spiced Cauliflower with Peas
- Green Beans with Tomatoes and Olives
- Multigrain Seeded Loaf

# PSORIASIS

### FOODS THAT HARM

Products with gluten, for those who are allergic

### FOODS THAT HEAL

Asparagus

Spinach

Avocados

Chickpeas

Lentils

Flaxseeds

Oranges

Salmon

Mackerel

Herring

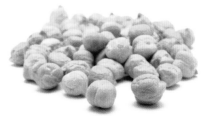

## HOW TO EAT

Boosting your immune system with a healthy diet can keep your skin looking better.

**Lace your diet with folate.** Good sources are listed at left.

**Befriend flax.** Seeds and oil are rich in anti-inflammatory essential fatty acids that may calm skin conditions.

**Opt for omega-3s.** In one study, eating 5.5 oz (156 g) of fatty fish a day improved symptoms.

### SAMPLE MEAL PLAN

**Breakfast:** 2 whole grain waffles with 2 tsp of reduced-calorie syrup; 1 cup low-fat yogurt sprinkled with 1 tsp of ground flaxseeds

**Lunch:** 1 can of wild salmon, drained and flaked, with 2 Tbsp low-fat mayonnaise on a pumpernickel bagel; 8 steamed asparagus spears

**Snack:** ¼ cup of hummus spread on 2 rice cakes

**Dinner:** 2 mini crab cakes made with fresh lump crabmeat; *Papaya and Avocado Salad* (page 178); ½ cup of cooked orzo

**Dessert:** 1 orange

### OTHER RECIPES TO TRY

- Grilled Salmon Salad
- Spinach Salad with Chickpeas
- Avocado, Jicama, and Orange Salad
- Salmon and Asparagus Farfalle with Walnut-Feta Sauce
- Brown Rice with Cabbage and Chickpeas
- Artichokes with Lentils and Lima Beans
- Orange Beets
- Whole Wheat Flaxseed Bread

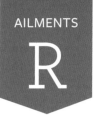

# RESPIRATORY DISORDERS

(Including bronchitis, emphysema, pneumonia, and sinusitis)

*See also* Colds and Flu, page 297; Asthma, page 284

### FOODS THAT HARM

Alcohol
Fatty and fried food

### FOODS THAT HEAL

Tomatoes
Cantaloupe
Leafy green vegetables
Lean meat
Oysters
Yogurt
Whole grains
Garlic
Chiles
Horseradish

### FOODS TO LIMIT

Milk
Beans
Legumes
Cabbage
Brussels sprouts
Broccoli
Onions

### HOW TO EAT

A nutritious and well-balanced diet can help prevent or reduce the severity of bronchitis, pneumonia, and other lung infections.

**Drink plenty of fluids,** especially warm liquids like chicken broth and hot tea, to help thin mucus and make breathing easier.

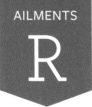

**Fill your plate with antioxidant foods.** Vitamins A, C, and beta-carotene, found in many fruits and vegetablese.

**Balance zinc content.** Up to 40 mg a day of this mineral (found in lean meat, oysters, yogurt, whole grain products, and seeds) boost immunity, but consuming more depresses your immune system.

**Get hot.** Spicy foods are natural decongestants.

**Pass on the gas.** Bloating and flatulence make breathing difficult. Avoid gas-producing foods like beans, eat slowly, and have small servings.

### SAMPLE MEAL PLAN

**Breakfast:** 1 poached egg; 1 whole wheat English muffin; 1 cup of cubed cantaloupe with ½ cup of low-fat yogurt

**Lunch:** *Chicken-Kale Soup with Roasted Pepper Puree* (page 135); 2 whole grain soft bread sticks

**Snack:** *Sweet and Spicy Snack Mix* (page 252)

**Dinner:** *Oysters with Tomato Salsa* (page 248); 8 baked whole grain tortilla chips with a ¼ cup of spicy guacamole

**Dessert:** 1 piece of fresh fruit

### OTHER RECIPES TO TRY

- Basic Chicken Stock
- Chunky Gazpacho with Garlicky Croutons
- Shrimp Ceviche with Avocado and Pumpkin Seeds
- Thai Roasted Shrimp
- Roasted Root Vegetables
- Carrot-Orange Juice

# ROSACEA

### FOODS THAT HEAL

Cucumbers

Ice water

### FOODS TO LIMIT

Specific trigger foods, such as alcohol and spicy foods

## HOW TO EAT

Follow these tips to avoid flare-ups.

**Chill out.** Eat cool foods from both a spice and temperature standpoint.

**Stay hydrated.** Choose water or non-caffeinated beverages, chilled or at room temperature. Drink more when it's hot out or when you're exercising.

**Keep a food diary** to figure out trigger foods.

### SAMPLE MEAL PLAN

**Breakfast:** ½ cup of chilled peach slices with ½ cup low-fat cottage cheese; 1 granola bar

**Lunch:** cheese sandwich with 1 Tbsp of low-fat mayonnaise, sliced cucumbers, grated carrots, and sprouts; 2 cups of mixed greens salad with 2 Tbsp low-fat dressing

**Snack:** a fruit smoothie

**Dinner:** *Poached Salmon with Cucumber-Dill Sauce* (page 200); 1 cup of chilled pasta salad; 1 whole grain roll

**Dessert:** 17 frozen grapes or a popsicle

### OTHER RECIPES TO TRY

- Berry Salad with Passion Fruit
- Cantaloupe and Orange Soup

- Japanese Sushi Rolls (cold)
- Tropical Fruit Salad
- Yogurt Parfait
- Tuna and Carrot Sandwich on Rye

# SEX DRIVE, DIMINISHED

## FOODS THAT HARM

Alcohol

## FOODS THAT HEAL

Citrus fruits
Skim milk and other dairy products
Green leafy vegetables
Wheat germ
Lean beef
Poultry
Liver
Fortified and enriched cereals
Oysters
Pine nuts
Beans
Garlic

## FOODS TO LIMIT

Red meat, butter, and other foods
with saturated fat

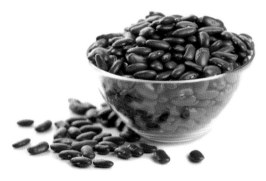

## HOW TO EAT

A healthy sex life depends on a balanced diet, good nerve function, healthy hormone levels, and an unobstructed blood flow to the pelvic area.

**Eat a diet high in complex carbs and low in saturated fats.** This is important for maintaining good blood circulation to your sex organs.

**Consume more zinc,** found in many of the foods listed at left, as well as eggs, nuts, and whole grains.

**Pump up iron.** Iron-deficiency anemia can dampen desire.

**Mix in some garlic.** It's high in allicin, which stimulates circulation and blood flow to sexual organs in both men and women.

**Get a daily dose of pine nuts.** They're a great source of arginine, the precursor for nitric oxide, a main ingredient in drugs like Viagra.

## SAMPLE MEAL PLAN

**Breakfast:** 1 serving of whole grain cereal (look for 16 g of whole grains per serving) with 1 cup of skim milk, a handful of berries, and 2 Tbsp of wheat germ

**Lunch:** quick chicken pasta salad: mix ¼ cup reduced-fat pesto (jarred variety is fine) with 1 cup cooked pasta, 1 cup of your favorite roasted, steamed or grilled vegetables, and 3 oz of sliced roasted chicken (without the skin)

**Snack:** 1 orange

**Dinner:** *Grilled Oysters with Fennel and Spinach* (page 247); 2 small ears of grilled corn on the cob; ½ cup of coleslaw made with low-fat mayonnaise

**Dessert:** 1 cup of low-fat ice cream with 2 Tbsp of crushed nuts

### OTHER RECIPES TO TRY

- Individual Breakfast Tortilla
- Wheat Germ Smoothie
- Beef Fillet Salad with Mustard Vinaigrette
- Endive, Apple, and Watercress Salad
- Braised Mixed Greens with Dried Currants
- Beef, Scallion, and Asparagus Roll-Ups
- Oysters with Tomato Salsa

# SHINGLES

### FOODS THAT HEAL

Nuts and seeds

Wheat germ

Vegetable oils

Seafood

Lean meat

Poultry

Milk

Yogurt

Beans

Whole grains

### HOW TO EAT

Good nutrition may help prevent postherpetic neuralgia, a long-term complication of shingles.

**Get plenty of E and C.** These antioxidants help prevent inflammation and boost immunity. Vitamin E is found in some of the foods above. Good sources for C include citrus, melons, and peppers.

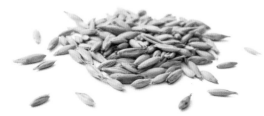

**Eat a little extra zinc.** It strengthens your immune system.

### SAMPLE MEAL PLAN

**Breakfast:** 2 buttermilk pancakes with 2 Tbsp reduced-calorie syrup; 1 slice of lean turkey bacon; ½ cup of fresh fruit

**Lunch:** *Green Pork Chili* (page 127); 2 cups mixed greens salad with 2 Tbsp reduced-fat dressing; 1 whole grain roll

**Snack:** 1 oz of nuts or seeds

**Dinner:** Stir-fry made with vegetables, brown rice, and shrimp, chicken, pork, or lean beef; garnish with fresh orange sections

**Dessert:** *Yogurt Parfait* (page 000)

### OTHER RECIPES TO TRY

- Broccoli and Pearl Barley Salad
- Orange Beef with Broccoli and Jicama
- Pork Chops and Cabbage
- Scallops Florentine
- Springtime Quinoa
- Rice Salad with Chicken and Grapes
- Rice-Stuffed Squash

# SINUSITIS

*See* Respiratory Disorders, page 345

# SLEEP DISORDERS

*See* Insomnia, page 321

# SORE THROAT

## FOODS THAT HARM
Alcohol
Caffeine

## FOODS THAT HEAL
Lemon
Honey
Yogurt
Eggs
Seafood
Lean meat
Whole grains
Fruit juice
Water
Tea

## HOW TO EAT

Prevent that initial sore throat from becoming a more serious condition with these tips.

**Switch to a liquid diet.** See the meal plan below to maintain nutrition without exacerbating throat pain.

**Aim for 5 to 10 servings of fruits and vegetables a day.** Initially, get them in smoothies and shakes. You can also stew fruits until they're very soft and mash cooked vegetables.

**Sip some lemon tea.** Squeeze the juice of a lemon—high in immune-boosting vitamin C—into a cup of boiling water and add a teaspoon of honey.

**Gargle with honey.** Stir 1 to 3 tsp (5 to 15 mL) of honey into 1 cup (250 mL) of warm water, and gargle two or three times a day.

## SAMPLE MEAL PLAN

**Breakfast:** 1 cup of oatmeal prepared with skim milk; ½ cup of stewed fruit; cup of hot water with lemon and honey

**Snack:** *Strawberry-Yogurt Smoothie* (page 131)

**Lunch:** *Vegetable Stock* (page 137) with your favorite vegetables, cooked grains, or soft noodles

**Snack:** 1 cup of fruit-flavored Jell-O

**Dinner:** *Carrot Soup with Dill* (page 138) with 2 Tbsp of grated cheese; 1 soft whole grain roll

**Dessert:** 8 oz protein shake

## OTHER RECIPES TO TRY

- Quick Chicken Noodle Soup
- Cod and Vegetable Stew
- Miso Soup with Tofu
- Cantaloupe and Orange Soup
- Zucchini-Carrot Crustless Quiche Squares
- Warm Kasha and Seafood Salad
- Mashed Turnips with Carrots and Potatoes

# STRESS

## FOODS THAT HEAL
Whole grains
Seafood
Lean meat
Poultry
Milk
Eggs
Nuts
Herbal tea

## FOODS TO LIMIT
Alcohol
Caffeinated drinks
Fatty foods
Hot or spicy foods

## HOW TO EAT

The right foods provide energy, while vitamins and minerals help your body maintain resistance to infection when under stress.

**Zap stress with zinc.** It helps keep your immune system strong. See foods on page 349.

**Eat four to six small meals.** Stress interferes with digestion, so small meals throughout the day are best.

**Enjoy carbs.** Studies have shown that a diet higher in carbohydrates and lower in protein can reduce your chance of stress-induced depression. See the meal plan below.

**Eat breakfast.** You'll handle stress much better if you're fueled.

**Munch slowly.** Eating quickly can promote more stress-related GI troubles.

**Sip chamomile or peppermint tea.** They have a calming effect.

### SAMPLE MEAL PLAN

**Mini Breakfast:** *Mushroom and Bell Pepper Frittata* (page 123)

**A.M. Mini Meal:** *Whole Wheat Flaxseed Bread* (page 242), toasted, with 1 tsp of jam; 1 cup peppermint tea

**Mini Lunch:** large baked potato topped with 1 Tbsp grated low-fat cheese and ¼ cup of salsa; small salad with 2 Tbsp low-fat dressing

**P.M. Mini Meal:** 1 piece of fresh fruit; 1 cup chamomile tea

**Mini Dinner:** *Pasta with Walnut Cream Sauce* (page 217).

**Dessert:** 8 oz milkshake

## OTHER RECIPES TO TRY

- Lamb Burgers with Fruit Relish
- Couscous-Stuffed Peppers
- Spinach-Stuffed Meat Loaf
- Twice Baked Stuffed Sweet Potatoes
- Spiced Almonds

# STROKE

### FOODS THAT HARM

Red meat, butter, and other foods with saturated fats

Palm and coconut oil

Salty foods, such as pickles

### FOODS THAT HEAL

Oats

Lentils

Flaxseeds

Whole grains

Grapes

Nuts

Red wine

Apples

Berries

Trout

Mackerel

Walnuts

Canola oil

Soybeans

Green leafy vegetables

Low-fat dairy products

Garlic

Onions

## HOW TO EAT

Diet plays an important role in reducing or eliminating stroke risk factors.

**Adopt a low-fat, low-sodium, high-fiber diet.** This will help to lower your chances of developing risk factors for a stroke such as high blood pressure, diabetes, or high cholesterol.

**Add important phytochemicals.** Resveratrol, found in grapes, nuts, and red wine, may inhibit blood clots and relax blood vessels. Quercetin, found in apples and berries, may reduce fat deposits in arteries.

**Eat fatty fish two or three times a week.** No fan of fish? Try walnuts, walnut oil, canola (rapeseed) oil, flaxseed oil, soybeans, and leafy greens.

**Cook with garlic and onions.** They boost the body's natural clot-dissolving mechanism.

**Get milk.** Nutrients such as calcium, potassium, magnesium, and vitamin D in low-fat dairy products help lower blood pressure.

## SAMPLE MEAL PLAN

**Breakfast:** *Buckwheat Pancakes with Fruit Sauce* (page 129); a cup of skim milk

**Lunch:** grilled chicken sandwich (without the skin) made on 2 slices of low-sodium whole grain bread with lettuce, tomato, and red onion; at least 1 cup steamed broccoli

**Snack:** 1 medium apple

**Dinner:** 3 oz of baked salmon; *Braised Mixed Greens with Dried Currants* (page 233); a small, baked sweet potato

**Dessert:** a glass of red wine

## OTHER RECIPES TO TRY

- Hot Cereal with Apples and Dates
- Salmon and Fennel Lettuce Wraps
- Grilled Salmon Salad
- Spinach Salad with Chickpeas
- Mediterranean Salad with Edamame
- Poached Salmon with Cucumber-Dill Sauce
- Fried Rice with Tofu and Vegetables
- Toasted Oat-Raisin Bread

# ULCERATIVE COLITIS

*See* Inflammatory Bowel Disease, page 320

# URINARY TRACT INFECTIONS

### FOODS THAT HARM

Caffeinated drinks

Alcohol

Spicy food

### FOODS THAT HEAL

Cranberries and cranberry juice

Water

Oranges

Tomatoes

Broccoli

Yogurt

## HOW TO EAT

You can speed healing and help prevent recurrences with these tips.

**Drink plenty of water,** at least 8 to 10 glasses a day to increase urine flow and flush out infectious material.

**Drink cranberry juice.** Research shows that cranberries and blueberries contain substances that speed the elimination of bacteria.

**Pump up vitamin C** to boost immunity and fight infection.

**Go for yogurt.** It can inhibit the growth of microorganisms that cause UTIs, and it can maintain healthy bacteria when you're taking antibiotics.

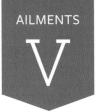
## SAMPLE MEAL PLAN

**Breakfast:** *Blueberry and Cranberry Granola* (page 120) with ½ cup of low-fat yogurt; 1 cup of cranberry juice

**Lunch:** cheese sandwich made with 2 slices of whole grain bread, 2 oz of low-fat colby cheese, a slice of tomato, and 1 Tbsp of low-fat mayonnaise or spread; *Green Beans with Tomatoes and Olives* (page 233)

**Snack:** 1 orange

**Dinner:** 3 oz of sliced turkey breast; half of a baked acorn squash; 1 cup of steamed broccoli

**Dessert:** 1 cup of low-fat yogurt with sliced fruit

### OTHER RECIPES TO TRY

- Yogurt Parfait
- Strawberry-Yogurt Smoothie
- Broccoli Potato Soup
- Avocado, Jicama, and Orange Salad
- Romaine Lettuce with Chunky Tomato Vinaigrette
- Pan-Seared Scallops with Oranges and Sun-Dried Tomatoes
- Penne with Fresh Tomato Sauce and Grilled Eggplant
- Savory Cranberry Chutney

# VARICOSE VEINS

### FOODS THAT HEAL

Oranges and other citrus fruits
Berries
Broccoli
Red peppers
Whole grain cereals
Whole wheat pasta
Popcorn
Grapes

## HOW TO EAT

A well-balanced diet that helps you maintain a healthy weight or lose weight is key since obesity is a risk factor for varicose veins. Some foods may even have an effect on blood vessels to minimize the problem. Here's how.

**Hit high C.** Getting lots of vitamin C strengthens blood vessels. Foods high in C also provide other healthy compounds. In fact, one small study showed that the flavonoid hesperidin in oranges improved varicose veins.

**Feast on fiber.** It can prevent constipation, which can make varicose veins worse by increasing pressure.

**Pick some berries.** Blueberries, raspberries, blackberries, and grapes contain antioxidants that help reduce blood vessel leakage.

## SAMPLE MEAL PLAN

**Breakfast:** *Blueberry-Oatmeal Muffins* (page 120); ½ cup of low-fat yogurt with strawberries

**Lunch:** veggie burger on a whole wheat roll with lettuce, tomato, and 2 Tbsp of low-fat dressing; 1 cup of minestrone soup; ½ cup of steamed broccoli

**Snack:** a small bunch of grapes

**Dinner:** *Pan-Seared Scallops with Oranges and Sun-Dried Tomatoes* (page 208); 1 cup of whole wheat pasta salad with added vegetables; 1 medium ear of grilled corn on the cob

**Snack:** 2 cups of air-popped popcorn

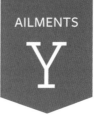
## OTHER RECIPES TO TRY

- Chicken Salad with Citrus
- Whole Wheat Noodles with Peanut Sauce and Chicken
- Mixed Berry and Stone Fruit Soup
- Fruity Granola Mix
- Orange-Walnut Broccoli
- Carrot-Orange Juice

# YEAST INFECTIONS

## FOODS THAT HARM

Sugary foods

## FOODS THAT HEAL

Yogurt with live cultures

Sauerkraut

Tempeh

Kefir

Miso

Cherries

Grapes

Apricots

## HOW TO EAT

Follow these tips to reduce your chance of getting a yeast infection or ease symptoms if you have one.

**Avoid sweetened yogurts.** Sugar can worsen symptoms.

**Get some garlic.** It's a powerful bacterial fighter. Aim for 2 raw cloves per day.

**Try fermented foods,** such as sauerkraut, tempeh (a fermented soy product), kefir (a yogurtlike drink), and miso. They contain probiotics that in theory could work against infections in the same way live cultures in yogurt do.

**Ditch the sweet stuff**—fruit juices, sweetened breakfast cereals, ice cream,

and desserts as well as anything made with high-fructose corn syrup. Satisfy your sweet tooth with cherries, grapes, fresh apricots, or carrots. Yeast thrives on sugar.

**Steer clear of yeast.** Choose yeast-free sprouted bread instead of regular.

## SAMPLE MEAL PLAN

**Breakfast:** 1 slice of toasted yeast-free bread with 1 tsp of trans fat free soft spread; *Strawberry-Yogurt Smoothie* (page 131)

**Lunch:** bowl of vegetable soup seasoned with miso; 1 cup of brown rice; 1 cup steamed vegetables; 2 Tbsp of sauerkraut

**Snack:** 2 rice cakes with 2 tsp of almond butter

**Dinner:** *Caraway-Coated Pepper Steak with Cherry Sauce* (page 181); ½ cup of mashed potatoes; ½ cup of cooked carrots

**Dessert:** 1 cup of grapes dipped in ½ cup low-fat yogurt made with live cultures

## OTHER RECIPES TO TRY

- Yogurt Parfait
- Strawberry-Yogurt Smoothie
- Miso Soup with Tofu
- Fruit Salad with Spiced Coconut
- Baked Pasta with Garlic and Greens
- Braised Mixed Greens with Dried Currants
- Turkey Bacon and Apricot Bites
- Cherry Crisp

# GLYCEMIC INDEX AND GLYCEMIC LOAD

To gauge how efficiently food works its way through your digestive system to affect your blood sugar, researchers at the University of Toronto developed the glycemic index (GI). The faster a food is digested and absorbed into your bloodstream, the higher its GI. High-GI foods cause a rapid increase in blood sugar, which is dangerous, especially for people with diabetes.

But GI was based on a standard measurement (50 g of carbohydrates) for all foods. In real life, people don't tend to eat the same amounts of sugar as they do pasta or carrots.

## GLYCEMIC INDEX VS. GLYCEMIC LOAD

Below are a few common foods and their GI and GL values. Note the differences and how the GL becomes a better way to look at the effect that foods have on blood sugar.

| FOOD | GI | SIZE | GL |
|---|---|---|---|
| **Grains and Cereals** | | | |
| Bagel, white | 72 | 2 ½ oz (70 g) | 25 |
| Barley, pearled | 25 | 5 oz (150 g) | 11 |
| Bread, white | 71 | 1 oz (30 g) | 10 |
| Bread, whole grain, pumpernickel | 46 | 1 oz (30 g) | 5 |
| Bread, whole wheat | 67 | 1 oz (30 g) | 8 |
| Cereal, All-Bran | 50 | 1 oz (30 g) | 9 |
| Cereal, cornflakes | 80 | 1 oz (30 g) | 21 |
| Cereal, muesli | 66 | 1 oz (30 g) | 16 |
| **Fruits** | | | |
| Apple | 39 | 4 oz (125 g) | 6 |
| Apple juice, unsweetened | 41 | 8 ½ oz (250 mL) | 12 |
| Banana | 46 | 4 oz (125 g) | 12 |
| Grapefruit | 25 | 4 oz (125 g) | 3 |
| Grapes | 43 | 4 oz (125 g) | 7 |
| Orange | 40 | 4 oz (125 g) | 4 |
| Peach | 42 | 4 oz (125 g) | 5 |
| Watermelon | 72 | 4 oz (125 g) | 4 |
| **Vegetables** | | | |
| Baked potato | 60 | 5 oz (150 g) | 18 |
| Baked potato, mashed | 74 | 5 oz (150 g) | 15 |
| Carrots | 92 | 3 oz (90 g) | 5 |
| Kidney beans | 29 | 5.2 oz (150 g) | 7 |
| Lentils | 29 | 5.2 oz (150 g) | 5 |
| Peas | 51 | 3 oz (90 g) | 4 |
| Soybeans | 15 | 5.2 oz (150 g) | 1 |
| Sweet potato | 48 | 5 oz (150 g) | 16 |

So scientists used a little math wizardry to translate the glycemic index into more practical terms. What emerged is the glycemic load (GL). This tool considers the type of carbohydrate in the food and the amount of carbohydrate in a standard serving. By this new criterion, sugar and starchy foods and some fruits have high GL values whereas most vegetables and fruits have low GL values, meaning they are less likely to make your blood sugar spike.

Both are useful—GI helps you choose better carbs while GL helps with portion sizes. Today, there are more than 750 published GI and GL values of various foods. However, you should take all GL lists as a general guide only. As it turns out, one person's glycemic response can differ from another's. It may vary even in the same person from day to day. Also, the state of food can change its GL.

For example, small differences in a banana's ripeness can double its GL. Plus, fat and protein slow down digestion, making the GL of a baked potato topped with sour cream and served with a steak different than the GL of the potato itself.

People who eat diets with a high GL have a higher rate of obesity, diabetes, heart disease, and cancer. One study found that swapping just one baked potato per week for a serving of brown rice could reduce a person's odds of developing type 2 diabetes by up to 30%.

# RECIPE INDEX

# INDEX